EXOTIC ANIMAL
MEDICINE
REVIEW & TEST

Commissioning Editor: *Robert Edwards*
Development Editor: *Veronika Watkins / Clive Hewat*
Project Manager: *Julie Taylor*
Designer/Design Direction: *Miles Hitchen*
Illustration Manager: *Jennifer Rose*
Illustrator: *Antbits Ltd*

EXOTIC ANIMAL MEDICINE
REVIEW & TEST

Edited by

Jaime Samour MVZ (Hons), PhD, Dip ECZM (Avian)

Director
Wildlife Division, Wrsan,
Abu Dhabi,
United Arab Emirates

Chairman of the Education Committee
European College of Zoological Medicine

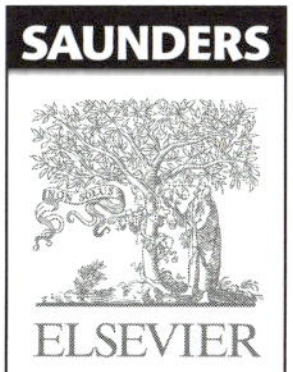

Edinburgh London New York Oxford Philadelphia St Louis Sydney Toronto 2012

ELSEVIER
SAUNDERS

ISBN 9780702044441

British Library Cataloguing in Publication Data
A catalogue record for this book is available from the British Library

Library of Congress Cataloging in Publication Data
A catalog record for this book is available from the Library of Congress

Notices

Knowledge and best practice in this field are constantly changing. As new research and experience broaden our understanding, changes in research methods, professional practices, or medical treatment may become necessary.

Practitioners and researchers must always rely on their own experience and knowledge in evaluating and using any information, methods, compounds, or experiments described herein. In using such information or methods they should be mindful of their own safety and the safety of others, including parties for whom they have a professional responsibility.

With respect to any drug or pharmaceutical products identified, readers are advised to check the most current information provided (i) on procedures featured or (ii) by the manufacturer of each product to be administered, to verify the recommended dose or formula, the method and duration of administration, and contraindications. It is the responsibility of practitioners, relying on their own experience and knowledge of their patients, to make diagnoses, to determine dosages and the best treatment for each individual patient, and to take all appropriate safety precautions.

To the fullest extent of the law, neither the Publisher nor the authors, contributors, or editors, assume any liability for any injury and/or damage to persons or property as a matter of products liability, negligence or otherwise, or from any use or operation of any methods, products, instructions, or ideas contained in the material herein.

Printed in China

Contents

Contributors

Thomas A. Bailey, BSc, BVSc, MRCVS, Cert Zoo Med, MSc (Wild Animal Health), PhD, Dip ECZM (Avian)
Falcon and Wildlife Veterinarian,
Dubai Falcon Hospital,
Dubai,
United Arab Emirates

John Chitty, BVetMed, Cert Zoo Med, CBiol, MSB, MRCVS
Director,
JC Exotic Pet Consultancy Ltd,
Salisbury,
United Kingdom

Peter Coutteel, DVM
Director,
Dierenartsencentru, TRIGENIO,
Nijlen,
Belgium

Lorenzo Crosta, Dr. med. vet., PhD
Co-Director, Avian,
Zoo and Exotic Animal Consulting,
Clinica Veterinaria Valcurone,
Missaglia (LC),
Italy

Robert J. Doneley, BVSc, FACVSc (Avian Medicine), CMAVA
Head of Service,
Small Animal Hospital,
Veterinary Medical Centre,
School of Veterinary Science,
University of Queensland, Gatton,
Australia

Gerry Dorrestein, Prof. dr dr hc, Dip ECZM (Hons)
Director,
Diagnostic Pathology Laboratory NOIVBD,
Veldhoven,
The Netherlands

Dominik Fischer, DVM
Resident Veterinarian,
Klinik für Vögel,
Reptilien, Amphibien und Fische,
Justus-Liebig-Universität Giessen,
Giessen,
Germany

Neil A. Forbes BVetMed, CBiol MIBiol, FRCVS, Dip ECZM (Avian)
Head of Exotics Service,
Great Western Exotic Vets,
Vets Now Referral Hospital,
Swindon,
United Kingdom

Brett Gartrell, BVSc, MACVSc (Avian), PhD
Associate Professor,
Institute of Veterinary,
Animal and Biomedical Sciences,
Massey University,
Palmerston North,
New Zealand

Jean-Michel Hatt, Prof., Dr. med. vet., MSc, Dip ACZM, Dip ECZM (Avian)
Director, Clinic for Zoo Animals,
Exotic Pets and Wildlife,
Vetsuisse Faculty,
University of Zurich,
Zurich,
Switzerland

Manfred Hochleithner, Dr. med. vet., Dip ECZM (Avian)
Co-Director,
Fachtierarzt für Kleintiere,
Tierklinik Strebersdorf,
Vienna,
Austria

Minh Huynh, DVM, MRCVS
Resident, European College of
Zoological Medicine (Avian),
Arcueil,
France

Lance Jepson, MA, VetMB, CBiol, MSB, MRCVS
Director, Vet4dragons,
Fenton Veterinary Practice,
Haverfordwest,
United Kingdom

Dominik Kaiser, Dr. med. vet.
Resident Veterinary Officer,
Kleintier-und Vogelpraxis,
Baden-Dättwil,
Switzerland

Angela Lennox, DVM, Dip ABVP (Avian)
Director, Avian and Exotic Animal Clinic
of Indianapolis,
Indianapolis,
United States of America

Michael Lierz, Prof. Dr., DZooMed, Dip ECZM, Dip ECPVS
Director, Klinik für Vögel,
Reptilien, Amphibien und Fische,
Justus-Liebig-Universität Giessen,
Giessen,
Germany

Christopher Lloyd, BVSc, MSc (Wild Animal Health), Cert Zoo Med, MRCVS
Medical Director,
Nad Al Shiba Veterinary Hospital,
Dubai,
United Arab Emirates

Andres Montesinos, DVM
Director,
Centro Veterinario los Sauces,
Madrid,
Spain

Jesus Naldo, DVM
Senior Veterinary Officer,
Wildlife Division,
Abu Dhabi,
United Arab Emirates

Mikel Sabater Gonzalez, LV, MRCVS
Resident, European College of Zoological
Medicine (Avian),
Valencia,
Spain

Jaime Samour, MVZ (Hons), PhD, Dip ECZM (Avian)
Director,
Wildlife Division,
Abu Dhabi,
United Arab Emirates

Peter Sandmeier, Dr. med. vet., Dip ECZM (Avian)
Director,
Kleintier-und Vogelpraxis,
Baden-Dättwil,
Switzerland

Paolo Zucca, DVM, PhD, BSc Psych
Veterinary Officer,
Zooantropology Unit,
Healthcare Services Agency,
Trieste,
Italy

Acknowledgements

I would like to express my most sincere gratitude to Mr David Jones, Mr John Knight, Professor James Kirkwood, the late Tony Fitzgerald, Jude Howlett, Robbie Hutton, John Finch, Janet Markham, Jane Lawrie, the late Dr Christine Hawkey, Mike Hart and David Spratt, former members of staff at the Veterinary Science Department, Institute of Zoology, Zoological Society of London for their friendship, understanding and encouragement during those glorious years I spent working among them at the London Zoo.

To HH Sheikh Sultan bin Zayed Al Nahyan for his continuing support to the clinical and research programme of the Veterinary Science Department, Wildlife Division, Wrsan.

Dedication

This book is dedicated to the memory of Dr Christine Hawkey for guiding me into the world of exotic animal medicine.

To my wife Merle for inspiring me to be a better man and to my children Omar, Miriam, Adam and Yasmeen for inspiring me to be a better father.

A real man is the one who is able to build a castle with the stones others have thrown at him

Jaime Samour
Abu Dhabi, United Arab Emirates, 2012

Preface

My professional life in the world of zoo and wild animal medicine started one cold November morning in 1981 at the main door of the Animal Hospital at the London Zoo. This was the opportunity I had been dreaming of since I was a small child… I was finally here and ready to begin my training as a zoo veterinarian.

I was born in El Salvador, Central America and from an early age I'd taken a deep interest in zoos and wildlife in general. There was a zoo in San Salvador, the capital of El Salvador, where I spent many afternoons watching the animals. I still have the small notebook where I used to write the scientific names of all the animals I saw and I dreamed of visiting the countries and habitats where they used to live. I was young and naïve then, but driven by enthusiasm; I started writing letters to the most important zoos in the world informing the Directors that I wanted to become a zoo veterinarian and to ask what was required. There were a few very polite responses telling me that before becoming a zoo veterinarian I needed to go first to a veterinary school and study medicine in domestic animals. I attended veterinary school in Veracruz, Mexico from where I graduated in 1978. With the degree under my arm, I restarted corresponding with zoos from all over the world. This time I received an encouraging response, from the Senior Veterinary Officer at London Zoo, informing me that I could come and spend some time studying and learning at the Veterinary Science Department. I took the opportunity eagerly and after overcoming some difficult obstacles, I was finally at the main door of the Animal Hospital at London Zoo ready to begin my training as a zoo veterinarian… This was a long time ago and a lot has happened since then. However, I am who I am and I am where I am due to the friendship, understanding and encouragement I received during those early years of my professional career without which I would probably still be in my native country working with domestic animals.

There were only a handful of individuals working full time with zoo and wild animals when I started my career, but I am very proud to say that I witnessed the development of exotic animal medicine as we now know it. Incidentally, allow me please to get this off my chest: for many, "exotic animal medicine" refers to the medical care of non-domesticated pets, "zoological medicine" refers to the medical care of animals maintained in zoological collections and "wildlife medicine" refers to the medical care of free-living animals. In my humble opinion, this is a matter of semantics and all these terms refer to the same thing.

The title of this book is divided in two: "Exotic animal medicine" and "Review and test". The first part, "Exotic animal medicine", refers to the five main zoological groups kept as pets or maintained in zoological collections or commonly seen in rescue and rehabilitation centres throughout the world. The second part of the title, "Review and test", implies that the book contains material in the form of real-life clinical cases to test the clinical and diagnostic skills of professionals and students alike.

The cases are presented in a systematic and comprehensive manner using descriptive and diagnostic images, together with relevant clinical history information, clinical diagnostic or post-mortem findings and laboratory results. The reader is then challenged to formulate a differential diagnosis, to suggest a recommended therapy pathway, to provide an educated prognosis and propose ways of prevention. The final diagnosis together with information relevant to the therapy, prognosis and prevention is presented at the end of each case.

Exotic Animal Medicine: Review and test has gone one step further to achieve its ultimate goal by producing a pedagogic interactive website using selected clinical cases from the original book. The material used has been modified slightly to conform to the design of the website and to ease interaction with the cases presented. It can be accessed and used as easily on a mobile phone or tablet as on computer. The website was conceived and created parallel to the book in order to keep abreast with the latest development in information technology and will, I believe, prove to be a great and exciting learning tool.

I sincerely hope this book will prove helpful to professionals and students interested in becoming specialists in the field of exotic animal medicine.

When you hear the applause of your success, listen as well to the laughter of your failure.

Jaime Samour
Abu Dhabi, United Arab Emirates, 2012

CHAPTER 1

Mammals

Case 1.1 *J. Chitty*

Clinical history

A 6-year-old neutered female rabbit (*Oryctolagus cuniculi*) was presented with a large oral mass. While this was not causing irritation, it had begun to interfere with the eating. The owner had first noticed the mass 3 weeks previously but had not taken it for examination as the rabbit appeared well.

Physical examination

The rabbit appeared well and in good body condition. The mass in the left cheek was easily palpable and could be visualized on oral examination with an auriscope. The surface appeared smooth with no ulceration (Fig. 1.1). There was no pain associated with the mass. Dental roots could not be palpated. Oral examination (as far as it allowed) detected no evidence of dental disease. The mass did not appear excoriated or ulcerated. There were no other masses detectable in the abdomen or on the skin.

Q *1. What are your differentials for this mass?*

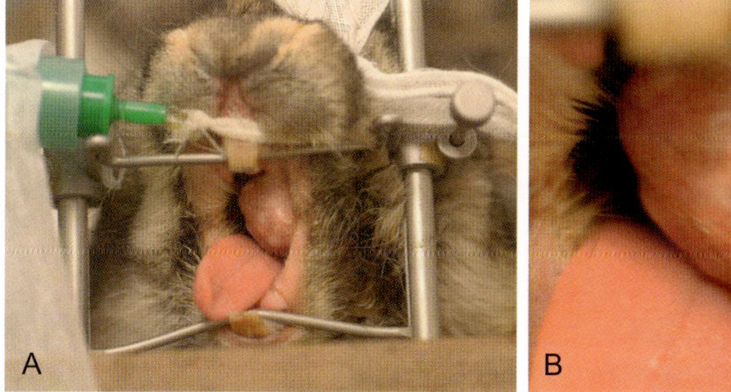

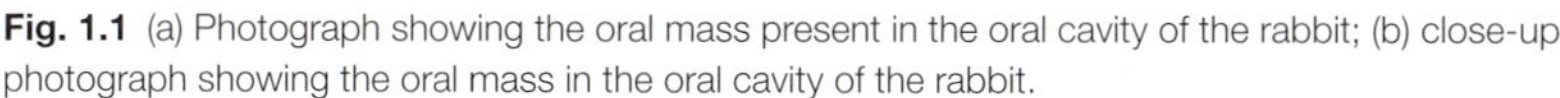

Fig. 1.1 (a) Photograph showing the oral mass present in the oral cavity of the rabbit; (b) close-up photograph showing the oral mass in the oral cavity of the rabbit.

Differential diagnoses

- ➤ Neoplasia
- ➤ Abscess associated with:
  - Dental root disease
  - Penetration of tooth crowns into the diastema
  - External injury

Q *2. How would you distinguish between these differentials?*

- ➤ Radiography
  - Skull (Fig. 1.2)
  - Thorax (checking metastatic disease of either tumour or abscess – Fig. 1.3)
- ➤ Biopsy

Q *3. What biopsy technique would you recommend?*

Laboratory diagnosis

Biopsy

Wedge punch or excision biopsies would be difficult to perform and to close the oral wound. Leaving an open wound in the mouth would almost certainly result in pain and reduced appetite. Fine needle aspirate would be less traumatic but may be less likely to achieve a diagnosis as it gives no clues as to tissue architecture. It was therefore decided to perform Trucut biopsy as a compromise between iatrogenic trauma and diagnostic capability.

Biopsy results

Mass in mouth (five sections). Within these sections, there is a non-encapsulated, moderately well-demarcated neoplastic mass that extensively effaces the normal architecture of the submucosa. This mass is composed of multiple lobules of

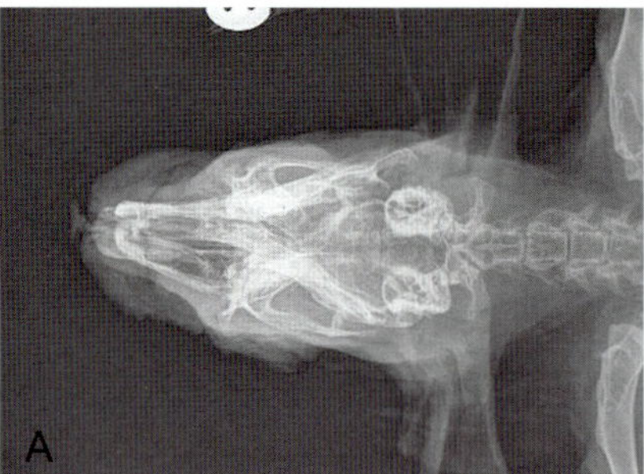

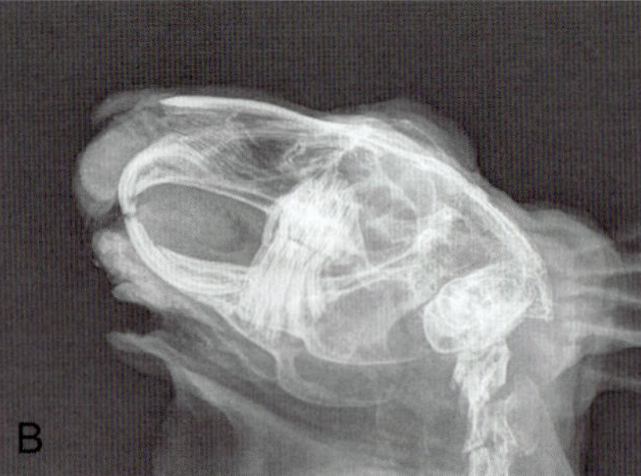

Fig. 1.2 (a) Ventrodorsal survey radiograph of the head of the rabbit; (b) latero-lateral radiograph of the head of the rabbit.

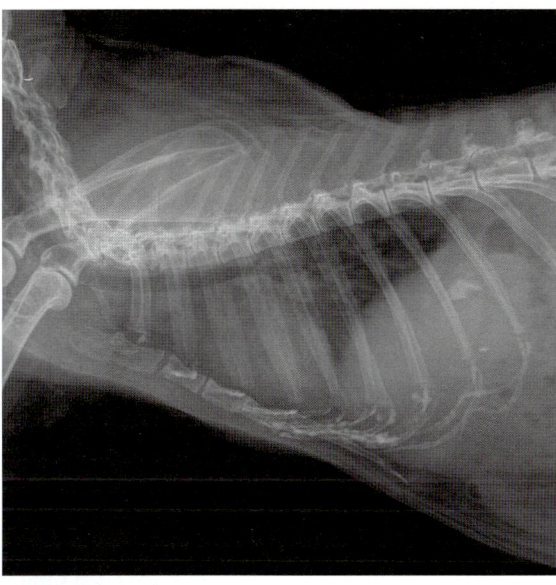

Fig. 1.3 Latero-lateral survey radiograph of the thoracic cavity of the rabbit.

neoplastic cells supported by moderate amounts of fibrovascular stroma. These lobules consist of a single layer of peripherally palisading, tall columnar cells that have moderate amounts of cytoplasm with variably distinct borders and these cells exhibit basal clearing and an apical nucleus, round to oval, with finely stippled chromatin. In the middle of this lobule, there is a population of stellate cells that form loose sheets embedded in a faintly basophilic matrix. These stellate cells have small amounts of cytoplasm with an indistinct border and their nuclei are oval to angular and have finely stippled chromatin. There are, in addition, multifocal islands that have a central cystic cavity filled with laminar keratin and that are lined by a stratified squamous epithelium. There are multifocal areas of mineralization within the mass. The supportive stroma is either relatively bland fibrous fibrovascular stroma or, in some areas, contains abundant spindle-shaped cells with indistinct borders and moderate amounts of cytoplasm and their nucleus is oval elongated with finely stippled chromatin. Mitoses are less than 1 per 10 high power fields in this population.

Radiography results

Radiographs taken at the same time as biopsy (under isoflurane anaesthesia) confirmed there was no evidence of dental disease or bony involvement. The chest appeared clear of metastases.

Histological diagnosis

- Odontogenic tumour, oral mass

Comments

The submitted mass contains an odontogenic epithelium that exhibits the characteristic palisading, basilar clearing, apical nuclear polarity and a population of loose stellate cells within the middle of these trabeculae. There are, in addition, in this mass, multiple areas of squamous metaplasia and keratinization as well as multifocal mineralization. The epithelial component appears to be the predominant component of this mass and these features are most consistent of a keratinizing ameloblastoma. There is little information in the literature as to odontogenic tumour in rabbit but, in other species, ameloblastoma is expected to behave in a locally infiltrative manner but metastasis is not expected. Excision would be expected to be curative for this mass.

Therapy

On the basis of these results, the mass was removed during a second anaesthetic (sevoflurane induction: isoflurane maintenance).

The mass was removed using radiosurgery (Fig. 1.4). It was well encapsulated – histopathology confirmed it had been completely removed. The wound was sutured using 4/0 Vicryl (Ethicon) and covered with Orabase gel.

4. What postoperative care would you recommend?

Postoperative medical management

- Antibiosis – trimethoprim–sulphonamide at 30 mg/kg BID for 7 days
- Analgesia – meloxicam at 1 mg/kg BID for 5 days
- Support feeding using Critical Care (Oxbow) until feeding well for herself
- Metoclopramide at 1 mg/kg BID subcutaneously until faeces passed normally – the rabbit was hospitalized until this stage

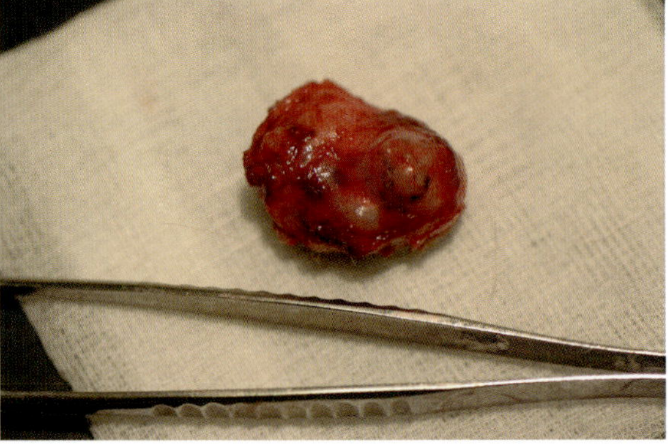

Fig. 1.4 Oral mass after removal using radiosurgery.

Further reading

Flecknell, P., 2006. Anaesthesia and perioperative care. In: Flecknell, E., Meredith, A. (Eds.), BSAVA Manual of Rabbit Medicine and Surgery, second ed. British Small Animal Veterinary Association, Gloucester, pp. 154–165.

Harcourt-Brown, F., 2002. Textbook of Rabbit Medicine. Butterworth Heinemann, Oxford.

Oglesbee, B.L., 2006. The 5-Minute Veterinary Consult: Ferret and Rabbit. Wiley Blackwell, Ames.

Case 1.2 *J. Chitty*

Clinical history

A 6-month-old female rabbit (*Oryctolagus cuniculi*) was presented with crusting around the nose and eyes and an ocular discharge. The rabbit had been purchased from a shelter a few weeks previously and there was no history of vaccination.

Physical examination

The rabbit appeared well on examination. There was hair loss and crusting around the eyes with evidence of a serous ocular discharge though there were no signs of conjunctivitis (Fig. 1.5). There were many scabs around the nose with associated purulent discharge (Fig. 1.6). These appeared partially to occlude the nares, resulting in an increased respiratory effort, and nose. Other than referred noise there were no abnormalities on thoracic auscultation. There was also crusting around the vent (Fig. 1.7). There were no other signs on examination.

Q *1. What are your differentials?*

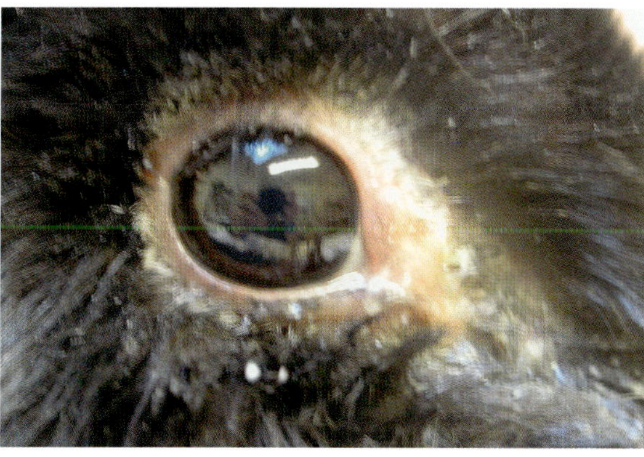

Fig. 1.5 Close-up photograph of the rabbit showing hair loss and crusting around the eye with evidence of serous discharge.

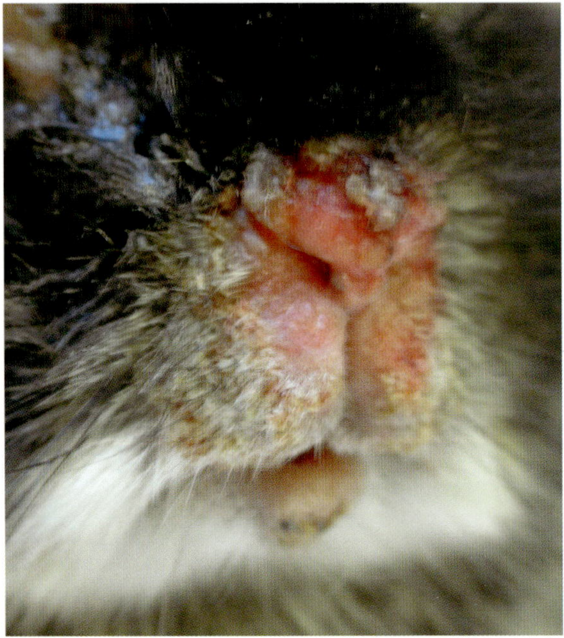

Fig. 1.6 Close-up view of the nose showing scabbing with associated purulent discharge.

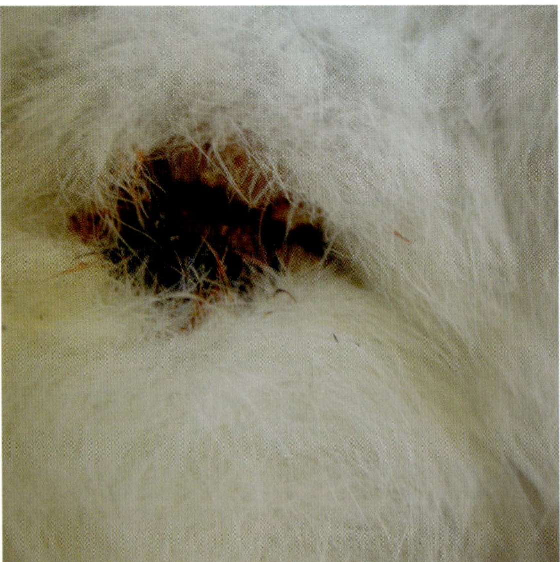

Fig. 1.7 Close-up image showing some crusting around the perimeter of the vent.

Differential diagnoses

- Respiratory disease with skin excoriation/scalding
- Infection
  - Treponemiasis
  - Bacterial pyoderma
    - Particularly secondary to trauma
  - Cutaneous myxomatosis

 *2. How would you investigate?*

Diagnostic plan

- Skin cytology – especially impression smears
- Bacteriology of the lesions
- Skin biopsy
- Radiography of the skull

Given cost constraints and the unlikelihood of vent lesions being linked to respiratory disease the owner decided against skull radiography.

Cytology

Impression smears of the lesions showed heterophils and mixed bacteria though a swab submitted for culture produced no growth.

 *3. Why do you feel the swab gave no growth in culture?*

- Submission of swab for aerobic culture only
- Presence of inhibitory factors preventing growth in the laboratory

Biopsy

The biopsy confirmed the presence of a superficial to deep bacterial infection and a heterophilic response. Silver stains did not reveal the presence of *Treponema cuniculi*.

Initial therapy

Following the biopsy, the rabbit was placed on enrofloxacin at 30 mg/kg daily by mouth pending the results.

By the time results returned (7 days) the lesions had worsened.

Q *4. Why do you feel this was the case?*

- Underlying lesions not detected in the biopsies
- Insufficient time for response
- Failure of antibiotics to penetrate lesions

- Resistance to fluoroquinolones
- Owner non-compliance
- Bacterial infection and cellular response swamping original lesions

Presumptive diagnosis

The most likely diagnosis from clinical signs and history is treponemiasis. Even though special stains were used, it is still not unusual for the organisms to be undetected on biopsy or cytology, especially if there is a concurrent bacterial pyoderma.

5. What other diagnostics may be used?

Additional diagnostic laboratory testing

- Serology. However, this may indicate past exposure only as it does not confirm current infection. False negatives are also possible as lesions may appear before seroconversion
- Trial therapy

Trial therapy

Trial therapy using amoxicillin at 50 mg/kg weekly SC on three occasions was started. Prior to therapy, the rabbit was placed on a grass and hay only diet (to preserve gut pH) and reduce the chances of alteration of gut flora when using a penicillin. A week later, the lesions had 75% resolved and were fully resolved by the final injection. This generally gives a presumptive diagnosis of treponemiasis.

There were no other rabbits in the household (it is generally advised to treat all in-contacts) but the owner was instructed to alert the rescue shelter. Benzyl or benzathine penicillin preparations are more normally used in the treatment of treponemiasis. However, this drug is currently unavailable other than in preparations containing antibiotics toxic to rabbits. However, long-acting amoxicillin preparations appear equally effective. This case illustrates that diagnostic testing is susceptible to error and that clinical medicine still has a role for acumen and trial therapies.

Further reading

Harcourt-Brown, F., 2002. Textbook of Rabbit Medicine. Butterworth Heinemann, Oxford.

Meredith, A., 2006. Dermatoses. In: Keeble, E., Meredith, A. (Eds.), BSAVA Manual of Rabbit Medicine and Surgery, second ed. British Small Animal Veterinary Association, Gloucester, pp. 129–136.

Oglesbee, B.L., 2006. The 5-Minute Veterinary Consult: Ferret and Rabbit. Wiley Blackwell, Ames.

Case 1.3 *A. Lennox*

Clinical history

A 7-year-old female lop rabbit weighing 2.5 kg was presented with the following clinical signs and symptoms of one week's duration:

- Decreased appetite
- Scratching at the right ear
- Slight clear ocular discharge.

Clinical examination

On presentation, the rabbit was a good weight and bright and alert. Abnormalities included white exudate in the right ear canal, and thickening of the base of the ear. The left ear canal was stenotic and could not be visualized beyond the horizontal portion. There was scant dried ocular discharge associated with the right eye. The rest of the examination was unremarkable. A blood sample was collected for haematology, which was unremarkable, and chemistry analysis, which is presented in Table 1.1. The rabbit was then sedated for survey radiographs of the skull, and collection of a sample from the right ear canal for culture and sensitivity.

Radiology

1. What is your interpretation of the radiographs in Fig. 1.8a–d?

Table 1.1 Blood chemistry results of the rabbit

Analysis	Results	Reference values
Albumin (g/l)	3.24	2.4–4.6
ALP (U/l)	20	4–16
ALT (U/l)	54	48–80
Bilirubin (mg/dl)	0.2	0.0–0.7
Calcium (mg/dl)	12.0	5.6–12.5
Phosphorus (mg/dl)	5.2	4.0–6.9
Creatinine (µmol/l)	0.8	0.5–2.5
BUN	14	13–29
Glucose (mg/dl)	144	75–155
Total protein (g/l)	6.7	5.4–8.3
Globulin (g/dl)	3.46	1.5–2.8

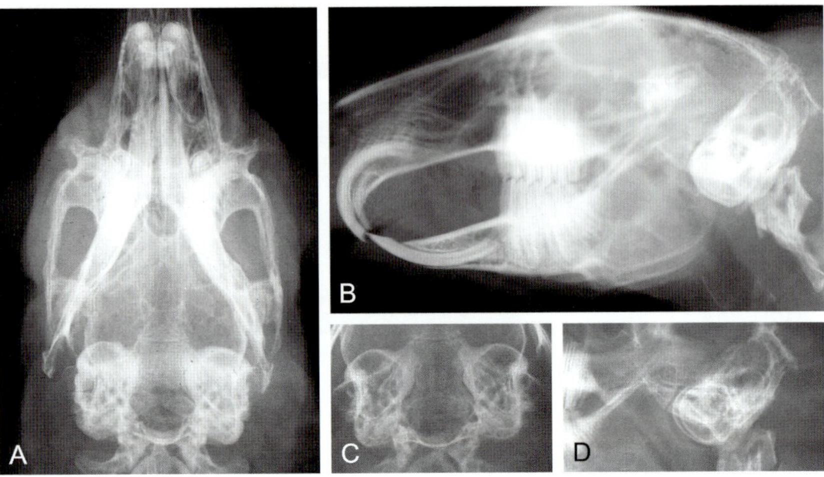

Fig. 1.8 Radiographs of the skulls of two rabbits. (a,b) Ventrodorsal and latero-lateral radiographs of the skull of the affected rabbit; (c,d) close-ups of normal osseous bullae in an unaffected rabbit.

Radiography interpretation

- Radiographic quality and positioning is fair to good, which is important for interpretation of the skull, and in particular the tympanic bullae
  - Radiographic findings include increased density of both tympanic bullae. Increased thickness of cortical bone and periosteal proliferation. The margins of the acoustic meati are irregular. These findings are indicative of chronic bilateral otitis media and possible empyema of the bullae
  - There is increased radiodensity of the bullae; however, this is less certain due to superimposition of the bullae in this view. There is no evidence of dental disease

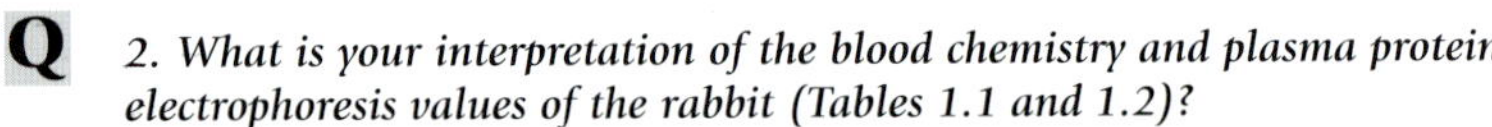

Q *2. What is your interpretation of the blood chemistry and plasma protein electrophoresis values of the rabbit (Tables 1.1 and 1.2)?*

Results

- Mild elevation of globulins, increase in beta globulins which may reflect an underlying acute inflammatory process
- Mild elevation of alkaline phosphatase (ALP) is unlikely to be of significance

Please evaluate the clinical history, Fig. 1.8a–d, the results of the physical examination and clinical diagnosis laboratory tests.

Q *3. List your differential diagnoses.*

Q *4. List your therapeutic strategy, and suggestions for additional diagnostic testing, if indicated.*

Table 1.2 Plasma protein electrophoresis of the rabbit

Parameters (g/dl)	Level	Range
Total protein	5.6	4–6
Albumin	2.89	1.7–3.6
Alpha 1 globulins	0.22	0.2–0.6
Alpha 2 globulins	0.69	0.2–0.8
Beta globulins	1.14	0.6–1.1
Gamma globulins	0.66	0.6–1.0
A:G ratio	1.07	0.8–1.3

Differential diagnoses

- Inflammation, possibly acute
- Otitis externa, right ear
- Otitis media, possibly bilateral

Therapy (Table 1.3)

Table 1.3 Therapy

Enrofloxacin, pending results of culture and sensitivity	5–15 mg/kg PO S-BID
Endoscopic-guided flushing of the ear canal under anaesthesia	
Support feeding	Oxbow Critical Care, approximately 100 ml in small frequent feedings; decreases as rabbit's appetite improves

Additional diagnostic testing

- Bilateral diagnostic otoscopy
- Computed tomography of the skull or limited to tympanic bullae

Culture and sensitivity of the ear canal revealed no growth of organisms. The owner elected to take the rabbit home on long-term antibiotic therapy without further evaluation or treatment of the ear canal. Two months later, the rabbit developed a mild left head tilt and horizontal nystagmus. The owner agreed to additional diagnostic testing at that time. The rabbit was anaesthetized for otoscopy of both ears and computed tomography of the skull. Otoscopy revealed bilateral otitis externa with an apparent intact tympanic membrane on the right side; the left could not be visualized due to marked stenosis of the horizontal ear canal.

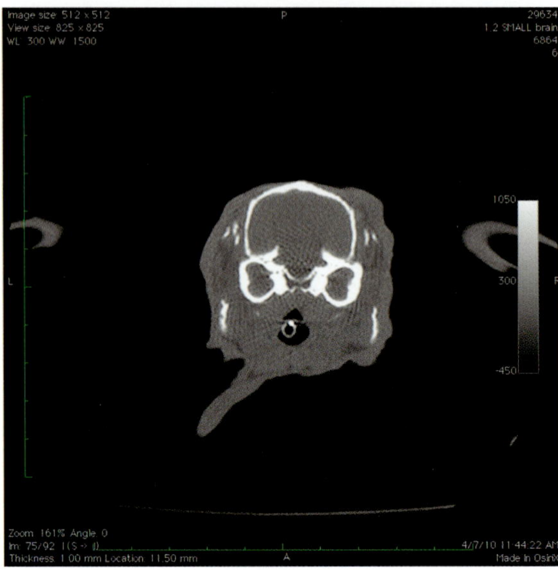

Fig. 1.9 Computed tomography. Axial view of the tympanic bullae, bone and soft tissue window.

Q *5. What is your interpretation of the computed tomography image presented in Fig. 1.9?*

➤ Bilateral otitis media with empyema of both tympanic bullae

Complete evaluation of the scan by a radiologist confirmed bilateral otitis media and externa; there were no other abnormalities noted.

Q *6. What are your recommendations for further therapy for this patient?*

➤ Total ear canal ablation and bulla osteotomy surgery with antibiotic impregnated bead placement

The rabbit was referred to a university-based veterinary surgeon with significant experience with this surgery in the rabbit. The surgery site was implanted with gentamicin and cefazolin impregnated beads at the time of surgery. Post-surgical care included meloxicam (0.2 mg/kg once daily PRN, enrofloxacin 10 mg/kg PO once daily, cisapride 0.5 mg/kg BID and support feeding.

Final diagnosis

➤ Bilateral otitis externa and media
➤ Secondary peripheral vestibular syndrome

Discussion

Otitis is a common disease in older rabbits, especially in lop varieties due to the abnormal anatomy of the external ear canal. Flexion and stenosis of the external ear canal can predispose to infection, which can progress to otitis media. Otitis media is also thought to originate from single or multiple foci of infection of the skull as a result of dental disease and/or sinusitis. Symptoms seldom develop until late in the course of the disease, and can include tilting of the head to one side, head shaking, scratching of the ears, inappetence, and depression. In cases where infection produces inflammation of the associated cranial nerves, a variety of neurological abnormalities can be seen: peripheral vestibular diseases, nystagmus, and facial nerve paralysis and Horner's syndrome. Antibiotics do not penetrate well into the infected osseous bullae due to vascular compromise, therefore, medical therapy is often only partially effective to completely unrewarding. In cases where abnormalities of the bullae are confirmed, osteotomy is recommended. It should be noted that computed tomography is a superior diagnostic imaging for evaluation of the bullae when compared to radiography.

Further reading

Chow, E.P., Bennett, R.A., Dustin, L., 2009. Ventral bulla osteotomy for treatment of otitis media in the rabbit. J. Exot. Pet Med. 18 (4), 299–305.

Deeb, B.J., Carpenter, J.W., 2004. Neurologic and musculoskeletal diseases. In: Quesenberry, K.E., Carpenter, J.W. (Eds.), Ferrets, Rabbits and Rodents, Clinical Medicine and Surgery, second ed. Saunders, St Louis, pp. 203–210.

Case 1.4 *A. Lennox*

Clinical history

A 4-year-old male rabbit weighing 5.71 kg was presented with the following clinical signs and symptoms:

- Decreased appetite
- Reduction of stool production
- Marked depression
- Abdominal distention.

The rabbit had been cared for by a rescue organization for 3 years, and had no previous medical history. A normal wellness exam was performed 6 months prior and was unremarkable. Diet was grass-based commercial pellets, grass hay and limited greens.

Clinical examination

On presentation, the rabbit was a good weight, but clinically dehydrated based on skin turgor. The abdomen was painful upon palpation. Stomach was fluid-filled and enlarged, and there was gas palpable in the caudal abdomen. The rabbit was depressed, but responsive to handling. The rabbit was administered midazolam at 0.25 mg/kg and hydromorphone at 0.1 mg/kg for sedation and analgesia. Radiographs were obtained using manual restraint only.

Radiology

1. What is your interpretation of the radiographs in Fig. 1.10a, b? Note that patient size precluded inclusion of the entire abdomen in a single view.

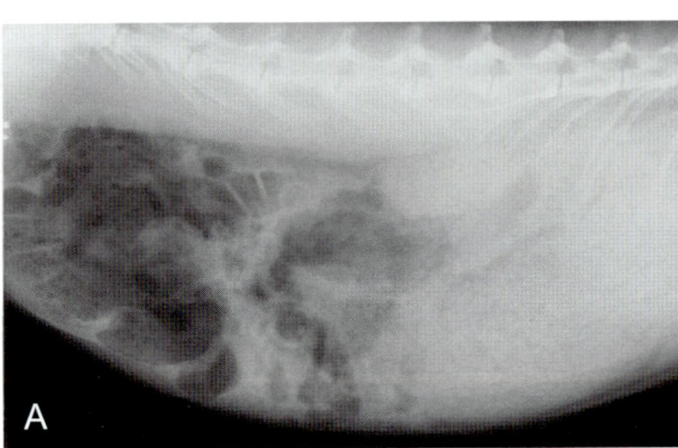

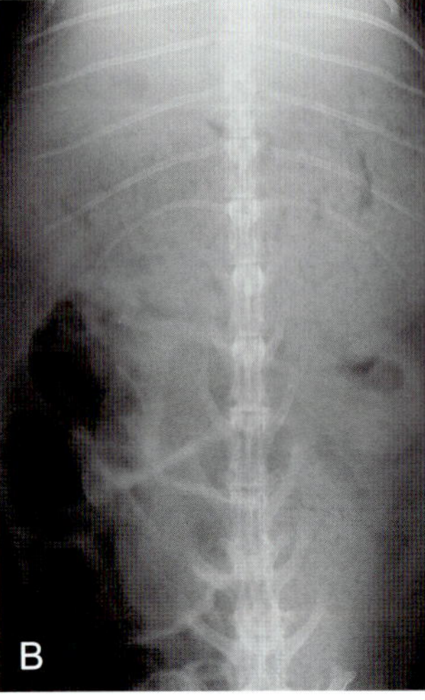

Fig. 1.10 (a) Lateral radiograph of portions of the abdomen of the rabbit; (b) ventrodorsal radiograph of portions of the abdomen of the rabbit.

Radiology interpretation

- Enlarged, fluid-filled stomach
- Gas-filled caecum and lower intestine

Clinical diagnosis laboratory examination

Blood was obtained from the lateral saphenous vein, and an in-house biochemistry was obtained, along with a blood film and haematocrit. Evaluation of the blood film, and the haematocrit were unremarkable (Table 1.4).

2. What is your interpretation of the findings of the results of blood analysis?

Summary of blood chemistry results

- Marked elevation of ALT with mild elevation of ALP
- Mild elevation of blood urea nitrogen (BUN)
- Mild elevation of calcium
- Moderate elevation of glucose

Q *3. List your differential diagnoses.*

Q *4. List your therapeutic strategy.*

Table 1.4 Blood chemistry values of the rabbit

Analysis	Results	Reference values
Albumin (g/l)	4.4	2.4–4.6
ALP (U/l)	25	4–16
ALT (U/l)	1025	48–80
Bilirubin (mg/dl)	0.6	0.0–0.7
Calcium (mg/dl)	13.8	5.6–12.5
Phosphorus (mg/dl)	6.2	4.0–6.9
Creatinine (μmol/l)	2.1	0.5–2.5
BUN	30	13–29
Glucose (mg/dl)	235	75–155
Total protein (g/l)	6.0	5.4–8.3
Globulin (g/dl)	1.6	1.5–2.8

Differential diagnoses

- Stress hypoglycaemia likely
- Gastrointestinal obstruction with secondary ileus
- Gastrointestinal stasis secondary to another disease process
- Hepatic disease
- Primary gastrointestinal disease – enteritis

Therapy (Table 1.5)

Table 1.5 Therapy

Analgesia	Buprenorphine: 0.01–0.05 mg/kg
	Butorphanol: 0.2–0.4 mg/kg
	Hydromorphone: 0.1 mg/kg
	As gastrointestinal disease can produce pain in rabbits, analgesia is an important part of therapy. Opioids appear beneficial for this purpose. While there is concern opioids may negatively impact the gastrointestinal tract, it should be kept in mind that pain and discomfort are potent inhibitors of motility
Fluid therapy	Place IV catheter and determine crystalloid fluid rate based on estimated dehydration with addition of maintenance requirements. Replace dehydration needs over 12 hours, as losses are assumed to be acute. Re-evaluate fluid needs every 8–12 hours
Motility modifiers	Cisapride: 0.5 mg/kg PO GID
	Trimebutine
Support feeding	Oxbow Critical Care 300 ml/24 hours in small frequent meals

Additional diagnostics

After 12 hours of therapy, condition had not improved. Repeat radiographs were obtained after re-administration of midazolam for sedation.

5. What is your interpretation of the radiographs in Fig. 1.11a, b?

Radiology interpretation

- Increasing size of fluid-filled stomach; stomach is taking a more rounded appearance
- Increasing amounts of gas in caecum and lower intestine, which is more apparent in the lateral view

At this point abdominal ultrasound and exploratory surgery were declined and euthanasia elected.

Post-mortem findings

The rabbit was euthanased and necropsy performed in-house (Fig. 1.12). The stomach was enlarged, and fluid-filled with mild serosal haemorrhages. The lower GI was partially filled with gas. There was no evidence of obstruction.

6. What additional lesions can you observe in the post-mortem image (see Fig. 1.12)?

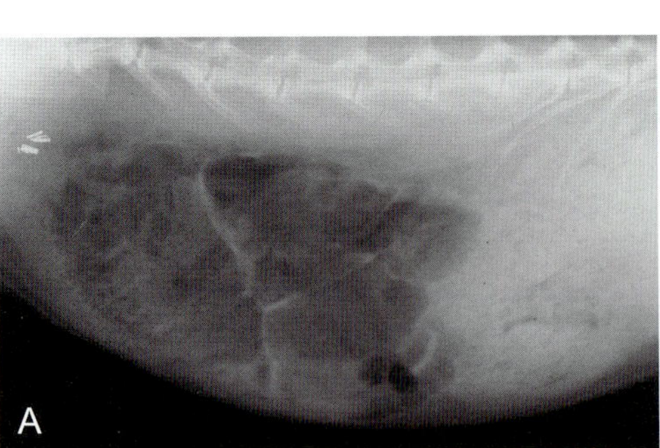

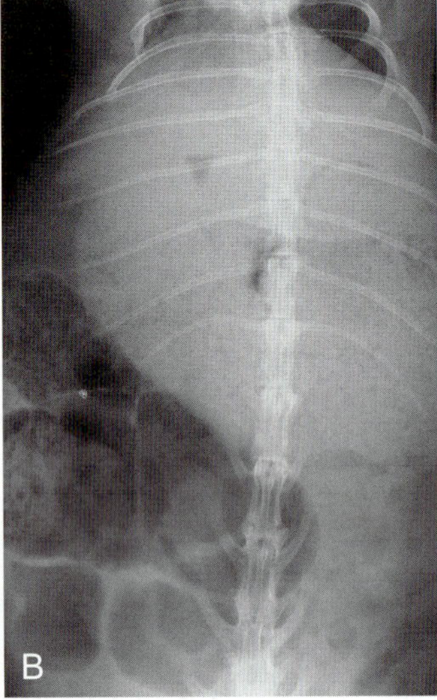

Fig. 1.11 (a) Lateral radiograph of portions of the abdomen of the rabbit, 12 hours post-presentation; (b) ventrodorsal radiograph of portions of the abdomen of the rabbit, 12 hours post-presentation.

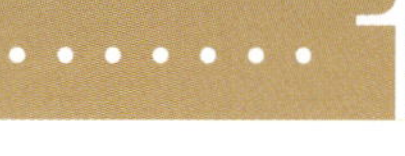

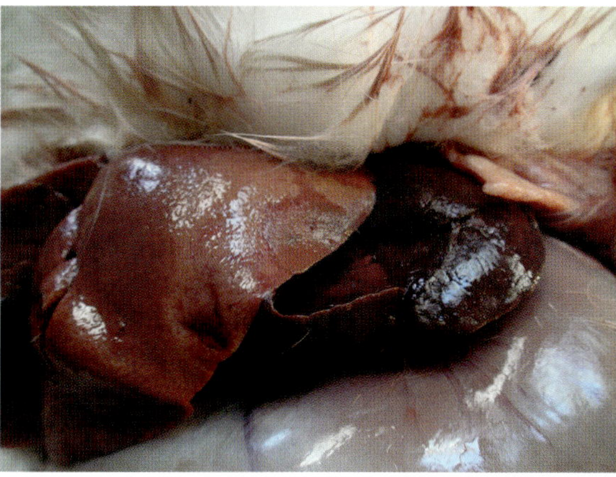

Fig. 1.12 Post-mortem examination of the rabbit.

Summary of post-mortem examination findings

- Liver: enlarged with torsion of right caudal liver lobe
- Stomach: enlarged and fluid-filled with mild serosal haemorrhage
- Intestines: mixture of food and gas
- Caecum: enlarged and gas distended

Final diagnosis

- Liver lobe torsion
- Secondary gastrointestinal stasis and ileus

Discussion

Gastrointestinal stasis is a common finding in ill rabbits. While in occasional cases stasis is a result of primary gastrointestinal disease, this syndrome can accompany many underlying conditions, including physiological and psychological stress, and worsens with anorexia and dehydration.

In this case, clinical condition and radiographic appearance of the gastrointestinal tract worsened despite therapy. This is often the most important indicator for surgical intervention. Liver torsion is common in rabbits, and involves the right caudate lobe of the liver, which is small with a narrow attachment to the hilar region. All documented cases of liver torsion involve this lobe. It is uncertain what predisposes liver to torsion, however, many affected rabbits are larger breeds, as in this case.

Diagnosis can be challenging and rabbits can present with variable, sometimes vague symptoms. However, many present with evidence of abdominal distress and show marked elevation in ALP. Disease is acute, and there is often no specific radiographic evidence of torsion. Ultrasound may be useful. Confirmation is at exploratory surgery.

There are several reports of successful surgical management of this condition when it is identified early in the course of the disease. Treatment consists of surgical removal of the affected liver lobe, and aggressive supportive care.

Further reading

Lichtenberger, M., Lennox, A.M., 2010. Updates and advanced therapies for gastrointestinal stasis in rabbits. Vet. Clin. North Am. Exot. Anim. Pract. 13 (3), 525–541.

Redrobe, S., 2010. Liver torsion in rabbits. In: Proceedings North American Veterinary Conference. Orlando, p. 1781.

Case 1.5 *A. Lennox*

Clinical history

A 5-month-old rabbit weighing 1.8 kg was presented with the following clinical signs and symptoms:

- Decreased appetite and reluctance to eat hay or greens
- Visible overgrowth of the incisors that were protruding from the mouth.

The rabbit was acquired one month previously from a pet store, and seemed otherwise healthy. Diet was commercial pellets, hay and occasional greens.

Physical examination

On presentation, the rabbit was slightly thin, but bright and alert. The mandibular incisors were elongated and deviated rostrally, protruding from the mouth. The maxillary incisors were elongated and curving caudodorsally. A cursory examination of the oral cavity with an otoscope in the conscious patient was attempted, and clinical information was minimal, but unremarkable. There were no other significant clinical findings. Blood was obtained for pre-anaesthetic work up (haematocrit and biochemistry panel) and was unremarkable. The rabbit was anaesthetized for complete oral examination and radiography of the skull.

Clinical diagnosis examination

Radiology

Q *1. What is your interpretation of the radiograph in Fig. 1.13a, b?*

Oral examination and endoscopy

Q *2. What is your interpretation of both the radiographs and the findings from endoscopy in Fig. 1.14a–c?*

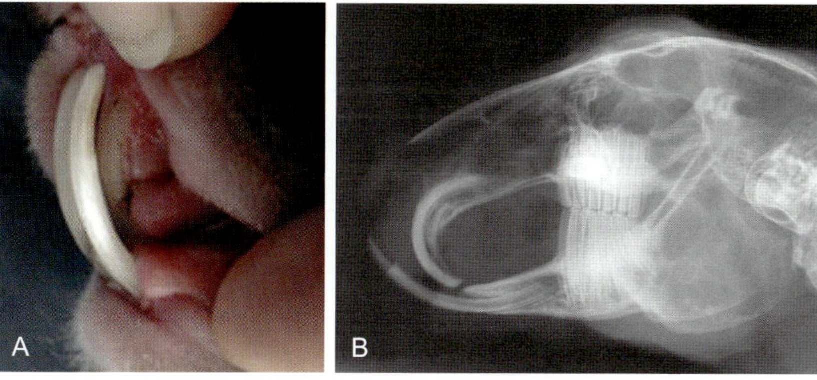

Fig. 1.13 (a) Photograph of the rabbit showing the overgrown incisors and (b) lateral radiograph of the skull of the rabbit.

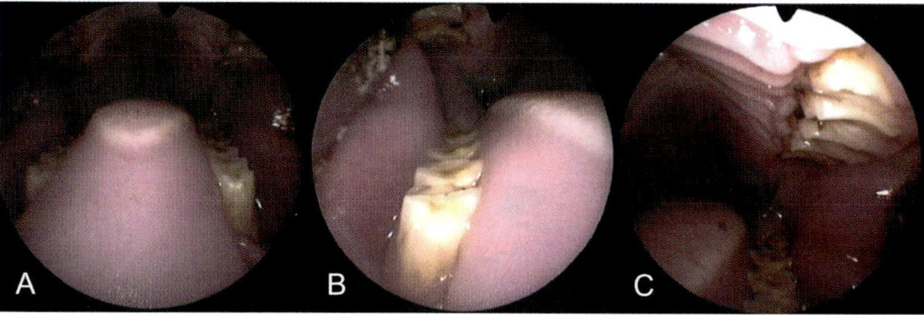

Fig. 1.14 Multiple endoscopic images of the oral cavity of the rabbit.

Results

- Radiographs demonstrate elongation and malocclusion of the primary maxillary and mandibular incisors. Cheek teeth arcades are unremarkable
- Oral endoscopic evaluation is normal

Q *3. List your differential diagnoses.*

Q *4. List your therapeutic strategy.*

Differential diagnoses

- Congenital malformation of the jaw (brachygnathism of the mandible or enognathism of the maxilla with resulting incisor malocclusion)
- Traumatic incisor malocclusion

Therapy (Table 1.6)

Table 1.6 Therapy

Incisor extraction	
Assist feeding	Herbivore Critical Care (Oxbow Pet Products, Murdock NE) as needed after surgery and into healing period until eating well on own
Analgesia	Opioid as part of pre-anaesthesia and during immediate post-surgery period for up to 24 hours
	Buprenorphine: 0.06 mg/kg q6–8 h
	Hydromorphone: 0.10 mg/kg q6–8 h
	Meloxicam 0.4 mg/kg PO for 2–3 days post-surgery, and then PRN

Discussion

Congenital jaw malformation is well described in rabbits and may represent a mandibular prognathism or maxillary brachygnathism. This malformation results in an abnormal occlusal plane and the inability of the incisors to wear normally upon each other, resulting in elongation, which can be extreme. Patterns of elongation vary but, in the rabbit, mandibular incisors typically elongate rostrally while maxillary incisors begin to curve caudally as they encounter the elongated mandibular incisors. Elongation may or may not result in perforation of soft tissues. Rabbits readily adapt to malocclusion and will continue to eat until the disease is severe. The best option for treatment of this condition is extraction of the incisors (Fig. 1.15). The technique is well described, and generally tolerated well. Prehension of food is performed with

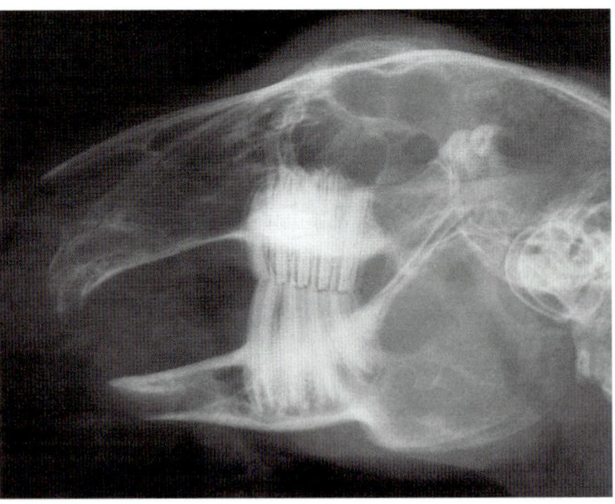

Fig. 1.15 Radiographs of the skull of the rabbit post-extraction of the incisors.

the lips and tongue; therefore rabbits are able to eat a normal diet, including hay. The loss of incisors, however, results in inability to cut larger food items into small pieces for prehension, for example whole carrots and large greens. These rabbits are also unable to cut naturally growing greens from the ground when foraging outdoors. These disabilities are minor and do not result in impacted quality of life.

Complications of extraction include bleeding, iatrogenic fracture and incomplete extraction. Teeth that are fractured or incompletely extracted may not re-erupt, or can be re-extracted when they erupt later.

One commonly utilized but inappropriate option for treatment of this condition is repeated reduction of the length of the incisors. As a normal occlusal plane cannot be achieved in this rabbit, the procedure will not be curative and will need to be repeated for the life of the patient. This must be performed under anaesthesia with a high-speed dental bur. The use of a cutting device, especially in the conscious patient is linked with risk of pain, soft tissue injury, vertical tooth fracture and damage to the apical germinal tissues including infection and abscess.

Elongation and malocclusion of the incisors is often a result of acquired dental disease of the cheek teeth. In this case, the young age of the animal and lack of abnormalities of cheek teeth make this unlikely. However, it is still possible for rabbits with congenital jaw malformation to develop acquired dental disease later in life.

Further reading

Capello, V., Gracic, M., 2005. Dental Procedures. In: Lennox, A.M. (Ed.), Handbook of Rabbit and Rodent Dentistry. Wiley Blackwell, Ames, pp. 213–248.

Case 1.6 *P. Zucca*

Clinical history

An adult rabbit developed alopecia associated with several crusty lesions on its face and toes that led the animal to heavy scratching and licking the affected areas. The rabbit is housed outdoors in a cage located in the garden and during the previous year it was vaccinated against myxomatosis.

Physical examination

The rabbit was in extreme distress due to an intense pruritus. Mobility was reduced due to the painful lesions on the face (Fig. 1.16) and toes and the rabbit was anorexic and dehydrated.

Clinical diagnosis examination

The skin was thickened and heavily encrusted; lesions were located mainly around the lips, nose, mouth, toes and they had an unpleasant smell. The areas surrounding the nail on the forelimbs seemed to be the most affected anatomical areas as shown in Fig. 1.17a, b.

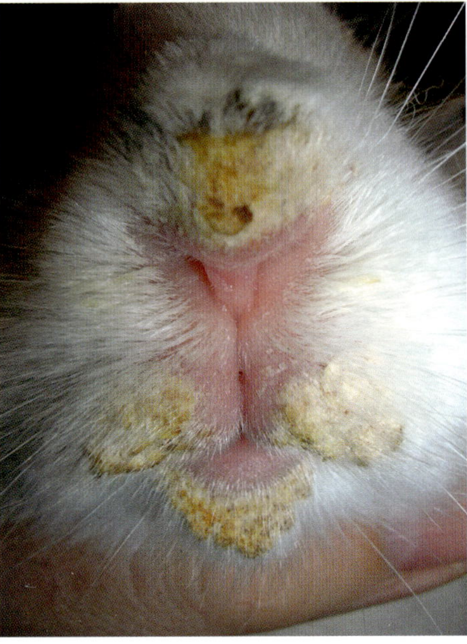

Fig. 1.16 The crusty lesions on the lips, mouth and nose are quite painful for the rabbit and a reduction in daily food/water intake is observed.

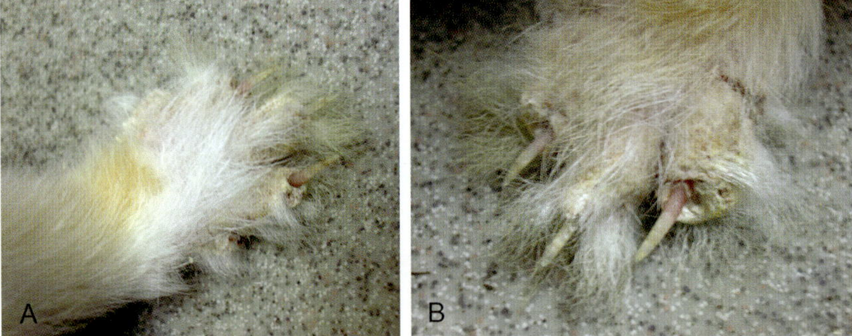

Fig. 1.17 If untreated, the pathological condition will progress until crusty lesions cover all digital skin causing secondary bacterial and/or fungal infections that lead to nail/claw avulsion.

Clinical diagnosis laboratory examination

- Deep skin scrapings from several alopecic locations were examined in 10% potassium hydroxide (KOH)

Summary of diagnostic results

- Distress behavioural patterns
- Pruritus
- Reduced mobility
- Anorexia
- Dehydration
- Crusty lesions around the face and toes
- Mites were found microscopically from skin scraping samples

 *1. List your differential diagnoses.*

 *2. List your therapeutic strategy.*

Differential diagnoses

- Dermatophytosis
- Myxomatosis (early stage in vaccinated rabbits or exposed to a low virulence viral strain)
- Bacterial dermatitis
- *Cheyletiella* spp.
- *Notoedres* spp.

Therapy

Mange in rabbits is usually treated as follows:

- Ivermectin (0.4 mg/kg SC q14d for 3 treatments)
- If crusty lesions are causing distress and pain to the animal a topical therapy with a corticosteroid/antibiotic could be administered in association with the parenteral therapy
- Environmental treatment by means of antiparasitic spray or powder that should be repeated with the same therapeutic schedule of rabbit treatment.

Final diagnosis

- Sarcoptic mange (*Sarcoptes scabiei*)

Discussion

Sarcoptic mange due to the *Sarcoptes scabiei* mite is a common pathological condition of rabbits all over the world. Mites burrow into the skin causing a painful and itching reaction. A similar pathological condition can also be caused by other mite species like *Psoroptes cuniculi*, which is the aetiological agent of ear mange, or by *Cheyletiella* spp. mite, which cause the fur mange. It is important also to associate to the pet treatment an environmental prophylaxis because mites can survive a long time far from the host and re-infections are quite common. The owner has to be informed that this parasitic disease has a secondary zoonotic potential.

Further reading

Harcourt-Brown, F., 2002. Textbook of Rabbit Medicine. Butterworth-Heinemann, Oxford.

Oglesbee, B.L., 2006. The 5-Minute Veterinary Consult: Ferret and Rabbit. Blackwell Publishing, Ames.

Quesenberry, K.E., Carpenter, J.W., 2004. Ferrets, Rabbits and Rodents: Clinical Medicine and Surgery, second ed. Saunders Elsevier, St Louis.

Case 1.7 *A. Lennox*

Clinical history

A 4-year-old female guinea pig weighing 1230g was presented with the following clinical signs and symptoms:

- Decreased appetite
- Red-tinged urine noted on the bedding
- Slightly decreased activity.

The guinea pig was acquired at 3 months of age from the pet store. Diet was commercial pellets, grass hay, daily vitamin C tablets and occasional greens.

Clinical examination

On presentation, the guinea pig was slightly thin, but bright and alert and well hydrated. The caudal abdomen appeared painful during palpation.

Q *1. What is the differential diagnosis for red-tinged urine in the guinea pig?*

- Plant pigment/porphyrin in the urine
- Urinary tract disease, including urolithiasis
- Reproductive disease in the intact female
- Contamination of urine with blood from another source (toenail, laceration)

During the examination, the guinea pig produced clear urine with a slight pink to red colour. Urinalysis was performed (urinalysis test strip and spun cytologic specimen) which confirmed the presence of blood.

2. The most likely sources of blood in this female guinea pig are the urinary and reproductive tracts. How can the two be distinguished in this species? How likely is urinalysis to confirm the source?

Like most rodent species, the guinea pig possesses two separate external urogenital orifices, vaginal and urethral. Careful observation during gentle caudal palpation often results in expression of blood-tinged fluid from either urogenital orifice. Urinalysis may not confirm diagnosis. Normal voided urine may be contaminated with blood exiting the vaginal orifice, complicating diagnosis. Urine obtained via cystocentesis can also be a source of error, as an enlarged blood-filled uterus may inadvertently be tapped instead. Supporting evidence for urinary versus reproductive disease may be obtained with additional diagnostic tests, including radiography and endoscopy (vaginoscopy/urethroscopy).

The guinea pig was sedated with midazolam and butorphanol. Careful expression of the bladder revealed blood-tinged urine emerging from the urinary orifice, and not the vaginal orifice. Radiographs were obtained.

Clinical diagnosis examination

Radiology

 *3. What is your interpretation of the radiographs in Fig. 1.18a, b?*

Radiology interpretation

- Presence of a single irregular urethrolith
- There is a moderate amount of gas in the stomach, and smaller accumulations in the caecum and intestines

Re-examination of the patient revealed that the tip of the urethrolith could be palpated with some difficulty in the proximal urethra.

Clinical diagnosis laboratory examination

Blood was obtained from the lateral saphenous vein, and an in-house biochemistry was obtained, along with a blood film and haematocrit, which were within normal limits.

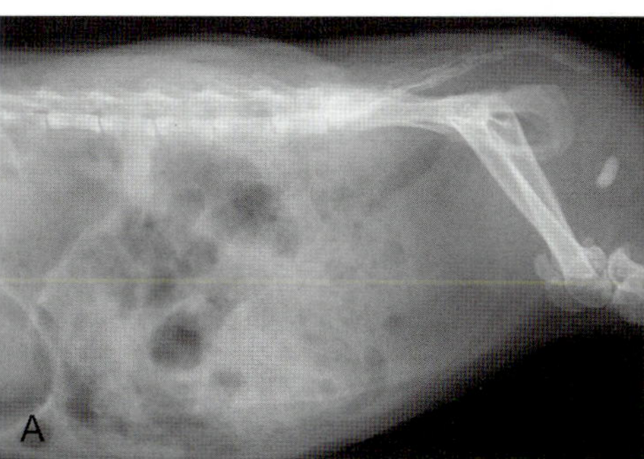

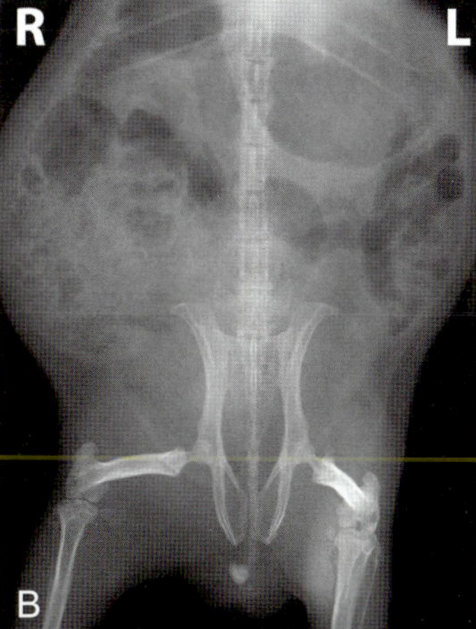

Fig. 1.18 (a) Lateral view of the abdomen of the guinea pig; (b) ventrodorsal radiograph of the abdomen of the guinea pig.

Q *4. What are the treatment options for this patient? What are the advantages and disadvantages of each?*

Treatment options

- Removal of the urethrolith. Options for removal include:
  - Urethrotomy
  - Manual removal via the urinary orifice
  - Retrieval via urethroscopy
  - Retrograde displacement of the urolith within the urinary bladder and removal via cystotomy.

Urethrotomy carries the risk of secondary stenosis of the surgical site and partial to complete obstruction. The proximal position of the stone makes manual removal less likely. Endoscopic removal may be possible if the stone can be visualized and manipulated out with retrieval instruments; however, some uroliths may be tightly adhered to the mucosa. Repositioning of the urethrolith within the bladder is likely possible, but necessitates an abdominal surgery.

The guinea pig was administered pre-anaesthetic medications (midazolam, hydromorphone and ketamine), and induced and maintained via facemask with isoflurane and oxygen. The patient was positioned in dorsal recumbency and prepared for urethral endoscopy. Lidocaine and bupivacaine were administered circumferentially around the urethral orifice. The urethral orifice was dilated using a hook and ring retractor system. At this point, the tip of the urolith was clearly visible. It was gently removed using a fine haemostat (Fig. 1.19). A sample for bacterial culture and sensitivity was collected from the urethra, which was then gently flushed with sterile saline. The patient recovered uneventfully.

 *5. What additional therapeutic options can be offered for the patient at this point?*

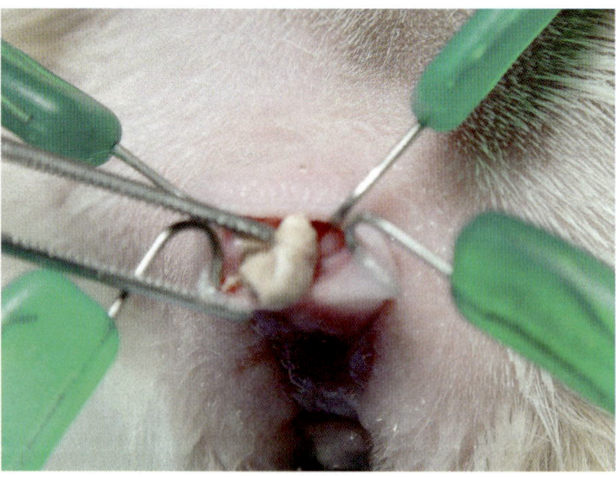

Fig. 1.19 The urolith was removed using a pair of fine haemostats.

Therapy

- Analgesia for 3–4 days following the procedure, modified based on patient behaviour and attitude
- Antibiotics pending results of culture and sensitivity
- Hand feeding if the patient is unwilling to eat normally following the procedure

The patient was sent home the same evening of the procedure, and the owner reported appetite was decreased for 24 hours. At this point, the guinea pig exhibited normal behaviour and appetite, and there was no more blood observed in the urine. Culture and sensitivity revealed no growth of bacterial organisms. Antibiotics were discontinued after 5 days.

Final diagnosis

- Urethrolithiasis
- Urethritis

Discussion

Urolithiasis is common in guinea pigs, and uroliths can be found in all portions of the urinary tract. Urethral stones can produce obstruction in male guinea pigs, but seldom do in female pigs due to the relative size of the urethra and the presence of the preputium clitoridis.

The cause of urolithiasis in guinea pigs is uncertain. While current recommendations include reduction of calcium-rich foods in the diet, including alfalfa, medical manipulation of diet and/or urine pH has not been uniformly successful. A recent survey of pet-owned guinea pigs with and without uroliths revealed a very slight decrease in incidence in pigs consuming less pellets, more hay and more greens, which may be a reflection of increased water intake.

Since reproductive disease in females can produce bloody discharge, which can be found mixed with voided urine, reliance on urinalysis to confirm urinary disease is problematic; diagnosis should be based on additional work up and confirmation.

Further reading

Capello, V., Lennox, A.M., 2008. Guinea pigs: abnormalities of the abdomen. Clinical Radiology of Exotic Companion Mammals. Wiley Blackwell, Ames, pp. 198–211.

Flecknell, P., 2005. Guinea pigs. In: Meredith, A., Redrobe, S. (Eds.), BSAVA Manual of Exotic Pets, fourth ed. British Small Animal Veterinary Association, Gloucester, pp. 28–62.

Hawkins, M.G., Drazenovich, T.L., Kass, P.H., Westropp, J.L., 2008. Risk factors associated with the development of urolithiasis in pet guinea pigs (*Cavia porcellus*). In: Proceedings of the Association of Exotic Animal Veterinarians. Atlanta.

Case 1.8 *M. Hochleithner*

Clinical history

A 3-year-old female guinea pig (*Cavia porcellus*) was referred to the clinic with a history of blood in the urine one month ago; this was treated with antibiotics for 6 days with good success. For two days, the owner has monitored polydipsia and, again, blood in the urine, also loss of appetite for 1 day.

Clinical examination

The guinea pig was active during clinical investigation. The bodyweight was 980 g and the teeth were normal. At abdominal palpation, two round enlargements, about 2.5–3 cm, on each side next to the kidneys could be palpated. The guinea pig showed pain during palpation.

Q *1. What diagnostic tests can and/or should be considered?*

Clinical diagnosis examination

- Radiology
- Ultrasound
- Computed tomography

Q *2. What are the advantages and disadvantages of each of these in this particular case?*

- *Radiology*: good information about mineralization, dental problems and possible fractures, soft tissue within abdomen might be difficult to identify, stones in the urinary tract could be seen but also missed
- *Ultrasound*: good information about soft tissue and organs within abdomen
- *Computed tomography*: expensive and anaesthesia necessary

Q *3. What would be the next diagnostic step when only one procedure is allowed by the owner?*

We recommended ultrasound for identifying the structures within the abdomen.

Result

Ultrasound

The bladder was very small and a large hyperechoic 1.2 cm structure with distal extinction of the ultrasound could be visualized; craniodorsal of the urinary bladder, a small structure with a 1 mm thick hyperechoic wall and hypoechoic lumen with a total diameter of 6 mm could be identified and followed craniolateral on both sides

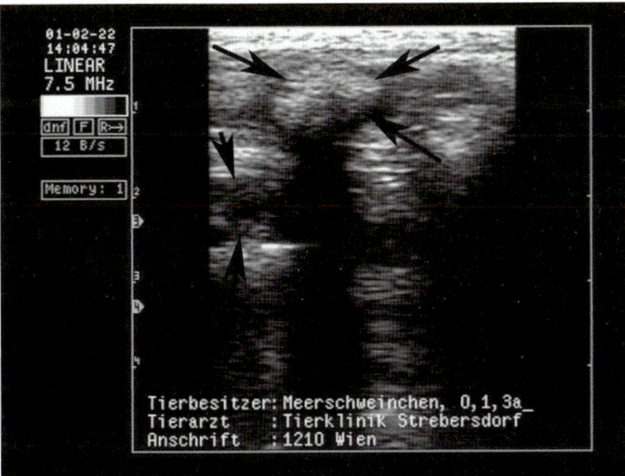

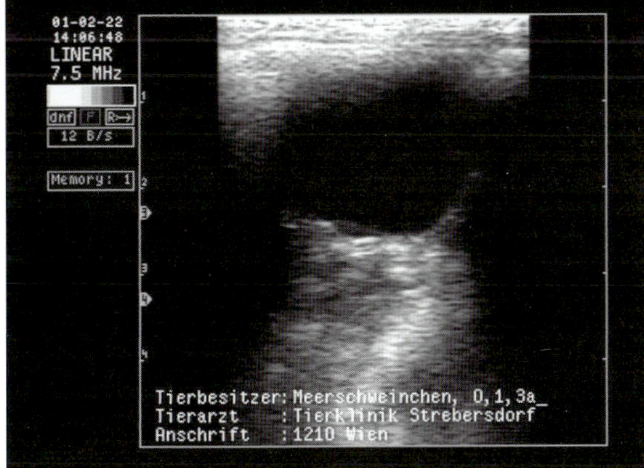

Fig. 1.20 Ultrasound images of the guinea pig.

to the region of the kidneys; laterally to the kidneys a hypoechoic round to oval-shaped structure with a small hyperechoic wall and some hyperechoic clasps inside, the right one measuring 2.5 × 2.3 cm and the left measuring 3.2 × 2.8 cm.

In ultrasound, it is essential always to have at least two views like in radiographs – a longitudinal and a transverse view. In guinea pigs and rabbits, ultrasound is not easy to perform when the GI tract is filled with a lot of gas (Fig. 1.20a, b).

Q *4. What is your interpretation of the ultrasound?*

Result

➤ Urinary bladder stone, suspected pyo-hydrometra and ovarian cysts

Q *5. What would you recommend for treatment?*

Therapy

- Antibiotics, fluids, dietary change, no surgery necessary
- Pain management, fluids, antibiotics, surgery to remove the stone
- Pain management, fluids, antibiotics, surgery with ovario-hysterectomy and removing the stone

Pain management with meloxicam 1 mg/kg and fluid therapy, antibiotics (enrofloxacin 5 mg/kg) prior to surgery with ovario-hysterectomy and stone removal (Fig. 1.21a, b).

Q *6. Is it necessary to analyse the stone?*

Yes. Female guinea pigs older than three years seem to be predisposed for cystitis and cystic calculi. Most of the stones contain calcium carbonate, calcium phosphate

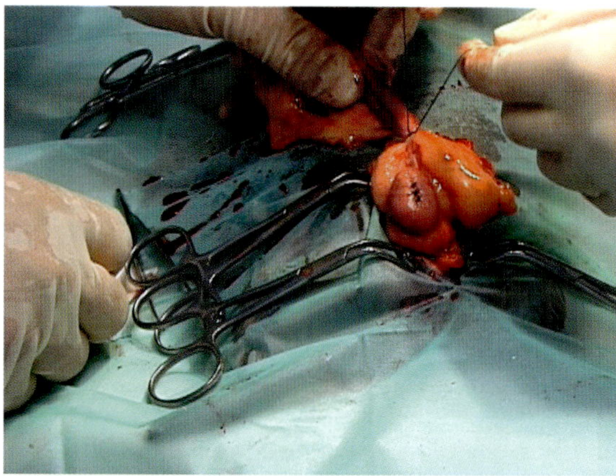

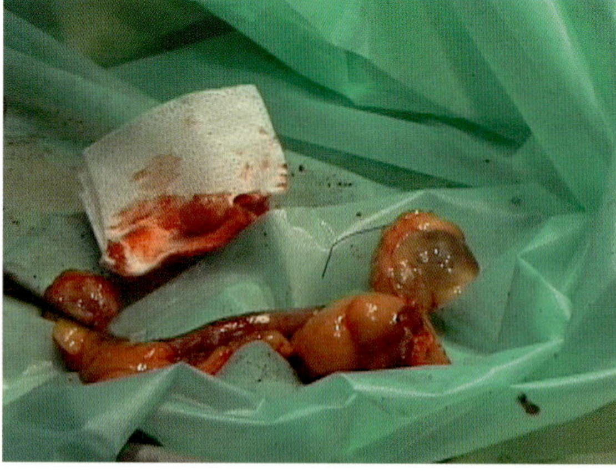

Fig. 1.21 Ovario-hysterectomy and stone removal in the guinea pig.

and, sometimes, calcium oxalate. Most of the urethra stones contain struvit due to urease-producing bacteria.

➤ Urolithiasis analysis: calcium carbonate

7. Can there be anything done to prevent stone production?

Check if owner gives mineral supplement and, if so, care has to be taken that calcium and phosphate are not too high. Also vitamin supplement (too high vitamin D) can be a problem. Feed soft diets like carrots and salad to increase urinary production. Analysis for the content of alfalfa is recommended as this is high in calcium. Extra calcium supplementation, as often suggested in pet shops and dry foods, should be avoided. Encourage more water consumption.

8. Is it necessary to recheck the guinea pig?

As uroliths are often recurrent, it is suggested to recheck the guinea pig with ultrasound 6 months after surgery.

9. Is it common in guinea pigs that there are also pathological changes in the ovaries and the uterus?

At the age of three and older, the incidence of ovarian cysts and tumours of the uterus increases. In this case, beside the ovary cysts also a pyometra and endometritis was diagnosed.

Discussion

In guinea pigs (and rabbits) with a history of blood in the urine it always has to be in mind that there might not only be infection, but urolithiasis as the primary cause. In all animals, there is always the chance that there can be two diseases at the same time. Blood in urine therefore can be a problem of the genital tract. So it is always recommended to investigate the whole animal and not only the symptom that is significant!

Further reading

Hesse, A., Neiger, R., 2008. Harnsteine bei Kleintieren. Enke, Stuttgart, Germany.

Meredith, A., Redrobe, S., 2002. BSAVA Manual of Exotic Pets, fourth ed. British Small Animal Veterinary Association, Gloucester.

Quesenberry, K.E., Carpenter, J.W., 2004. Ferrets, Rabbits and Rodents: Clinical Medicine and Surgery, second ed. Saunders Elsevier, St Louis.

Case 1.9 *M. Sabater*

Clinical history

A 4-year-old entire female tricolour English guinea pig (*Cavia porcellus*) is presented for examination after some days of lethargy and anorexia. The animal lives alone in an indoor cage and is fed a mix of guinea pig pellets (*ad libitum*), fresh greens and small amounts of fruit. The patient has never been vaccinated or dewormed. During the last month, she started showing progressive reduction of appetite until becoming completely anorectic for over the past 3 days. She has also not been passing faeces for the last 24 hours. The owner reports that the animal is urinating normally. A non-healing skin ulcer has also been present in the right flank for the last 5 months. Time for exercise out of the cage was provided twice a week.

Physical examination

On examination, the guinea pig was found relatively alert and responsive. The body condition score was 2/5 and she was markedly dehydrated. Capillary refill time was less than 2 seconds. Pulmonary and cardiac auscultation were normal. There were no evident signs of ocular or nasal discharge. No mandibular or maxilar abscesses could be palpated. Upper premolars and molars appeared to be slightly elongated. Intestinal hypoperistaltism was detected on abdominal auscultation. Mild abdominal tympanism without evident signs of pain was detected on palpation. Excessive laxity of abdominal musculature was found. Abdominal palpation also revealed the presence of two intra-abdominal masses (2 and 3 cm diameter) in the mid abdomen. The left mass appeared irregular on palpation. The urinary bladder was empty. A follicular abscess and 1 cm diameter ulceration were present in the right flank. No signs of pruritus were evident. No other abnormalities could be detected on physical examination.

Q *1. After evaluating the clinical history, Fig. 1.22a, b and the results of the physical examination, list the diagnostic tests that could be useful for this case.*

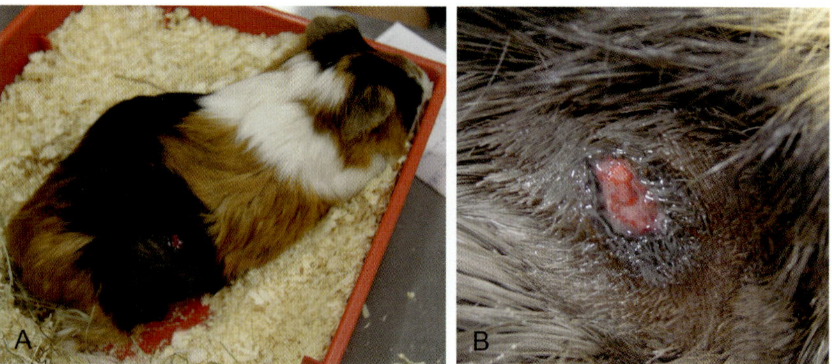

Fig. 1.22 (a,b) Images showing skin lesions on the right flank of the female guinea pig.

Clinical diagnosis examination

Conscious survey radiographs and ultrasonographic examination were performed.

Radiology

2. What is your interpretation of the radiographs in Fig. 1.23a, b?

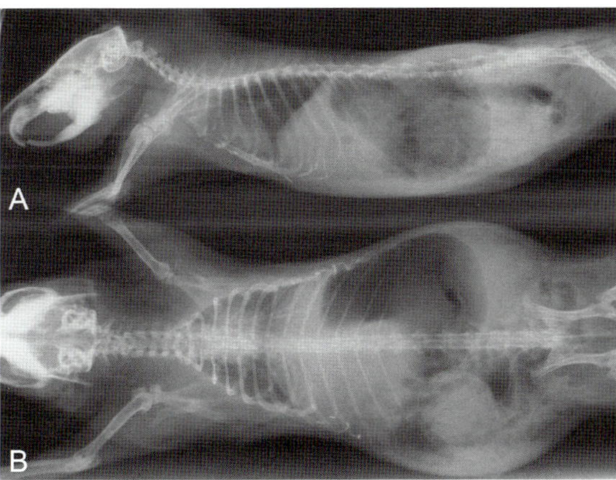

Fig. 1.23 (a) Ventrodorsal and (b) right-lateral survey radiographs of a 4-year-old female entire guinea pig.

Ultrasonography (Fig. 1.24)

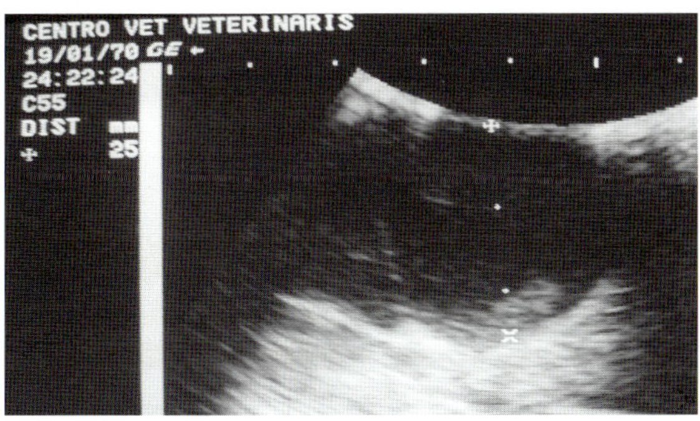

Fig. 1.24 Ultrasonographic appearance of the right intra-abdominal mass.

Clinical diagnosis laboratory examination

A blood sample was collected for routine haematology, biochemistry and plasma protein electrophoresis analyses. A faecal sample was collected to check for the presence of endoparasites.

The results of the clinical diagnosis laboratory assays are noted in Tables 1.7–1.9.

Table 1.7 Haematology values of the guinea pig

Parameters	Results (absolute)	Results (%)	Reference values
RBC ($\times 10^{12}$/l)	5.34		4–7
Hb (g/dl)	13.9		11–17
Hct (l/l)	42.7		35–45
MCV (fl)	80		
MCH (pg)	26.1		
MCHC (g/dl)	32.6		
WBC ($\times 10^{9}$/l)	14.66		7–14
Neutrophils ($\times 10^{9}$/l)	5.13	35	20–60
Band	0.15	1	
Segmented	4.98	34	
Lymphocytes ($\times 10^{9}$/l)	7.7	53	30–80
Monocytes ($\times 10^{9}$/l)	0.44	3	2–20
Eosinophils ($\times 10^{9}$/l)	1.17	8	0–5
Basophils ($\times 10^{9}$/l)	0.15	1	0–1
Platelets ($\times 10^{9}$/l)	542		

Table 1.8 Blood chemistry values of the guinea pig

Analysis	Results	Reference values
ALKP (U/l)	78	
Calcium (mg/dl)	10.8	7.8–10.5
Cholesterol (mg/dl)	13	20–43
Creatinine (mg/dl)	0.2	0.6–2.2
ALT (U/l)	74	10–25
Glucose (mg/dl)	115	50–135
Phosphorus (mg/dl)	3.85	5.3
Triglycerides (mg/dl)	28	0–145
Urea (mg/dl)	51	9–32

Table 1.9 Plasma protein electrophoresis of the guinea pig

Parameters	Fractions (%)	Concentrations (g/l)	Reference values
Total protein		53	46–62
Albumin	66.8	35.4	21–39
Total globulins	33.2	17.6	17–26
Alpha 1 globulins	3	1.6	
Alpha 2 globulins	14.6	7.7	
Beta globulins	7.2	3.8	
Gamma globulins	8.4	4.5	
A:G ratio		2.01	

RBC, WBC and thrombocyte morphology

- No abnormalities detected

3. What is your interpretation of the haematology, blood chemistry and protein electrophoresis values shown in Tables 1.7–1.9?

Faecal examination

- Direct smear and flotation from faeces collected from the cage: no parasitic forms observed

Cytology

Cytology of the white content of the mass was performed in house and increased numbers of neutrophils, macrophages and bacteria were found confirming the presence of an infectious component. No parasitic, fungal or neoplastic forms were found. Mass removal and histopathological examination were offered but rejected by the owner.

Summary of diagnostic results

- Radiographic findings included the presence of abundant radiolucent gas density in the stomach and intestines, an enlarged liver and the presence of two radiodense soft tissue density masses in the abdomen. No other abnormal findings could be reported from radiographic examination
- Ultrasonographic examination confirmed the presence of two hyperechoic masses of 2 and 3 cm diameter in the ovarian/uterine projection region. The left one presented a trabeculated image. The liver appeared slightly hyperechogenic

- Haematology analysis showed minimal leucocytosis
- Blood chemistry analysis showed minimal elevations of total calcium levels, decreased levels of cholesterol and creatinine, and marked elevations of urea and ALT
- Plasma protein electrophoresis within normal limits
- Faecal examination was negative for the presence of endoparasites
- Cytology from the skin mass revealed a bacterial infectious component

Please evaluate the clinical history, Figs 1.22a, b, 1.23a, b, 1.24, the results of the physical examination and clinical and laboratory diagnostic tests.

4. List your differential diagnoses.

Differential diagnoses

- Ovarian cysts
- Neoplasia (trichofoliculoma) or abscess
- Minimal degree of acquired cheek teeth malocclusion of suspected nutritional origin due to an inadequate diet mainly based on pellets and a lack of fibre
- Tympanism that may be secondary to dental pathology, pain, lack of exercise, anorexia, dehydration, mechanic, organomegaly (ovarian cysts), intestinal obstruction, parasitism

5. List your therapeutic strategy.

Therapy

Ovario-hysterectomy and skin mass removal after stabilization of the patient were recommended to the owner but declined. The possibility of performing an echo-guided drainage of the ovarian cysts and the posterior application of a deslorelin implant were discussed with the owner and accepted. Benefits, risks and prognosis were also discussed with the owner. A total of 12 ml of transparent and non-cellular fluid was obtained from the left cyst (Fig. 1.25) (two punctures were necessary due to the presence of cavities within the mass) and 6 ml were obtained from the right one.

The therapeutic management of the guinea pig is given in Table 1.10.

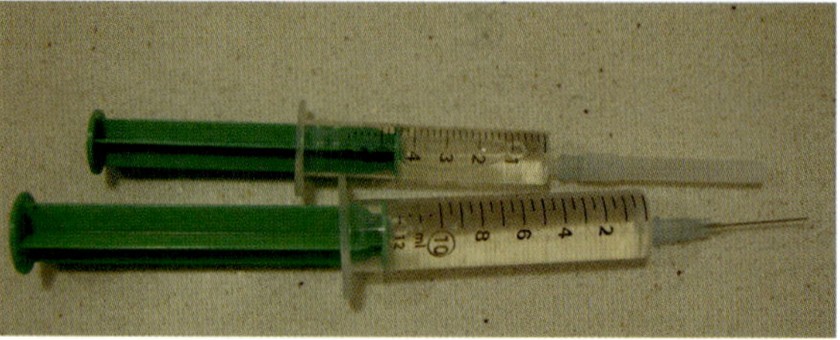

Fig. 1.25 A total of 12 ml of transparent non-cellular fluid was obtained from the left cyst.

Table 1.10 Therapy

Buprenorphine	0.05 mg/kg SC BID
Meloxicam oral suspension	0.2 mg/kg once a day for 3 days
Metoclopramide oral suspension	0.5 mg/kg PO TID
Fluids	Glu NaCl 0.9% 10 ml/kg SC BID
Forced feeding	6 ml of Oxbow Critical Care for herbivores PO QID
Wound management	Disinfection with diluted clorhexidine 0.05% and application of silver sulphadiazine cream topically BID

Evolution

The guinea pig started passing faeces after 16 hours of therapy and started eating by herself after 32 hours. The animal was sent home to continue with the treatment 3 days after admission. One week after and one month after, the animal was rechecked and no palpable masses were detected on physical examination. Appetite and faeces were normal.

Discussion

Rete-ovarii cysts have been identified in 76% of entire female guinea pigs between 18 months and 5 years old. Cysts develop spontaneously, varying in diameter from 0.5 to 7 cm and increasing their size with time. They could be simple or multilobulated and the content tends to be a clear and transparent fluid. In most cases, both ovaries are affected. Cysts could be functional or not. Affected individuals could present abdominal distension and occasionally fatigue, anorexia and depression. If cysts are functional, bilateral truncal alopecia is the most common clinical sign. The recommended treatment consists of ovario-hysterectomy. Percutaneous aspiration of the cysts tends to show recurrence. They could also be associated with fibroleiomyomas, endometrial cystic hyperplasia, mucometra and endometritis. Cysts could be associated with a decline in fertility. In this case, and despite no research studies being available at present for the guinea pig, the authors opted for a deslorelin implant to decrease the hormonal levels. Other medical therapeutic options reported in the literature are hormone therapy with leuprolide acetate injections (100 µg/kg SC every three weeks), gonadotrophin-releasing hormone (GnRH) (25 µg/guinea pig every two weeks for two injections), or human chorionic gonadotrophin (HCG) (1000 USP repeated in 7–10 days) (allergic reactions and reduced effectiveness reported). In this case, the authors consider that the anorexia and gut stasis shown could be related to a mechanical effect due to the big size of the cysts.

Skin and subcutaneous tumours are the second most commonly reported neoplasia of guinea pigs. Benign trichoepitheliomas tend to be cystic structures arising from the body (usually dorsum) and may contain sebum, hair and keratin debris. The bacterial infection evidenced through cytology could have been secondary. Trichoepitheliomas could become ulcerated and may present discharge. The recommended treatment is the surgical excision of the mass.

Further reading

Carpenter, J., 2005. Exotic Animal Formulary, third ed. Saunders Elsevier, St Louis.
Keeble, E., Meredith, A., 2009. BSAVA Manual of Rodents and Ferrets. British Small Animal Veterinary Association, Gloucester.
Richardson, V., 2000. Diseases of the Guinea Pig, second ed. Blackwell, Ames.

Case 1.10 *A. Lennox*

Clinical history

An 18-month-old rat weighing 950 g was presented with the following symptoms:

- Decreased appetite and reduced stool production over the last 2 weeks
- Increasing respiratory effort noted over the last 48 hours
- Marked depression over the last 24 hours, with history of decreased activity for about 2 weeks.

The rat had a history of a mammary tumour surgically excised about 3 months ago. Diet was commercial rodent block plus about 20% table foods including fruits and vegetables. There was no other significant history.

Clinical examination

On presentation, the rat was thin, clinically dehydrated based on skin turgor, hypothermic and depressed. There was both increased respiratory rate and effort, with no nasal or ocular discharge. Dyspnoea increased with handling and stress. Upon auscultation of the thorax, cardiac sounds were obscured by harsh lung sounds. There were no abnormalities of the upper respiratory tract noted. The owner initially declined all diagnostic testing.

1. Without the benefit of additional diagnostics, what are your differential diagnoses? What can you offer for therapy at this point?

Differential diagnoses

- Pneumonia, bacterial most likely
- Cardiovascular disease
- Trauma – haemothorax, pulmonary oedema, diaphragmatic hernia
- Thoracic neoplasia

Without other confirmatory tests, this presentation is often assumed to be bacterial pneumonia, and trial therapeutics commonly offered.

Therapy (Table 1.11)

Table 1.11 Therapy

Fluid therapy	While intravenous or intraosseous fluids are ideal for depressed and dehydrated patients, obtaining vascular access in this patient necessitates increased risk, which should be considered When administering fluids subcutaneously, calculate fluid volume from estimated % dehydration added to maintenance requirements, and divide into 3 boluses. Replace dehydration needs over 24 hours, as losses are assumed to be chronic based on history. Re-evaluate fluid needs every 8–12 hours
Antibiotics	Enrofloxacin 5–15 mg/kg PO or IM; note multiple IM injections of this drug are associated with pain and muscle necrosis; PO administration may be difficult in patients with dyspnoea Enrofloxacin can also be administered via nebulization Doxycycline: 70–100 mg/kg IM q7d
Oxygen	
Restoration of normothermia	To prevent exacerbating dyspnoea, re-warming is performed gently
Support feeding	Dyspnoeic patients are often unwilling to eat. Some patients are able to take liquid nutrition administered by slow and patient hand feeding with products such as strained vegetable baby food, commercial hand-feeding products or ground rodent diets

Clinical re-evaluation

Demeanour and activity improved within 24 hours with correction of dehydration. However, respiratory symptoms were unchanged. Hand feeding was difficult, but possible with care. The owner elected to take the patient home with hand feeding and oral enrofloxacin. Long-acting doxycycline was injected intramuscularly after correction of dehydration.

Clinical recheck examination

The rat was presented 2 weeks after initial diagnosis. The respiratory symptoms had worsened, and the owner was experiencing increased difficulties related to hand feeding. Diagnostic testing was strongly recommended.

2. What additional diagnostic tests could be considered at this point? What are the limitations of each?

Diagnostic testing

- Thoracic radiographs
- Ultrasonography, including echocardiography

- Specific pathogen testing – serology and polymerase chain reaction (PCR)
- Culture and sensitivity

Thoracic radiography is the most practical next diagnostic step. Ultrasonography and/or echocardiography can be useful, but challenging in this small patient. Serology and PCR are available for some common rat respiratory pathogens, however, some organisms, in particular *Mycoplasma* spp., are ubiquitous in pet rats, therefore interpretation is problematic. Obtaining a sample for culture and sensitivity is extremely difficult in this small patient with marked dyspnoea. Methods include endotracheal wash, which is technically very difficult, and thoracocentesis, which is risky.

3. What are the problems related to obtaining radiographs of a patient in severe respiratory distress? What are the options, and what would you recommend?

Methods to obtain radiographs may represent serious risk in the dyspnoeic patient. Options include:

- Radiography utilizing general anaesthesia
- Radiography utilizing manual restraint only
- Radiography utilizing low dose sedation.

Choose radiography with low dose sedation. In humans and other companion species including rabbits, death rate for sedation is lower than that for general anaesthesia. General anaesthesia produces respiratory depression, with some drugs producing more potent effects than others. Low dose sedation has been shown to be extremely effective for facilitation of diagnostic testing and treatment in very sick animals, in particular those with respiratory distress.

Low dose midazolam (0.25 mg/ml) combined with an opioid such as butorphanol at 0.20 mg/ml has been shown to reduce anxiety related to respiratory distress, and even temporarily improve respiratory effort.

Radiology

Q ***4. What is your interpretation of the radiographs in Fig. 1.26a, b?***

- On the lateral view, the cardiac shadow is partially effaced by a pulmonary opacity occurring in the lung. The cranial part of the cardiac shadow can be seen and is rounded, but not enlarged
- On the ventrodorsal view, the left side of the cardiac shadow is effaced by the alveolar pattern in the left lung. The right side of the cardiac shadow is not well seen due to the pulmonary opacity
- Conclusion is alveolar disease consistent with pneumonia, non-cardiogenic oedema or haemorrhage; concurrent cardiac disease is less likely but cannot be absolutely ruled out

Due to worsening condition, and the severe radiographic lesions, euthanasia was elected.

Q ***5. What lesions can you observe in the post-mortem image of the lungs and heart of this rat (see Fig. 1.26a, b)?***

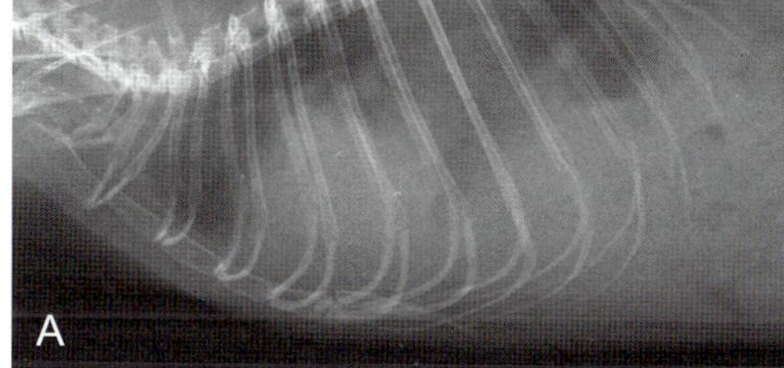

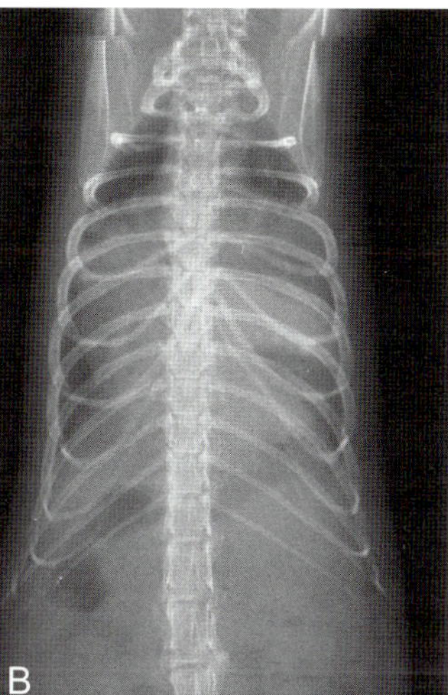

Fig. 1.26 (a) Lateral view of the thorax of the rat; (b) ventrodorsal view of the thorax of the rat.

Summary of post-mortem examination findings

- Collapsed, consolidated firm lungs; the left lobe is rounded
- Incised left lung lobe reveals a large pulmonary abscess

Final diagnosis

- Severe bacterial pneumonia with pulmonary abscess
- Exact aetiology uncertain, and is likely multifactorial; consider abscess-forming *Streptococcus* spp. as a co-pathogen

Discussion

Respiratory disease represents one of the most common presentations of the pet rat to the veterinarian. Symptoms may range from occasional sneezing and lethargy to respiratory distress with dehydration and shock. Aetiologies vary, and may include a number of bacterial or viral organisms, sometimes in combination. These most commonly include *Mycoplasma* spp., cilia-associated bacillus (CAR), *Pseudomonas aeruginosa*, *Corynebacterium kutscheri*, *Streptococcus* and others. Episodes of respiratory disease may be preceded by stressful events (change in social setting, for example, loss or addition of a companion) or other underlying illness.

Culture and sensitivity (c/s) for aid in diagnosis of bacterial respiratory disease in rats is problematic. Patient size prevents deep nasal culture or endotracheal wash. *Mycoplasma* spp., which are commonly implicated in respiratory disease of rats, are not identified with routine c/s (see below). In most cases, treatment of respiratory disease proceeds without benefit of culture and absolute identification of the primary pathogen.

Mycoplasma spp. (*M pulmonis* and *M arthritidis*) are commonly implicated in respiratory disease in pet rats. Strict biosurveillance through ELISA testing, elimination and biosecurity have dramatically reduced the incidence of this disease in laboratory colonies in the USA, Europe and Japan. A survey of more than 100 institutions in Europe revealed an infection rate of 3.6%. Conversely, a survey of caught wild rats in the USA demonstrated antibodies in 72.9% of animals. Disease is often subclinical.

Mice and rats serve as models for mycoplasmal pneumonia in humans. Studies indicate inflammation is an important component of pulmonary mycoplasmosis. Diagnostic testing for *Mycoplasma* spp. includes serology, PCR, culture and thorough histological identification of lesions. Culture is impractical due to the nature of the organism, however, serology and PCR are available to practitioners.

In the author's experience, radiographs are extremely helpful and aid in identification of cardiac disease, which is the primary differential for lower respiratory disease, and severe pulmonary changes, including pulmonary abscess. Rats with collapsed, infiltrated lungs and abscess are not likely to respond long term to any form of therapy, and prognosis should be relayed to the owner. In these cases, palliative care is attempted until quality of life is poor, at which point euthanasia should be strongly considered. The author strongly recommends thoracic radiographs for all rats with evidence of severe respiratory disease, or chronic disease responding temporarily or only partially to antibiotic therapy.

Treatment includes supportive care and treatment of concurrent or secondary conditions, and antibiotics administered parentally and via nebulization. For critical patients severely dehydrated or in shock, antibiotic administration is delayed until fluid deficits are mostly corrected. While delay is counterintuitive, it should be kept in mind that antibiotics may be harmful in patients with pre-renal insufficiency. As most respiratory disease is chronic, a delay of 6–12 hours for correction of fluid deficits is not associated with increased mortality.

Fluid therapy is based on correction of fluid deficits. Antibiotics currently favoured by the author and others are a combination of enrofloxacin 15–20 mg/kg SID or 10–15 mg/kg BID, and doxycycline hyclate 5 mg/kg PO q12h. The anti-inflammatory effects of tetracycline-class drugs may be beneficial. In some species, *Mycoplasma* directly stimulates histamine production; therefore, antihistamines may be beneficial as well. Furosemide may be helpful in cases of thoracic fluid. The author has not attempted thoracocentesis in a rat.

The author has found that failure to respond is usually associated with the presence of firm or collapsed lung lobes or pulmonary abscess in cases for which necropsy was available. Since treatment of cardiac disease is markedly different from that of bacterial respiratory disease, distinguishing between the two is important. Diagnostic imaging techniques, such as radiography and ultrasonography, can be extremely useful. It should be noted that radiographic quality is of critical importance when working with very small patients. Careful technique, including mammography film, should be utilized.

Respiratory disease often responds to antimicrobial therapy. Failure to respond is often due to the nature of rat respiratory pathogens; *Mycoplasma* spp. tends to induce a severe inflammatory response, while *Streptococcus* tends to form pulmonary abscesses. Some rats respond to adjunct therapy such as bronchodilators and anti-inflammatory drugs, including steroids. Pulmonary abscesses cannot be resolved with antibiotic therapy, and often explain why some patients fail to respond, or only respond partially.

Further reading

Capello, V., Lennox, A.M., 2008. Radiographic equipment for the small exotic mammal patient. Clinical Radiology of Exotic Companion Mammals. Wiley Blackwell, Ames pp. 4–6.

Sayers, I., Smith, S., 2010. Mice, rats, hamsters and gerbils. In: Meredith, A., Redrobe, S. (Eds.), BSAVA Manual of Exotic Pets. British Small Animal Veterinary Association, Gloucester, pp. 1–27.

Case 1.11 *M. Sabater*

Clinical history

Two rats were presented for examination of tumoural masses. Rat 1 (Fig. 1.27): a 2.5-year-old entire female pet rat (*Rattus norvegicus*) is presented for examination with two masses that have been continuously growing for the past

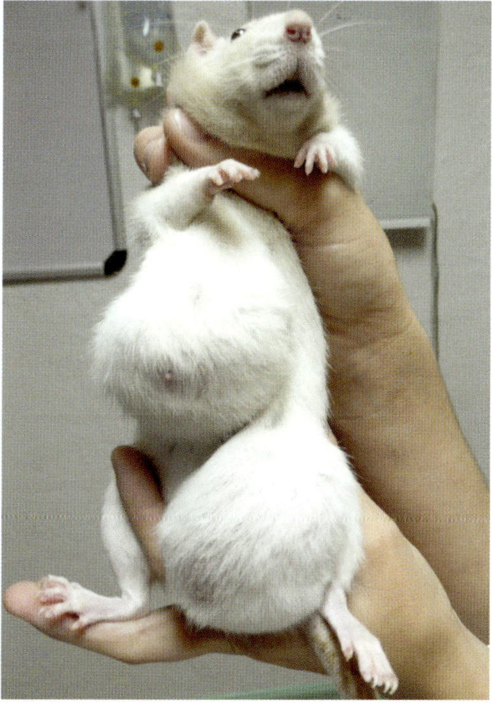

Fig. 1.27 Entire female rat presented with visible masses.

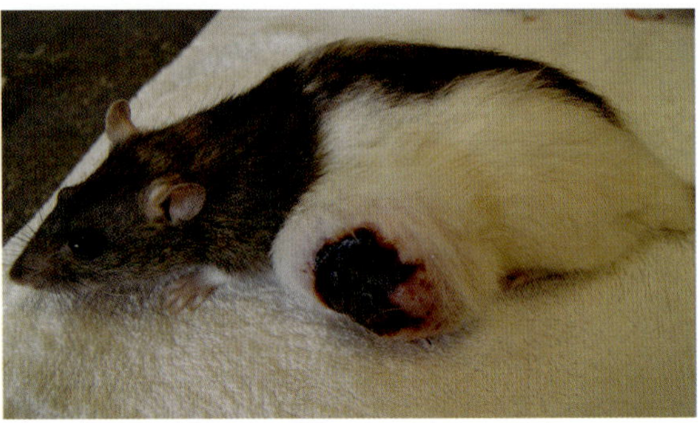

Fig. 1.28 Entire female rat presented with visible masses.

4 months. The rat shares the cage with another female rat and is fed a mix of laboratory rat pellets, nuts, fresh vegetables and fruits. The rat has never been vaccinated, however, and faecal tests to check for endoparasites were done 9 months before. The owner also reports that the animal is urinating and defaecating normally. Rat 2 (Fig. 1.28): a 2-year-old entire female rat is presented for examination of one mass that has been growing for the last 3 months. The rat lives in a cage with another two female rats and is fed on rat pellets, cereals, vegetables and fruit. The owner does not report signs of pruritus.

Physical examination

On examination, both rats were alert and responsive. The body condition score was 3/5 and the hydration status looked correct. Capillary refill time was less than 1.5 seconds. Pulmonary and cardiac auscultation was apparently normal. No signs of ocular or nasal discharge were evident. No abnormalities were detected on oral examination. The first rat presented two 4.5–5 cm diameter firm, non-ulcerated and non-attached to the muscle, round masses located in the right side of the thorax and in the left inguinal area. The second rat presented a unique 5×3 cm firm, non-attached to the underlying tissues, ulcerated and partially necrotic mass in the left side of the abdominal region. Abnormal findings were not detected on palpable lymph node examination. No signs of pruritus were evident in any of them. No porphyrins were detected under Wood's lamp examination. No other abnormalities could be detected on physical examination.

Q *1. After evaluating the clinical history, Figs 1.27 and 1.28, and the results of the physical examination, what is your presumptive diagnosis for this case?*

Q *2. What is your recommended diagnostic and therapeutic plan?*

Diagnosis

➤ Mammary gland tumours

Suggested therapeutic plan

Mastectomy and ovario-hysterectomy is the treatment of choice. The prognosis is favourable if the tumour is benign and the tumoural tissue is completely resected (including affected regional lymph nodes when necessary). Sometimes more than one surgery is required due to the recurrence of fibroadenomas.

Discussion

Mammary gland tumours are common in rodents. The distribution of mammary tissue in the rat is present on either side of the ventral midline from axillary to inguinal regions but tumours could also arise in the submandibular and scapular regions, the flanks and the base of the tail. Mammary tumours could be solitary or multiple. In rats, mammary tumours can develop in both males and females. Tumours tend to become very large so impairment of movement or eating, or even discomfort could be associated with them. Large tumours could become ulcerated and secondarily contaminated by bacteria. Benign fibroadenomas of the mammary glands are the more common subcutaneous tumours, but malignant tumours like adenocarcinomas have also been reported (less than 10% of mammary tumours in rats) so complete haematology and biochemistry, x-rays and ultrasonographic examination to check for metastasis are always recommended before surgical treatment. Mammary tumours tend to metastasize to regional lymph nodes, abdominal viscera or lungs.

Ovario-hysterectomy of young female rats may decrease the incidence of mammary tumours and should always be considered. Also the results from a study reported that restriction of the amount of food to 80% of *ad libitum* feeding reduced the incidence of mammary tumours in rats.

The use of the GnRH agonist deslorelin in healthy females in the form of subcutaneous implant should be considered as a possible option to reduce hormonal levels and maybe subsequently reduce the incidence of these tumours in the future (to the author's knowledge, no studies of deslorelin effects in rats are currently available).

Further reading

Donnelly, T., 2004. Disease problems of small rodents. In: Quesenberry, K., Carpenter, J. (Eds.), Ferrets, Rabbits and Rodents Clinical Medicine and Surgery, second ed. Saunders Elsevier, St Louis.

Orr, H., 2009. Rodents: neoplastic and endocrine diseases. In: Keeble, E., Meredith, A. (Eds.), BSAVA Manual of Rodents and Ferrets. British Small Animal Association, Gloucester, UK.

Case 1.12 *M. Huynh*

Clinical history

An 8-year-old male degu (*Octodon degus*) is presented for chronic respiratory distress for 2 weeks and for an acute episode of anorexia for 1 day. The degu is maintained in a standard vertical cage with several platforms. Over the last 2 weeks he has been reluctant to eat his pellet. His diet is mainly composed of alfalfa hay and mixed degu pellets. He has not produced any faeces for the last day.

Physical examination

On examination, the degu presented the following clinical signs:

- Sneezing and inspiratory dyspnoea
- Dehydrated
- Severely bloated.

1. List your differential diagnoses.

Causes of inspiratory dyspnoea and gastric bloat include any aetiological agent impairing the patency of the upper airway. Degus as well as rabbits and rodents are obligate nasal breathers, therefore gastric aerophagia appears rapidly with an upper airway obstruction.

Causes of obstruction include:

- Primary sinusitis (bacterial) or secondary to dental disease
- Foreign body
- Neoplasia
- Trauma.

Clinical diagnosis examination

A set of skull radiographs was obtained (Fig. 1.29a, b) as well as a whole body radiograph (Fig. 1.29c).

2. What is your interpretation of the images seen in Fig. 1.29a–c?

The skull radiograph shows some degree of severe dental disease with a strong alteration of the occlusal plane. A radiodense bony proliferation is visible on the sinus area on both sides and is consistent with an elodontoma. The whole body radiograph shows a generalized ileus with air-distended intestinal loop secondary to aerophagic respiratory pattern.

Final diagnosis

➤ Dental disease and elodontoma

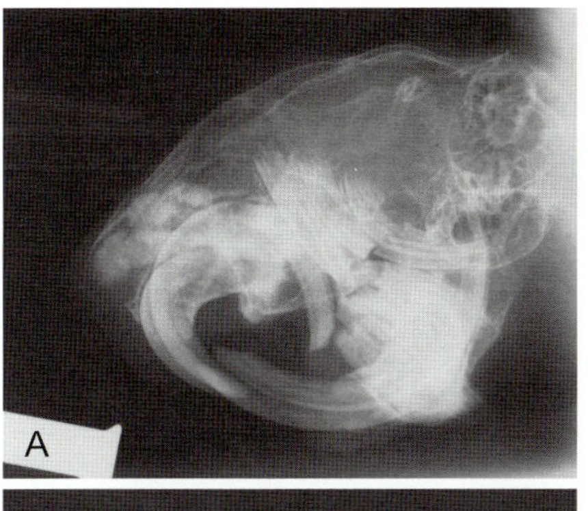

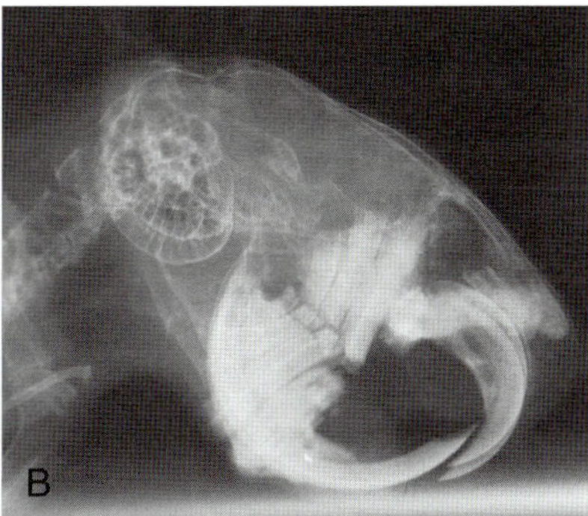

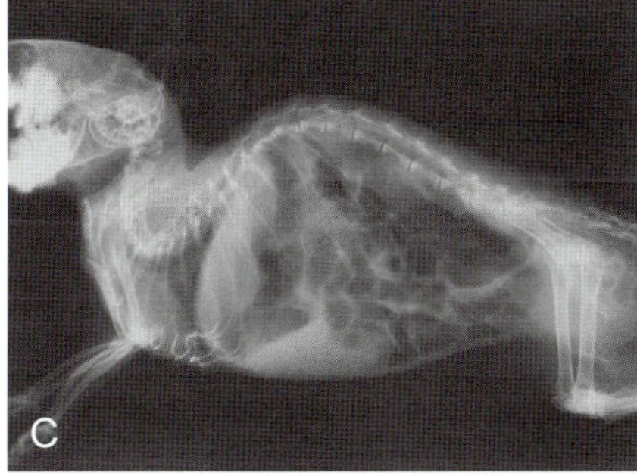

Fig. 1.29 (a) Oblique left radiographic view of the skull of the degu; (b) lateral right radiographic view of the skull of the degu; (c) whole body latero-lateral radiograph of the degu showing air distension of the intestinal tract.

Discussion

Odontoma-like tumours have been described in squirrel-like rodents and degus. Elodontoma is defined as hamartoma of continuous developing odontogenic tissue at the apex of elodont teeth. The aetiology remains unknown but repeated trauma and dental malocclusion have been implicated. The neoplastic tissue forms a space-occupying mass obstructing the nasal cavity. Secondary bacterial infection of the sinus is common. The prognosis of this tumour is poor and euthanasia should be advised in such advanced cases. Dental disease represents a wide majority (60%) of health disorders in degus. Acquired dental disease is related to the feeding behaviour of the species, preferring young and tender leaves in an optimal environment. These diets have less abrasive properties compared to shrubs, barks and green grass that are available in the wild. An appropriate degu diet should include hay, fresh vegetables and chinchilla pellets excluding all sources of sugar.

Further reading

Capello, V., Gracic, M., 2005. Dental procedures. In: Lennox, A.M. (Ed.), Handbook of Rabbit and Rodent Dentistry. Wiley Blackwell, Ames, pp. 213–248.

Jekl, V., Hauptman, K., Knotek, Z., 2011. Diseases in pet degus: a retrospective study in 300 animals. J. Small Anim. Pract. 52 (2), 107–112.

Jekl, V., Hauptman, K., Skoric, M., et al., 2008. Elodontoma in a degu (*Octodon degus*). J. Exot. Pet Med. 17 (3), 216–220.

Case 1.13 *A. Montesinos*

Clinical history

A 3.5-year-old castrated ferret (*Mustela putorius furo*) weighing 1200 g was presented with the following clinical signs of 3 days' duration:

- Anorexia
- Vomiting
- Green diarrhoea.

The ferret was kept in an open cage and was allowed free access to the house. The diet of the ferret was based on commercial ferret food *ad libitum* and treats were offered twice a week. The referral veterinarian sent a whole body radiograph with a presumptive diagnosis of foreign body ingestion.

Clinical examination

On presentation, the ferret had a poor body condition of 2/5 and was inactive and lethargic. There was severe dehydration and he was aggressive. Bilateral cataracts were evident with a tacky white punctuate in both corneas. Abdominal palpation showed acute pain. Whole body radiographs were taken and blood samples were collected for haematology, blood gases and blood chemistry.

Radiology

1. What is your interpretation of the radiographs in Fig. 1.30a–c?

Clinical diagnosis laboratory

The results of the clinical diagnosis laboratory assays are given in Tables 1.12–1.14.

RBC, WBC and thrombocyte morphology

➤ Normal WBC morphology, regular population of red blood cells

2. What is your interpretation of the haematology, blood chemistry and blood gases values shown in Tables 1.12–1.14?

Results

➤ Radiographic findings from the referring clinician were limited due to the presence of a processing artefact. Nevertheless, there was a small amount of gas in the stomach and a radiodense image in the small intestine. There was no dilatation of the intestinal loops

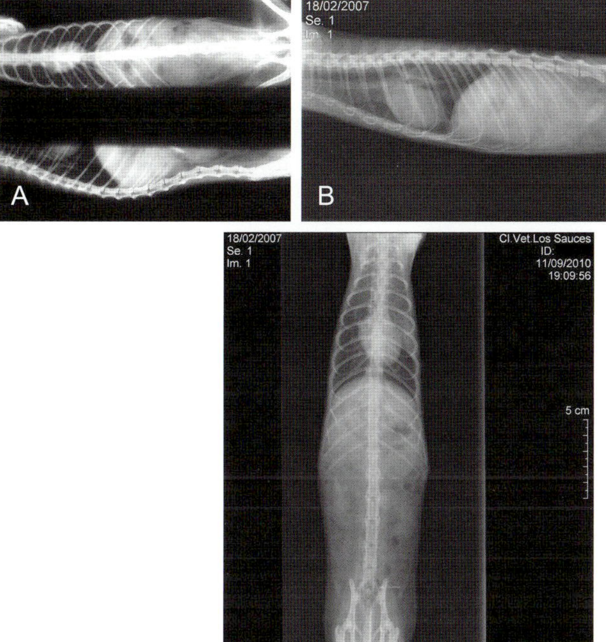

Fig. 1.30 (a) Ventrodorsal and latero-lateral survey radiograph of a 3-year-old ferret sent by the referring veterinarian; (b) latero-lateral survey radiograph of a 3-year-old ferret with vomiting of 3 days' duration; (c) ventrodorsal survey radiograph of a 3-year-old ferret with vomiting of 3 days' duration.

Table 1.12 Haematology values for the ferret

Parameters	Results (absolute)	Results (%)	Reference values
Hb (g/dl)	16.7		12–16.9
Hct (l/l)	0.54	54	0.33–0.47
WBC ($\times10^9$/l)	7.2		4.9–13.8
Neutrophils ($\times10^9$/l)	6.04	84	24–78%
Banded neutrophils	0.36	5	0–2.2%
Lymphocytes ($\times10^9$/l)	0.432	6	28–69%
Eosinophils ($\times10^9$/l)	0.0072	1	0–7%
Basophils ($\times10^9$/l)	0	0	0–1%
Monocytes ($\times10^9$/l)	0.288	4	3.4–8.2%

Table 1.13 Blood chemistry values of the ferret

Analysis	Results	Reference values
BUN (mg/dl)	17	12–43
Cl (mmol/l)	102	103–121
Creatinine	0.2	0.2–0.6
GGT (U/l)	11	0–5
GPT (U/l)	315	82–289
Glucose (mg/dl)	111	62.5–134
Potassium (mmol/l)	3.2	4.3–5.3
Sodium (mmol/l)	133	146–160
Total protein (g/l)	68	53–72

Table 1.14 Blood gases status of the ferret

Parameters	Results	Reference values
pH	7.296	7.277–7.409
pCO_2 (mmHg)	56.1	30.4±0.6
TCO_2 (mmol/l)	29	20–28
HCO_3 (mmol/l)	27.4	15.7±0.7
Exc base (mmol/l)	1	0±2
Anion gap (mmol/l)	26	22.8±3.5
Total plasmatic osmolality (calculated)	268.1	295–329

- Radiographic findings in the second and third radiographs included the presence of a radiodense object in the jejunum–ileum area. There was also an increased density on the left lung field and a fractured *os penis*
- Haematology analyses showed neutrophilia and left shift, suggesting a non-specific acute process. The high haematocrit value was consistent with severe dehydration
- Blood chemistry analysis showed elevated levels of glutamic pyruvic transaminase (GPT), gamma-glutamyl transpeptidase (GGT), suggesting a liver implication in an acute inflammatory process
- Blood gases showed:
  - Normal pH, although the values of TCO_2 and HCO_3 were over the limits of a compensatory response suggesting a mixed acid–base disequilibrium
  - Low levels of Na. This is a normal finding in ferrets with gastrointestinal disease and respiratory acidosis. Other causes of hyponatraemia are renal failure, endocrine disorders (diabetes mellitus, hypoadrenocorticism, diabetes

insipidus) and congestive heart failure. These causes were ruled out on the basis of the analytical laboratory results, clinical history and physical examination findings

- Low levels of Cl and K. The more obvious cause of this low level is vomiting. Hypochloraemia and metabolic alkaloses results in hypokalaemia
- Low osmolality due to the loss of salts with vomiting

Please evaluate the clinical history, Fig. 1.30a–c, the results of the physical examination and clinical diagnostic tests.

 *3. List your differential diagnoses.*

 *4. List your diagnostic strategy and possible diagnostic test.*

Differential diagnoses

- Intestinal obstruction
- Pancreatitis
- Aspiration pneumonia due to acute onset of vomiting

Diagnostic plan

More imaging techniques were necessary to confirm the presumptive diagnosis of intestinal obstruction in preparation for surgery. The owner agreed to make an ultrasound study.

Echography

 *5. What is your interpretation of the ultrasound image of Fig. 1.31?*

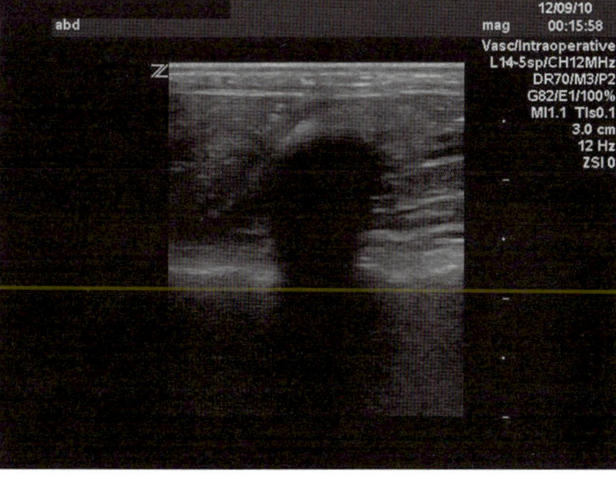

Fig. 1.31 Ultrasound view of a section of the small intestine of the ferret.

Results of the ultrasound study

- A foreign body is casting a shadow over the bottom of the image, confirming the diagnosis of intestinal obstruction

Therapy (Table 1.15)

Table 1.15 Therapy

Amoxicillin clavulanic acid 140 mg/ml	25 mg/kg SC BID, 10 days
Metronidazole 5 mg/ml	25 mg/kg IV BID, 3 days, then PO BID
Fluids	NaCl 50 ml/kg/day IV IRC during surgery and 3 days after, 20 mEq/l of fluids were added as potassium supplement

Because the ferret was dehydrated, an IV catheter was placed in the cephalic vein and saline solution was administered for 1 hour prior to the surgery. Antibiotics were given before the surgical procedure. Because the hypochloraemia and hypokalaemia were not severe, potassium supplement was administered for maintenance.

Anaesthesia and analgesia

The ferret was classified as an ASAII patient and was sedated using midazolam 0.5 mg/kg IV and induced with metomidate 1 mg/kg IV. After intubation with a 2 mm non-cuffed endotracheal tube, anaesthesia was maintained with sevofluorane 2–3 %. Rectal temperature, haemoglobin saturation, blood pressure and end tidal CO_2 concentration were monitored during the surgical procedure. A drop in blood pressure (60 mmHg) was detected when the abdominal cavity was opened but the blood pressure was raised using a bolus of hydroxietil starch 6%, 5 ml/kg. After the bolus and during surgery, the blood pressure was kept between 160 and 150 mmHg. After the surgical procedure was completed, midazolam was reversed using flumazenil 0.1 mg/kg IV and the surgical site was infiltrated using a mixture of lidocaine (2 mg/kg) and bupivacaine (2 mg/kg). One hour after the end of the surgery, an irc of ketamine (0.1 mg/kg) and fentanyl (0.01 mg/kg) was added to the supporting fluids. Meloxicam 0.1 mg/kg SC was also added to the analgesic treatment.

Surgery

The ferret was positioned in dorsal recumbency and a standard laparotomy was carried out. Longitudinal incision of the intestine over the obstruction was made (Fig. 1.32). A rubber piece was removed and the intestine closed horizontally, trying to avoid the risk of post-surgery stenosis. The intestine was sutured with 6/0 monofilament suture using a Lembert inverting pattern (Fig. 1.33). A flap of the omentum was used to cover the intestinal surgical wound (Fig. 1.34). The laparotomy was closed using routine techniques and the ferret recovered from anaesthesia uneventfully.

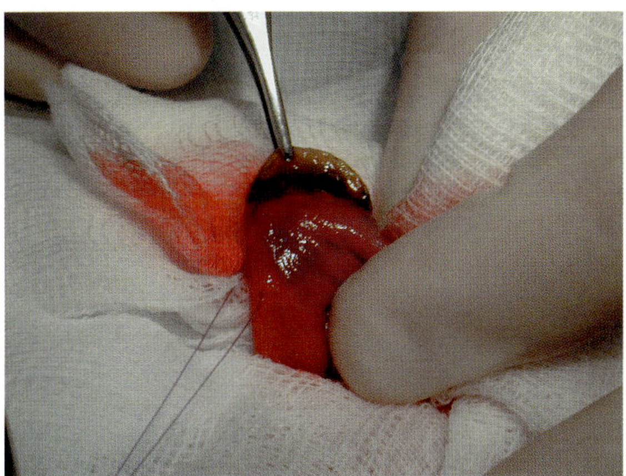

Fig. 1.32 View of the intestine of the ferret after the incision over the foreign body.

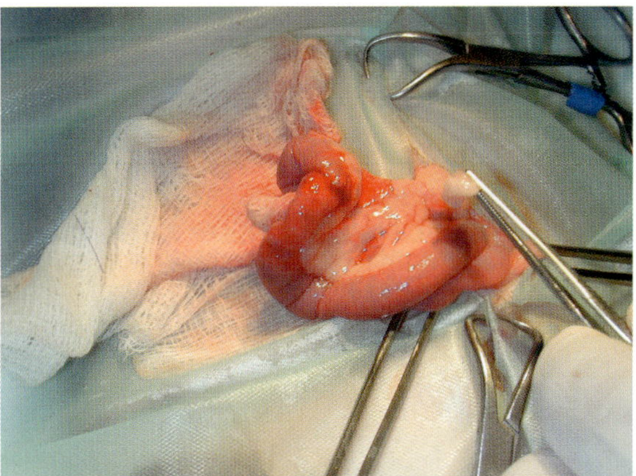

Fig. 1.33 After removal of the foreign body a Lembert inverting suture pattern was used to close the intestine.

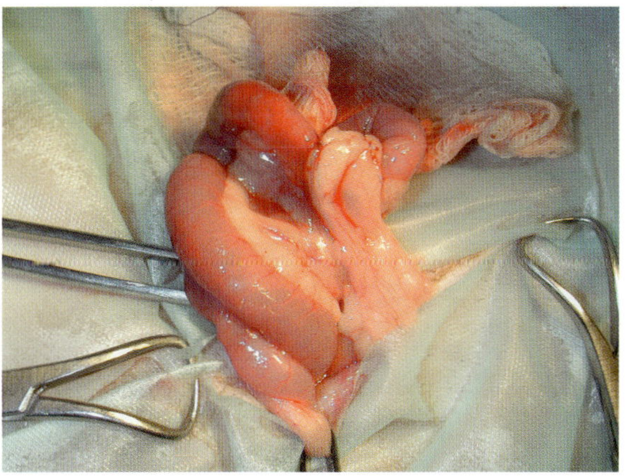

Fig. 1.34 An omentum flap was used to cover the intestinal surgical wound in order to obtain complete sealing of the intestine and to promote faster healing.

Final diagnosis

- Intestinal obstruction
- Aspiration pneumonia

Follow up

After 1 day of hospitalization, the ferret was fed with liquid feeding formula. Ten days after surgery the ferret was discharged with antibiotics for 2 weeks. Radiographs after 4 weeks (Fig. 1.35a, b) showed complete resolution of the pneumonia. The fractured *os penis* was an incidental finding and the ferret did not show any signs of pain or dysuria.

Discussion

Intestinal obstruction is often seen in ferret practice. The differential diagnoses include foreign body/trichobezoar obstruction, neoplasia, pancreatitis, adhesions of previous surgeries, faecal impaction and sepsis/peritonitis. The clinical picture includes vomiting, abdominal pain and lack of passing stools. Radiographs are the preferred diagnostic imaging method, showing dilatation of intestinal loops cranial to the obstruction. Ultrasound studies are useful in cases where the ileum is not visible in the radiographs. It also is useful to evaluate the status of the intestinal walls and the presence of perforation and free fluids in the abdominal cavity. Oesophagitis, electrolytic disorders and pain are the most common complications. Surgery is always indicated and recovery is good if there is not peritonitis. In this particular case, the foreign object was a piece of garment belonging to the owner.

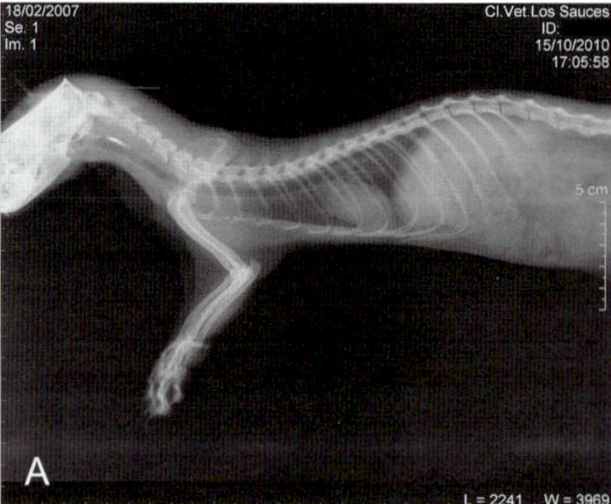

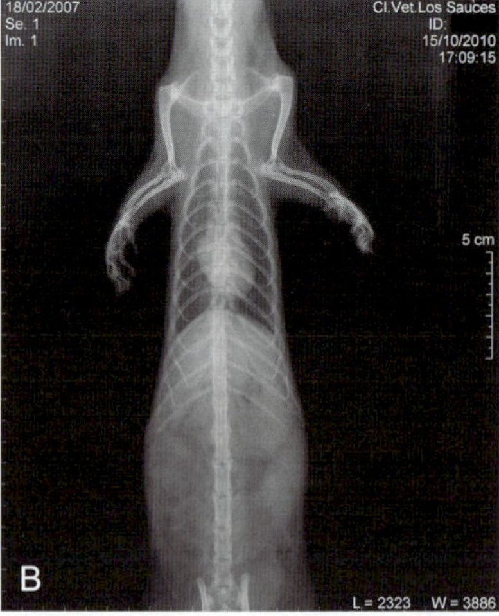

Fig. 1.35 (a) Latero-lateral survey radiograph of a 3-year-old ferret 4 weeks after surgery; (b) ventrodorsal survey radiograph of a 3-year-old ferret 4 weeks after surgery.

Further reading

Bateman, S.W., 2008. Make sense of blood gases results. Vet. Clin. North Am. Exot. Anim. Pract. 38, 559–575.

Capello, V., 2009. Common surgical procedures. In: Keeble, E., Meredith, A. (Eds.), BSAVA Manual of Ferrets and Rodents. British Small Animal Veterinary Association, Gloucester, pp. 254–260.

Dibartola, S.P., 2006. Introduction to acid–base disorders. In: Dibartola, S.P. (Ed.), Fluid, Electrolyte and Acid–base Disorders in Small Animal Practice, third ed. Elsevier, London, pp. 229–251.

Fox, J.G., 1998. Clinical pathology. In: Fox, J.G. (Ed.), Biology and Diseases of the Ferret, second ed. Saunders, Philadelphia, pp. 124–140.

Hoefer, H.L., Bell, J.A., 2003. Gastrointestinal diseases of the ferret. In: Quesenberry, K.E., Carpenter, J.W. (Eds.), Ferrets, Rabbits and Rodents Clinical Medicine and Surgery, second ed. Saunders, Philadelphia, pp. 25–40.

Case 1.14 *J. Chitty*

Clinical history

A 5-year-old neutered male ferret (*Mustela putorius furo*) was presented slightly thin (weight 850 g) and lethargic though eating normally. Previously he had a history of liver disease though this had apparently resolved more than 6 months ago (both clinically and on monitoring blood samples). Drinking and urination were normal.

Physical examination

On examination, the ferret was bright and alert, but slightly thin. There was no evidence of neurological deficits nor were any masses palpable. Oral examination showed no evidence of dental disease and mucus membranes appeared normal. Peripheral lymph nodes were not palpable. The hair coat appeared normal. There were no discharges apparent from nose, eyes or mouth. There was a Grade 1 pansystolic murmur on auscultation of the thorax. Faeces passed in the travelling box appeared normal.

1. What are your differential diagnoses?

Differential diagnoses

At this stage with non-specific signs, there are many differential diagnoses including:

- Neoplasia – especially adrenal disease or lymphoma
- Gastrointestinal disease
  - Endoparasitism
  - Neoplasia
  - Chronic inflammatory bowel diseases
  - Oral cavity lesions
  - Gastric ulceration – especially secondary to neoplasia or *Helicobacter* infection

- Renal failure
- Hepatic disease
- Cardiac disease
- Infection – chronic viral infection, e.g. human influenza virus or Aleutian disease.

2. How would you investigate this case?

Clinical diagnosis examination

Survey whole body radiographs were obtained and abdominal and cardiac ultrasonography was carried out.

Clinical diagnosis laboratory examination

Blood samples were obtained for haematology and biochemistry analyses. A faecal sample was analysed for the presence of endoparasites and a urinalysis was carried out (Tables 1.16 and 1.17).

Table 1.16 Results of the biochemistry analyses of the ferret

Analysis	Results	Reference range
Total protein	58 g/l	53–72
Albumin	33 g/l	33–44
Globulin	25 g/l	15–35
Albumin:globulin ratio	1.3	
Sodium	155 mmol/l	146–160
Potassium	4.9 mmol/l	4.5–7.7
Na:K ratio	32	
Chloride	114 mmol/l	102–121
Total calcium	2.17 mmol/l	2.0–2.95
Phosphate	2.0 mmol/l	1.3–2.9
Urea	13.9 mmol/l	3.6–16.0
Creatinine	64 μmol/l	35–80
Alk Phos	519 U/l	30–120
GLDH	1	U/L <10
Total bilirubin	3.1 μmol/l	0.1–17.1

Table 1.17 Results of the haematology analyses of the ferret

Analysis	Results (absolute)	Results	Reference range
RBC	7.07 $\times 10^{12}$/l		7.5–11.9
Hb	12.3 g/dl		12.0–20.8
HCT		43.7 %	36–68
MCV	62.0 fl		42.4–88.4
MCH	17.4 pg		15–20
MCHC	28.1 g/dl		26.2–38.6
Platelets	444 $\times 10^{12}$/l		180–800
WBC	5.42 $\times 10^{12}$/l		3.5–7.0
Neutrophils	2.76 $\times 10^{12}$/l	51%	1.9–5.9
Lymphocytes	2.60 $\times 10^{12}$/l	48%	1.7–2.9
Monocytes	0.00 $\times 10^{12}$/l	0%	
Eosinophils	0.05 $\times 10^{12}$/l	1%	0.0–0.35
Basophils	0.00 $\times 10^{12}$/l	0%	

Blood film examination

Two fresh blood smears and a film made from the submitted EDTA were examined. No abnormal white cells were seen. Red cells appeared normocytic and normochromic. Platelet morphology and numbers appeared normal with no evidence of platelet clumping or clots on the EDTA smear.

3. How would you interpret these blood results?

Summary of diagnostic results

Urinalysis

- SG 1.015 – otherwise NAD

Faecal parasitology

- No parasites detected

Electrophoresis

- Results were entirely in normal range (Fig. 1.36)

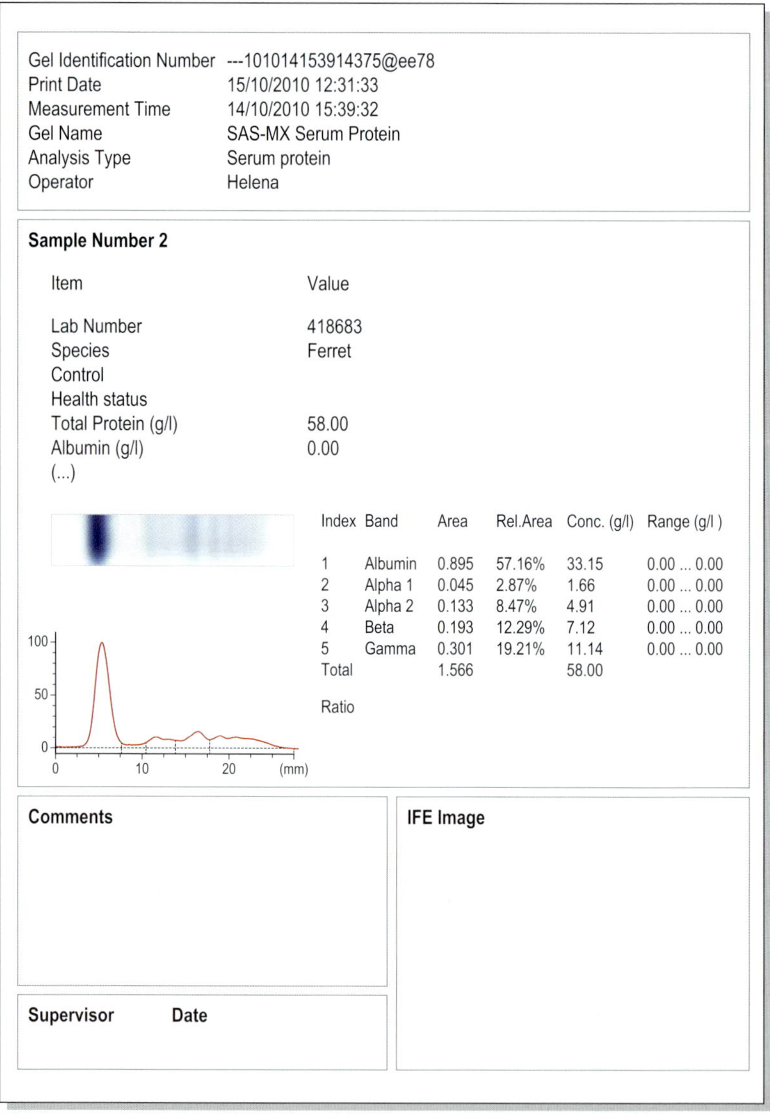

Gel Identification Number ---101014153914375@ee78
Print Date 15/10/2010 12:31:33
Measurement Time 14/10/2010 15:39:32
Gel Name SAS-MX Serum Protein
Analysis Type Serum protein
Operator Helena

Sample Number 2

Item	Value
Lab Number	418683
Species	Ferret
Control	
Health status	
Total Protein (g/l)	58.00
Albumin (g/l)	0.00
(...)	

Index	Band	Area	Rel.Area	Conc. (g/l)	Range (g/l)
1	Albumin	0.895	57.16%	33.15	0.00 ... 0.00
2	Alpha 1	0.045	2.87%	1.66	0.00 ... 0.00
3	Alpha 2	0.133	8.47%	4.91	0.00 ... 0.00
4	Beta	0.193	12.29%	7.12	0.00 ... 0.00
5	Gamma	0.301	19.21%	11.14	0.00 ... 0.00
Total		1.566		58.00	
Ratio					

Comments

IFE Image

Supervisor **Date**

Fig. 1.36 Electrophoresis results.

Blood analyses

- ➤ A mild non-regenerative anaemia may be associated with chronic disease
- ➤ ALKP is relatively non-specific but may be associated with hepatocellular damage, muscle damage or gut disease
- ➤ The absence of a gammopathy rules out Aleutian disease

Radiographs (Fig. 1.37a, b)

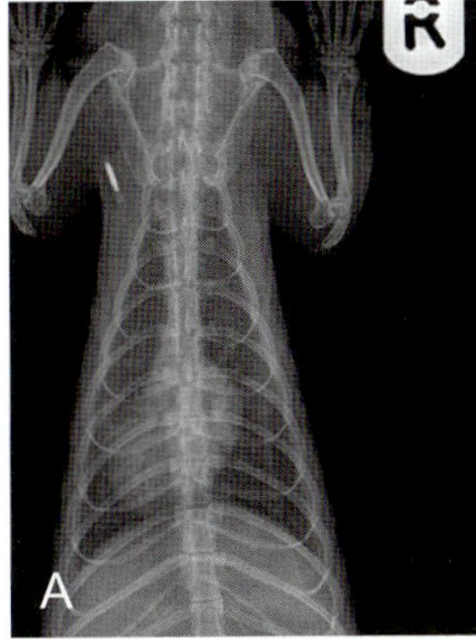

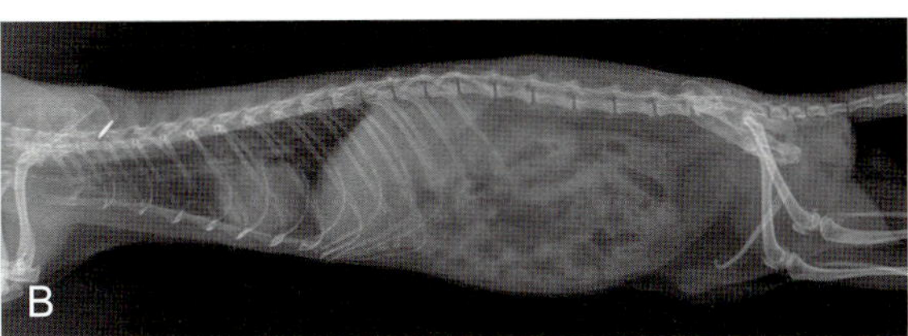

Fig. 1.37 (a) Ventrodorsal survey radiograph of the ferret; (b) latero-lateral survey radiograph of the ferret.

Q *4. What abnormalities can be seen in the radiographs?*

- The cardiac silhouette is rounded and enlarged
- Other organs appear of normal size

Ultrasonography

- Abdominal organs appeared structurally normal

Echocardiography revealed:

- Left ventricular wall thickness (4.1–7.3 mm – increased)
- Inter-ventricular septum 2.9 mm (normal)
- No evidence of pericardial effusion.

Q *5. What is your diagnosis?*

Final diagnosis

- Hypertrophic cardiomyopathy

Q *6. What is your therapy?*

Therapy

Angiotensin-converting enzyme (ACE) inhibitors and pimobendan may be helpful in these cases. Where there is evidence of congestion or effusion, furosemide may be helpful. In this case, imidapril (Prilium, Vetoquinol) was given at 0.25 mg/kg SID. The ferret increased activity levels quite quickly and there was a slight increase in bodyweight over the next month (920 g).

Discussion

Cardiomyopathy carries a guarded to poor prognosis in ferrets though management is possible in the short to medium term. Clinical signs are normally nebulous and murmurs rarely heard. Certainly it should be considered as a differential in any poor-doing or thin mid-aged to older ferret.

Further reading

Lewington, J.H., 2007. Ferret Husbandry Medicine and Surgery, second ed. Saunders Elsevier, St Louis.

Oglesbee, B.L., 2006. The 5-Minute Veterinary Consult: Ferret and Rabbit. Wiley Blackwell, Ames.

Orcutt, C., Malakoff, R., 2009. Ferrets: cardiovascular and respiratory system disorders. In: Keeble, E., Meredith, A. (Eds.), BSAVA Manual of Rodents & Ferrets. British Small Animal Veterinary Association, Gloucester, pp. 282–290.

Case 1.15 *M. Huynh*

Clinical history

A 2-year-old male ferret was presented for anorexia for 5 days. The ferret was vaccinated and living indoors with another ferret who did not show any signs. His diet is constituted exclusively of ferret pellets. No previous medical history was recorded.

Physical examination

On clinical examination, he showed the following symptoms:

- Lethargy
- Severe dehydration (>5% BW)
- A pale icterous mucous membrane
- Mild diarrhoea.

Clinical diagnostic laboratory examination

Blood samples were collected for haematology and blood chemistry analyses.

The results of the clinical diagnosis laboratory assays are shown in Tables 1.18 and 1.19.

RBC, WBC and thrombocyte morphology

Nothing abnormal detected.

 *1. What is your interpretation of haematology and biochemistry shown in Tables 1.18 and 1.19?*

Elevation of the ALT, ALKP and total bilirubin shows some degree of hepatic damage. CBC is uneventful and rules out a pre-hepatic cause of icterus.

Table 1.18 Haematology values of the ferret

Parameters	Results (absolute)	Results (%)	Reference values
RBC ($\times 10^{12}$/l)	10.53		10.2 (7.3–12.2)
Hb (g/dl)	17.5		17.8 (16.3–18.2)
Hct (l/l)	0.51		0.55 (0.36–0.50)
MCV (fl)	48.3		135.83±3.59 (106.18–162.36)
MCH (pg)	16.6		49.44±1.32 (39.17–59.67)
MCHC (g/dl)	34.4		36.41±0.16 (35.47–37.84)
WBC ($\times 10^{9}$/l)	4.47		9.7 (4.4–19.1)
Neutrophils (%)	46	57	57 (11–82)
Lymphocytes (%)	20.1	36	35.6 (12–54)
Monocytes (%)	0.28	4	4.4 (0–9)
Eosinophils (%)	6.2	2	2.4 (0–7)
Basophils (%)	0.06	0.1	0.1 (0–2)
Thrombocytes ($\times 10^{9}$/μl)	1346		453 (297–730)

Table 1.19 Blood chemistry values of the ferret

Analysis	Results	Reference values
ALKP (U/l)	297	-
Bilirubin (μmol/l)	44	4.6 (1.7)
Creatinine (mg/l)	4	38 (14)
ALT (U/l)	865	135 (125)
Glucose (mmol/l)	11.7	20.4 (1.7)
Total protein (g/l)	50	25.0 (8.7)
Total urea (mmol/l)	0.23	3.6 (2.2)

Clinical diagnosis examination

An abdominal ultrasound was performed.

Ultrasonography

2. What is your interpretation of the images seen in Fig. 1.38a, b?

The liver has a round shape, homogeneous and hypoechogenic compared to the surrounding fat tissue.

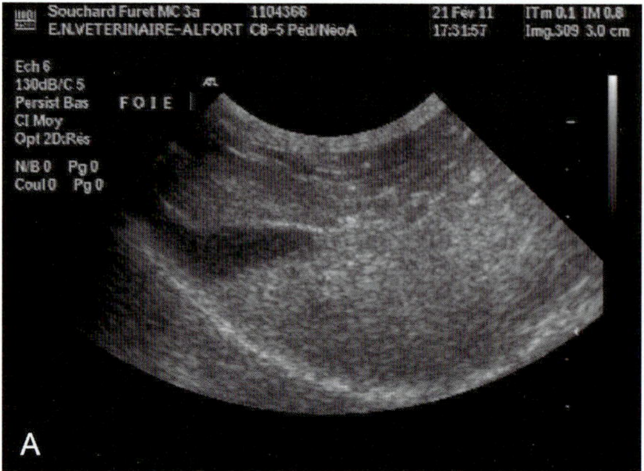

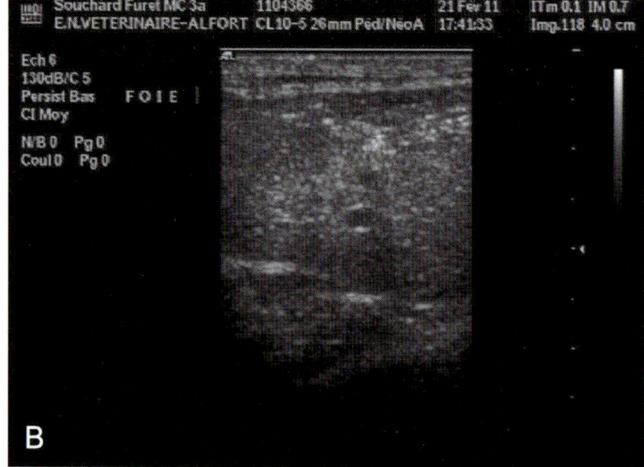

Fig. 1.38 (a) Ultrasonographic examination of the liver. Homogeneous aspect of the liver and round shape; (b) ultrasonographic examination of the liver. Notice the hyperechoic aspect of the liver compared to the surrounding fat tissue.

Please evaluate the clinical history and the results of the clinical and laboratory diagnostic tests.

Q *3. List your differential diagnoses.*

Q *4. Would you request any additional exam?*

Q *5. List your therapeutic strategy.*

Differential diagnoses

- Prehepatic causes of icterus have been ruled out by the haematology analysis results
- Hepatic causes of icterus: hepatitis (viral, bacterial, toxic), hepatic lipidosis, neoplasia
- Post-hepatic causes of icterus: cholecystitis, gallbladder calculi, parasitic cyst, neoplasia

Additional examination

An ultrasound-guided fine needle aspirate was performed in order to characterize the hepatic lesion.

Cytology

➤ The result of the cytology (Fig. 1.39) shows lipidic vacuole in the hepatocyte and is consistent with a hepatic lipidosis

Bacteriology

➤ Bacteriology culture of the liver sample revealed no growth

Therapy

The ferret was placed on the following therapeutic management:

- Amoxicillin clavulanate 12.5 mg/kg BID × 2 weeks
- NaCl 0.9% and Glc 5% 5 ml/kg IV
- Force feeding 5 ml of critical care carnivorous (Oxbow®) 5 times a day
- Ranitidine 4 mg/kg IV TID.

Final diagnosis

➤ Idiopathic hepatic lipidosis

Discussion

Hepatic lipidosis remains a subclinical disease and the presenting signs are related to the cause of weight loss. Any concurrent disease causing anorexia can induce hepatic lipidosis such as coronavirus infection, suppurative hepatitis, neoplasia, sepsis etc.

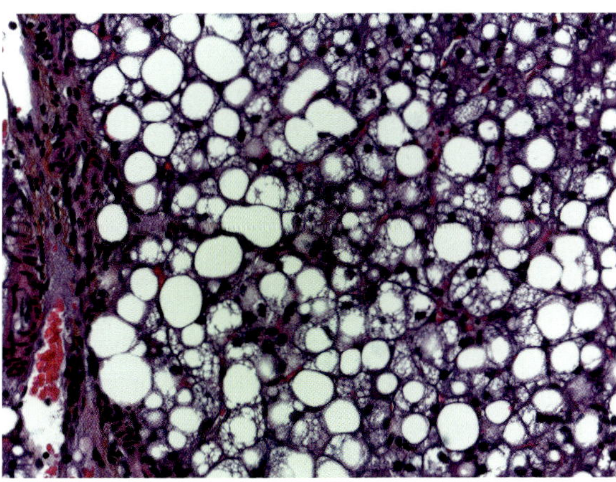

Fig. 1.39 Cytologic examination of the liver after HE stains. Notice the numerous lipidic vacuolization in the cytoplasm of hepatocytes.

Hepatic disorders are common in ferrets and remain underdiagnosed. Lymphocytic hepatitis and suppurative hepatitis are other potential differentials. Icterus is rare in ferrets, because of the efficient ability of the kidney to eliminate the bile pigment. Post-hepatic diseases have been reported in ferrets such as biliary cyst adenoma, biliary coccidiosis and cholecystitis.

Treatment of hepatic lipidosis relies on diagnosing the underlying cause and supportive care. Nutritional support is crucial. Milk thistle and S-adenosyl methionine have shown some benefits in some cases. Prognosis is generally good provided that the underlying cause is identified and solved.

Further reading

Burgess, M., 2007. Ferret gastrointestinal and hepatic diseases. In: Lewington, J. (Ed.), Ferret Husbandry, Medicine and Surgery. Saunders Elsevier, St Louis, pp. 203–223.

Hoefer, H.L., Bell, J.A., 2003. Gastrointestinal diseases. In: Quesenberry, K.E., Carpenter, J.W. (Eds.), Ferrets, Rabbits and Rodents: Clinical Medicine and Surgery. Saunders Elsevier, St Louis, pp. 25–40.

Mustonen, A.M., et al., 2009. Response to fasting in an unnaturally obese carnivore, the captive European polecat *Mustela putorius*. Exp. Biol. Med. 234 (11), 1287–1295.

Case 1.16 *M. Huynh*

Clinical history

A 4-month-old male ferret (*Mustela putorius*) was presented for severe lethargy, lack of appetite and fever. Some mild ocular discharges are seen. The ferret is alone in a household environment, he is not vaccinated. He was bought from a pet shop the previous week. On clinical examination the following findings were observed:

- Lateral recumbency
- Profound stupor
- Ocular discharge
- Hyperthermia (39.4°C).

Physical examination

On examination, the ferret is unresponsive and shows proprioceptive deficit on all four limbs with normal reflexes (Fig. 1.40). He also has an intermittent flexion of the neck. Fluoresceine test shows some mild ulceration on both corneas (Fig. 1.41).

1. List your differential diagnoses.

Differential diagnoses

The clinical examination (decreased proprioception and decreased mentation) is consistent with a multifocal neurologic disease such as meningitis.

➤ Viral : Aleutian mink disease, distemper, coronavirus

➤ Infectious: *Toxoplasma, Neospora, Cryptococcus*

- Inflammatory: lymphocytic meningitis
- Neoplastic: lymphoma
- Toxic
- Trauma

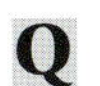 *2. Which test would you ask to rule out the different diseases?*

A cerebrospinal fluid (CSF) tap can be recommended to explore the different causes of meningitis. The sample can be more easily collected from the cisterna magna in ferrets (Fig. 1.42).

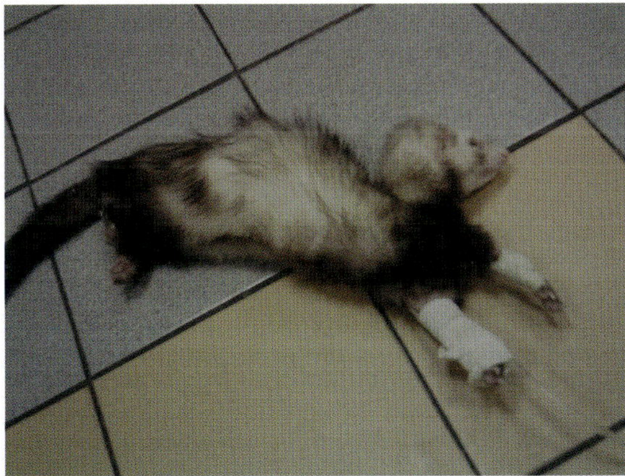

Fig. 1.40 Ferret in lateral recumbency and cervical flexion.

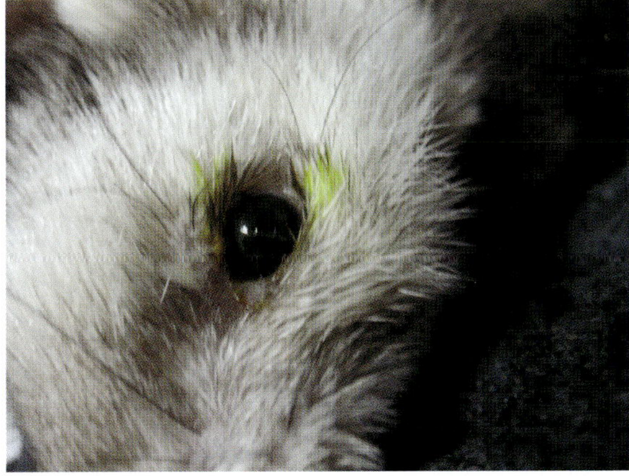

Fig. 1.41 Bilateral corneal ulceration in the eye of the ferret.

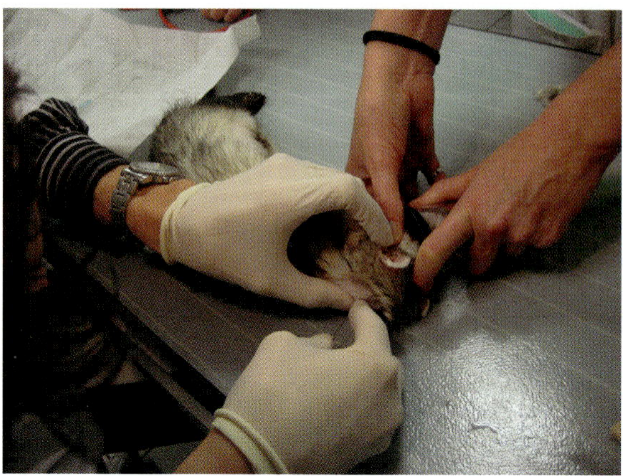

Fig. 1.42 Cerebrospinal fluid tap in the cisterna magna. Landmarks such as the atlas wings and the occiput are similar in small mammals.

Cerebrospinal fluid analysis

- CSF tap showed no abnormalities

Haematology

- Erythrocytes 76×10^6 /l
- Leucocytes 6×10^6 /l

Blood chemistry

- Protein 0.13 g/l (0.10–0.33)

Cytology

Within the serous fluid the cell differential is as follows:

- 65% lymphocytes
- 35% monocytes.

Clinical diagnosis laboratory results

- Within normal limits

Additional diagnostic testing

- RT-PCR was performed on the CSF and showed a positive result to distemper disease (Fig. 1.43)

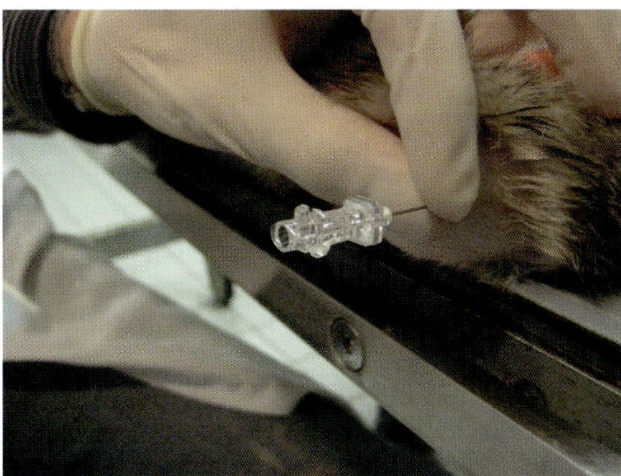

Fig. 1.43 The sample collected is analysed for cytology and RT-PCR.

Discussion

Distemper is caused by a large RNA paramyxovirus. Transmission can occur through airborne virus or direct contact with body fluid of an infected animal. The incubation period is 7 to 10 days. The virus enters the host via the nose or the mouth and then migrates to the lymph node of the lung. By the 6th day, the virus has migrated to the spleen, stomach, small intestine and liver. Fever develops at this point. Depending on the host's immune response, the virus can trigger only a few mild symptoms or a whole syndrome combination before death. Occasionally, dogs with CNS distemper do not have an inflammatory CSF as in this case (Ettinger and Feldman 2005).

Q *3. What other clinical signs can be seen in this disease?*

- Dermatological signs: reddening and thickening of the skin of the chin, lip progressing into crusting (Fig. 1.44a). Hyperkeratosis of the footpad is also observed commonly (Fig. 1.44b). Those signs are pathognomonic of distemper
- Gastrointestinal signs: diarrhoea
- Respiratory signs: pneumonia
- Ocular signs: keratitis

Q *4. What other diagnostic tests can we run to diagnose this disease?*

- Antibody titres can be run and show prior exposure to the virus (infection or vaccination). This test can be performed on blood or CSF. A positive antibody titre in the CSF is very significant as the vaccine-induced antibodies do not cross the brain barrier
- Fluorescent antibody test can be performed on infected tissue (differentiating vaccination antibody and infection). However, this test is not very sensitive
- RT-PCR can be performed on infected tissue, CSF, ocular swab, choanal/anal swab
- On cytology, some inclusion bodies can be seen on infected cells

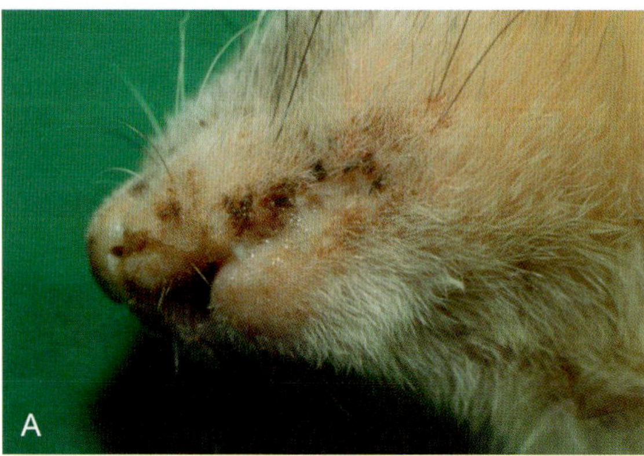

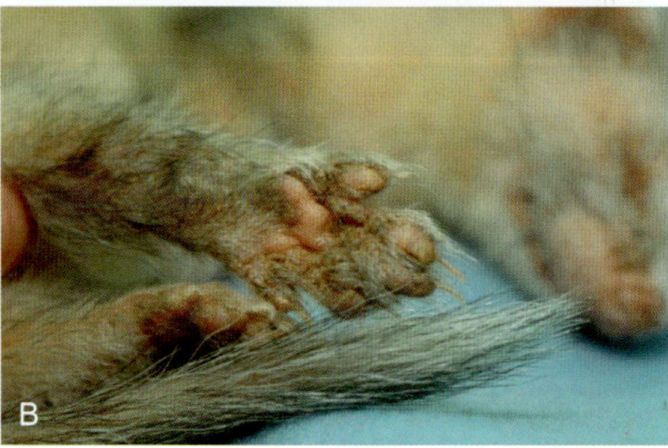

Fig. 1.44 (a) Dermatological signs of distemper: reddening and thickening of the skin of the chin, crust on the lips (courtesy of Jan Declercq); (b) dermatological sign of distemper: footpad hyperkeratosis (courtesy of Jan Declercq).

Q *5. What preventive measure can we advise?*

There is no treatment of distemper in ferrets. Therefore vaccination is crucial to prevent this disease. The use of a modified live vaccine (Purevax MERIAL™ or Galaxy D Schering Plough™) is preferred over a killed vaccine for longer protection time. In ferrets, anaphylactic reaction to the vaccine is a potential threat; therefore a single vaccinating agent is preferred over multivalent canine vaccines.

Further reading

Ettinger, S.J., Feldman, E.C., 2005. Textbook of Veterinary Internal Medicine, sixth ed. Saunders Elsevier, Philadelphia.

Langlois, I., 2005. Viral diseases of ferrets. Vet. Clin. North Am. Exot. Anim. Pract. 8 (1), 139–160.

Perpinan, D., Ramis, A., Tomas, A., et al., 2008. Outbreak of canine distemper in domestic ferrets (*Mustela putorius furo*). Vet. Rec. 163 (8), 246–250.

Welter, J., Taylor, J., Tartaglia, J., et al., 2000. Vaccination against canine distemper virus infection in infant ferrets with and without maternal antibody protection, using recombinant attenuated poxvirus vaccines. J. Virol. 74 (14), 6358–6367.

Case 1.17 *B. Gartrell*

Clinical history

Routine monitoring of a wild maternal roost of New Zealand short-tailed bats (Order: Microchiroptera) during the breeding season revealed large numbers of dead and dying bats. A selection of twenty dead bats and four live orphaned juveniles were presented to the wildlife clinic of the New Zealand Wildlife Health Centre.

The lesser short-tailed (ST) bat *Mystacina tuberculata* is the single surviving species of genus *Mystacina*, considered as endemic archaic remnant (~25 million years in NZ) with no close living relative in other countries. The bats are primarily insectivorous (beetles, moths, flies, cockroaches and weta) but they also eat nectar, pollen and fruit. They are considered to be an opportunistic forager that has an estimated daily food intake of ~40% of body mass (5–7 g). The bats use daily torpor to conserve energy during daylight hours. The bats are monoestrous, with a single pup born between December and January (southern hemisphere summer). The pups are usually born and reared in a maternity roost for 2–6 weeks.

Physical examination

Physical examination of the orphaned bats showed them to be of varying weights from 4.8 to 8.0 g. The young bats were unfurred, dehydrated as evidenced by skin turgor (Fig. 1.45).

Post-mortem examination

Post-mortem examination of the twenty dead bats showed only six adult bats and eight juveniles were in good condition for post-mortem examination (Fig. 1.46a). The rest were too decomposed for meaningful examination. All adult bats showed extensive haemorrhages in the subcutaneous tissues, peritoneal cavity and lungs

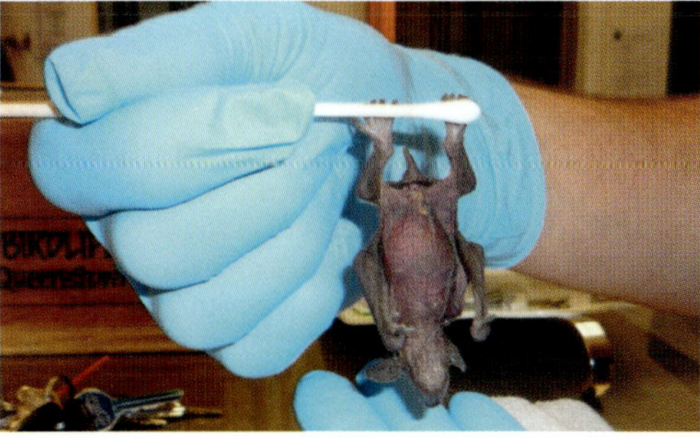

Fig. 1.45 Unfurred, dehydrated young bat showing skin turgor.

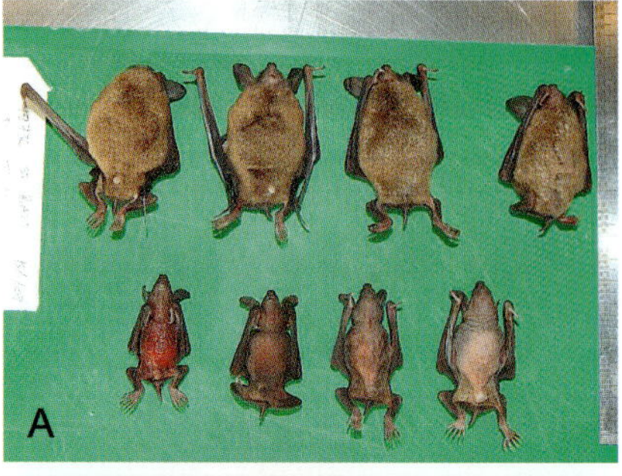

Fig. 1.46 (a, b) Post-mortem examination of adult bats.

(Fig. 1.46b). Adult female bats showed developed mammary glands. The juvenile bats were all unfurred and some showed empty gastrointestinal tracts, no fat reserves and muscle wasting. Some juveniles showed similar diffuse haemorrhages to the adults but others showed no haemorrhages at all.

1. What is your provisional post-mortem diagnosis?

Provisional post-mortem diagnosis

- Coagulopathy, suspected diphacinone toxicity
- Starvation and/or exposure in some juveniles

Summary of post-mortem examination findings

All the adult bats and some juveniles showed evidence of a coagulopathy. The anticoagulant poison diphacinone had been recently used in the area for rodent control. The unfurred stage of the juveniles means they were dependent on adults. Young bats are completely dependent on their mothers for milk and the colony for warmth. Some of the dead juvenile bats showed post-mortem findings indicative of starvation or exposure, suggesting some of the ones that died were orphaned animals.

Post-mortem laboratory findings

Aerobic cultures of lung and liver from the dead bats showed mixed organisms including *Hafnia alvei*, *Serratia* spp., non-haemolytic *Streptococcus*, *Proteus mirabilis* and *Escherichia coli*. These are likely to be opportunistic pathogens or post-mortem invaders rather than primary pathogens.

- Diphacinone concentrations in the liver from adults ranged from 0.20 to 0.45 µg/g (ppm)
- Diphacinone concentrations in the liver from juveniles ranged from 0.0 to 0.68 µg/g (ppm)

Summary of diagnostic results

Please evaluate the clinical history, Fig. 1.45, ***the results of the physical examination from the live bats and the post-mortem findings from the dead bats, Fig. 1.46a, b.***

2. List your differential diagnoses for the orphaned live juveniles.

3. List your therapeutic and husbandry strategy.

Differential diagnoses

- Coagulopathy due to anticoagulant poisoning
- Disseminated intravascular coagulopathy due to systemic bacterial or viral infection
- Primary coagulopathy

Therapy

Unfurred bat pups need thermal and nutritional support to survive. We postulated from the post-mortem findings that some pups were being exposed to anticoagulants through the mothers' milk and therefore we opted to treat presumptively for diphacinone toxicity.

- Supplementary syringe feeding with Wombaroo bat milk replacer 1–2 ml PO q3h (Fig. 1.47)
- Maintained in brooder at 35°C, 75% humidity with hanging polypropylene cloths as "perches"
- Vitamin K at 2 mg/kg PO SID for 4 weeks

As the pups became furred they were transferred to a temperature-controlled room to encourage flight and were given access to a nectar mix (Wombaroo Lorikeet and Honeyeater food) and live insects (mealworms) and leaf litter. Three of the four pups were successfully rehabilitated. One pup failed to fly well due to elbow arthritis and was euthanased. The cause of the elbow arthritis was not definitively determined but was postulated to be due to haemarthrosis.

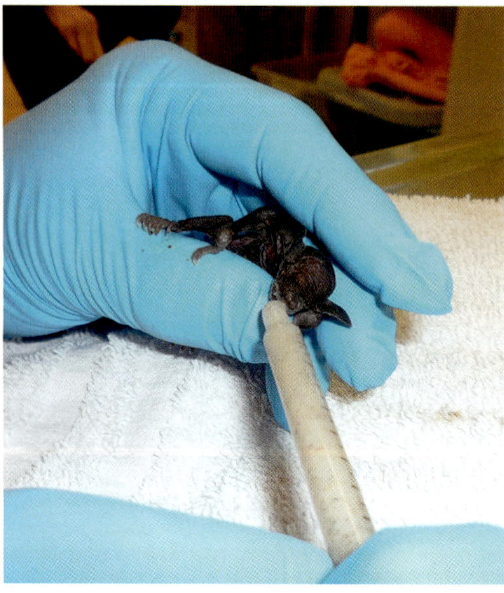

Fig. 1.47 Supplementary syringe feeding using Wombaroo bat milk replacer.

Final diagnosis

- Coagulopathy, diphacinone toxicity
- Starvation and/or exposure in some juveniles

Discussion

Bats are more sensitive to the effects of anticoagulant poisons than most mammals including rodents. The exact route of exposure of the bats is still to be determined but secondary poisoning via insects is more likely than direct consumption of baits. Weta in New Zealand have been shown to consume rat baits without ill effects and carry significant amounts of diphacinone in their guts. The juvenile bats presented with clinical signs and toxicology results suggesting a combined effect of the anticoagulant and starvation and exposure from becoming orphaned. Diphacinone is a second generation anticoagulant with a half-life in humans of up to 20 days. Extended treatment with the antidote vitamin K is therefore recommended. Hand-rearing bats poses the challenges of providing sufficient thermal and nutritional support and preventing zoonotic disease in the handlers. Gloves must always be worn when handling bats, and in countries with endemic rabies (and other Lyssaviruses) prophylactic vaccination of staff is highly recommended.

Further reading

Breed, A.C., 2008. Paramyxoviruses in bats. In: Fowler, M.E., Miller, R.E. (Eds.), Zoo and Wild Animal Medicine: Current Therapy, vol. 6. Saunders Elsevier, St Louis, pp. 225–235.

Lloyd, B.D., 2001. Advances in New Zealand mammalogy 1990–2000: Short-tailed bats. J. R. Soc. N. Z. 31 (1), 59–81.

Thompson, R.D., Mitchell, G.C., Burns, R.J., 1972. Vampire bat control by systemic treatment of livestock with an anticoagulant. Science 177 (4051), 806–808.

Case 1.18 *P. Zucca*

Clinical history

At the beginning of the autumn, three young European hedgehogs (*Erinaceus europaeus*) were found in a public garden during the daylight. A detailed survey of the surrounding area did not reveal the presence of any adult hedgehog (mother) and, after a while, the three hoglets were taken and deposited in a local wildlife rescue centre.

1. How do you evaluate if the hoglets are "genuine" orphans?

Physical examination

One subject was younger and more confident than the others with a bodyweight <100 g while the other two were shy and older with a bodyweight of around 150–200 g. The general body condition was good (Fig. 1.48). The hoglets reacted to external stimuli and they appeared both hungry and thirsty. None of the animals were carrying fly eggs on their body.

2. Why is it so important to relate the weight of the young hedgehogs to the season?

Clinical diagnosis examination

An "unrolling procedure" for performing the clinical diagnosis examination of the larger hedgehogs was required (Fig. 1.49). There are several techniques that can be used to "unroll" a hedgehog. The easiest one is placing the hedgehog in a normal

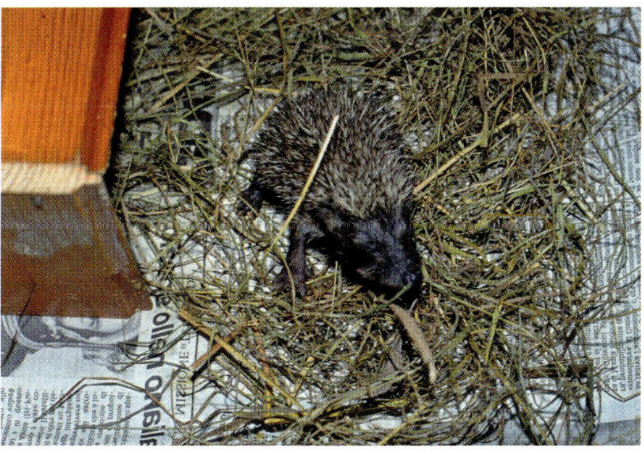

Fig. 1.48 Young hoglets should be hosted in a warm hospital box (28°C).

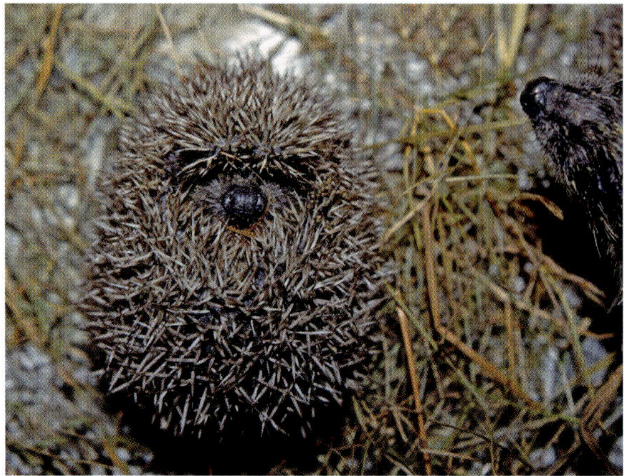

Fig. 1.49 It is not possible to perform a clinical examination without "unrolling" the hedgehog. For the same reason it is very difficult to administer oral medication if it is not pleasant tasting and well accepted by these spiny patients. However, drugs can be injected into mealworms (*Tenebrio molitor*), which are one of the favourite meals of hedgehogs.

standing position on a table; as soon as it extends the limbs, the hind legs are grasped and the hedgehog is held in a facedown position. The clinical diagnostic examination revealed that the older subjects were infected by ectoparasites (fleas) although no integument lesions were found.

Clinical diagnosis laboratory examination

A parasitological survey for endoparasites was performed by faecal flotation and the nematode egg count (*Capillaria* spp.) was high in the two subadult subjects.

Summary of clinical findings

- Young subjects rescued after the normal breeding season (autumn)
- Low bodyweight (one young hoglet and two subadult hoglets)
- Reactive to external stimuli
- Hungry and thirsty
- High burden of *Capillaria* spp. eggs in the faeces of the two subadults
- Fleas on the older hoglets

Q *3. List your therapeutic strategy.*

Therapy

- Warm hospitalization cages (28°C)
- Endoparasite treatment with fenbendazole 10 mg/kg PO q24h × 5 days
- Permethrine powder (1%) or Selamectine 6 mg/kg topically

- Hand feeding with a hedgehog milk replacement such as Esbilac Milk Replacer (Pet Ag – mix 1 part of Esbilac powder to 2 parts of warm boiled water) associated with abdominal and perineal manipulation for stimulating faecal elimination (younger hoglet), see also next paragraph
- Weaning of the two subadults with a mixed soft-wet diet, see also next paragraph

Raising hoglets

Hand rearing of young hedgehogs is frequently related to a high mortality especially during the first 2–3 weeks of life and diet is a key aspect of the care of sick, orphaned or underweight hedgehogs. If young hedgehogs are treated properly within a few hours after the rescue, the survival rate is high. The basic instructions for hand rearing hoglets are listed below:

- Handle young hedgehogs with cotton glove hands or pieces of soft cotton
- Keep them in a warm hospital box or use a heat pad to keep them warm
- Gently manipulate the abdomen and the perineal area for stimulating the faecal and urine excretion as soon as they are rescued and after each meal, until weaning
- A parasitological examination of the faeces using the flotation method should be performed as a routine examination to all the new rescued orphans
- Check carefully for wounds and external parasites such as fleas, ticks, fly eggs and maggots.

Several companion animal milk products have been used as milk replacements for raising hoglets. The best surrogate seems to be a canine milk replacement, Esbilac Milk Replacer (Pet Ag) added with a liquid multivitamin supplement. Data about the nutritional composition of the hedgehog milk are still controversial and the available reference values are shown in Table 1.20.

Never use cow milk for hand rearing hoglets because it is deficient in fat and protein.

Feeding schedule for neonate hoglets

- Bodyweight 5–30 g: 0.5–0.7 ml every 2–3 hours (6–7 hours overnight)
- Bodyweight 30–100 g: 1–2 ml every 4–5 hours (7–8 hours overnight)

Table 1.20 Basic nutritional analysis of the milk of the hedgehog, dog, goat and cow

Species	Water	Fat	Carbohydrate	Protein	Minerals
Hedgehog	79.4	10.1 (*25.5*)	2.0 (*trace*)	7.2 (*16.0*)	2.3
Dog	75.5	11.8	3.3	8.7	0.8
Goat	87.2	4.1	4.2	3.7	0.8
Cow	87.0	3.7	4.8	3.3	0.7

From Ben Shaul 1962 – first value and Landes et al. 1997 – second value in brackets.

Weaning should start once the teeth erupt and liquidized dog/cat food with added vitamins, mealworms and some fruits like mashed banana can be administered. Care is needed for not overfeeding hedgehogs and the maximum weight gain for a growing hedgehog should not exceed 50 g per week.

Final diagnosis

- Orphan hedgehogs (this is not a disease *per se* but a potential clinical condition involving a high mortality)

There are several reasons for which a litter of hedgehogs can be abandoned but the most frequent one is related to the death of their mother due to anthropic pressure (killed on a road, poisoned, etc).

Discussion

Hedgehogs are members of the Order Insectivora and they are most active at night when they prey on invertebrates such as earthworms and snails. The European hedgehog (*Erinaceus europaeus*) is not a companion animal although a homologous species, the African hedgehog (*Atelerix albiventris*) is becoming popular in the pet market. Nevertheless, hedgehogs have still to be considered as solitary, nocturnal wild animals. During the cold season, the European hedgehogs enter into a torpid state and this energy-demanding physiological state requires an individual weight of 400 g or more. In fact, sick or young subjects under 400 g body weight at the end of the summer do not survive the winter. Hedgehogs might carry several zoonotic diseases; among those we should mention is *Salmonella* spp. Transmission of these bacteria is facilitated because hedgehogs have a propensity for walking in their faeces and this behavioural pattern increases the environmental contamination of the cages and the facilities. The auto-insalivation (self-anointing) shown by this species might be mistaken as a sign of rabies although, like several other mammalian species, hedgehogs are sensitive to rabies infection and this aspect has to be always kept in mind every time a wild hedgehog from a rabies area is hospitalized. Young hedgehogs should be "rescued" only when it is certain that the animal is abandoned or ill and it needs human assistance. Underweight or orphan hoglets found during the autumn do not survive the winter and therefore they should be always considered as truly orphans.

Further reading

Ben Shaul, D.M., 1962. The composition of the milk of wild animals. International Zoo Yearbook 4, 333–342.

Landes, E., Zentek, J., Wolf, P., et al., 1997. Untersuchungen zur Zusammensetzung der Igelmilch und zur Entwicklung von Igelsäuglingen. Kleintierpraxis 42, 647–658.

Pesaro, S., Ressel, L., Zucca, P., 2002. "Pricking Medicine" a few physiological and therapeutic peculiarities of a spiny patient: *Erinaceus europaeus*. In: Proceedings of the 5th Conference of the European Hedgehog Research Group. April 5–6, Gemmano (RN), Italy, p. 20.

Peto, J., 2002. Hand Rearing Hoglets – The Early days. In: Proceedings of the 5th Conference of the European Hedgehog Research Group. April 5-6, Gemmano (RN), Italy, p. 21.
Quesenberry, K.E., Carpenter, J.W., 2004. Ferret, Rabbits and Rodents: Clinical Medicine and Surgery, second ed. WB Saunders, Philadelphia.
Reeve, N., 1994. Hedgehogs. T & AD Poyser Ltd, London.
Saupe, E., Poduschka, W., 1998. Hedgehogs. In: Gabrisch, K., Zwart, P. (Eds.), Krankheiten der Heimtiere, fourth ed. Exotische und heimische Tiere in der Tierarztpraxis. Schlutersche GmbH & Co., KG Verlag und Druckerei, Hannover, pp. 297–325.

Case 1.19 *C. Lloyd*

Clinical history

A 17-month-old captive-bred male, parent-raised cheetah *Acinonyx jubatus jubatus* was presented for persistent bilateral skin lesions of the medial aspect of the antebrachium. The cheetah had been vaccinated against feline leukaemia virus (Felo Vax PCT, Fort Dodge) every 2 weeks from 8 to 16 weeks old and again at 6 and 12 months old. The animal was housed with three other juvenile cheetah of mixed sex and fed a mixed diet of camel meat, goat and fowl. The animal had no previous clinical history other than a mild episode of sneezing and conjunctivitis at 13 months old.

Zoo staff had been treating the cheetah as follows; topical iodine solution (1:10 dilution povodine iodine) twice daily, clavulanic potentiated amoxicillin (10 mg/kg BID) × 21 days and prednisolone at 0.5 mg/kg SID with no sign of clinical improvement. A veterinary examination was requested as the lesions were progressing to affect the skin over the chest, a persistent unilateral ocular discharge had developed and proliferative lesions had appeared near the eye and nares.

The animal was anaesthetized with medetomidine and ketamine by remote injection, intubated and maintained on isoflurane for clinical examination.

Clinical findings

An area of localized hair loss with erythema, papules, ulceration and hyperkeratosis was present over the medial antebrachium on both legs. A white paste-like material could be expressed from the skin lesions (Fig. 1.50a). Hair loss, erythema and papules were also present over the chest and thoracic inlet. There was a mild bilateral conjunctivitis. Small proliferative skin lesions were present on the ventral aspect of the left nares and also at the lateral canthus of the left eye (Fig. 1.50b).

Haematology, biochemistry, hair plucks, skin scrapes, skin impressions and culture swabs were collected.

Results

Initial results were as follows:

- Haematology and biochemistry results were unremarkable
- Dermatophyte culture was negative

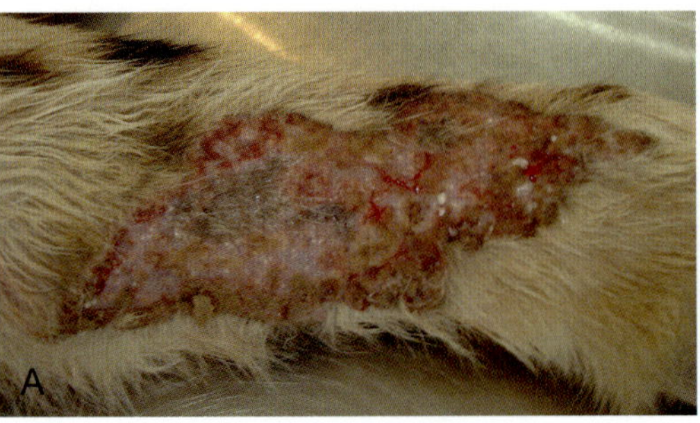

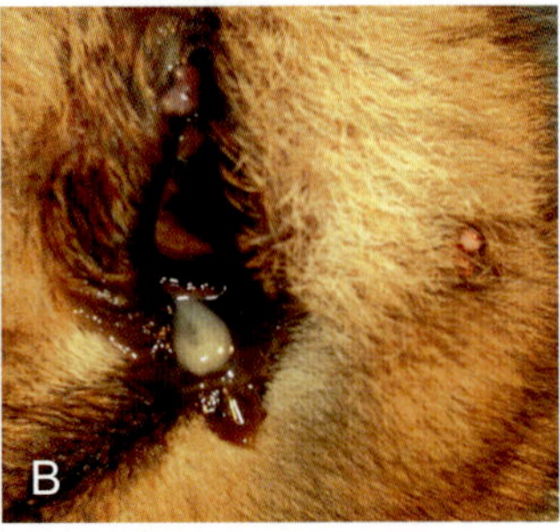

Fig. 1.50 (a) Erythematous, ulcerated, hyperkeratotic lesion on antebrachium. Note pasty white exudates; (b) conjunctivitis with proliferative lesion at lateral canthus.

- Fluid and exudates cultured from the leg lesions grew a *Staphylococcus* species sensitive to clindamycin, enrofloxacin and oxytetracycline
- Skin scrape: negative for parasites and fungal elements
- Skin impression (rapid stain): predominantly red blood cells and eosinophils with occasional lymphocytes. No parasite or fungal elements noticed.

Q *1. Please interpret the initial findings and produce a differential diagnosis list.*

➤ Chronic dermatitis associated with feline herpesvirus 1
➤ Insect bite hypersensitivity
➤ Eosinophilic granuloma complex
➤ Squamous cell carcinoma

Q *2. What other samples may aid in diagnosis?*

Other samples recommended would be:

- Multiple skin biopsies
- Oral and or conjunctival swabs for viral PCR and/or viral culture.

Results

Histopathology

Severe, chronic hyperplastic, ulcerative, perivascular dermatitis. The dermatitis is characterized by dense infiltrates of primarily plasma cells and secondarily eosinophils. There is occasional keratinocyte swelling, the nuclei containing round to oval amphophilic intranuclear material suspicious of intranuclear inclusion bodies.

PCR

➤ Moist swabs sent for PCR testing were positive for feline herpesvirus 1

Diagnosis

 Chronic dermatitis associated with feline herpesvirus 1 (FHV-1)

Q *3. Please formulate a treatment plan.*

Therapy

The cheetah was weaned off prednisolone over a course of 2 weeks and was placed on oral acyclovir (400 mg SID), clindamycin (12.5 mg/kg BID × 14 days) and L lysine (500 mg BID).

The acyclovir treatment continued for 3 months with no deleterious effects. At this time, the skin lesions on the chest, face and legs had fully recovered. A small scar remains on both front legs reflecting permanent damage to skin follicles.

Discussion

Chronic dermatitis associated with herpesvirus is a reported condition in cheetahs and has been recorded from North American zoos. Lesions characteristically affect the eyes, face, the inner aspects of the front legs, foot pads and chest. Lesions are typically raised with a white eosinophil-rich exudate. The histological appearance is characterized by dense infiltrates of eosinophils, mast cells, plasma cells and lymphocytes. Keratinocytes are often necrotic or swollen and may contain inclusion bodies, especially in samples from early lesions.

The lesions often spread centrifugally from a source of infection and are thought to be further spread by herpes-infected saliva and ocular secretions. This has also been hypothesized as the source of infection in cubs and hand rearing may be necessary to prevent infection. As in this case, vaccination does not prevent disease.

Treatment is reported as minimally responsive to topical or systemic antiviral drugs and surgical excision has been reported as successful. However, case studies are few and this animal appeared to respond to systemic antiviral therapy. The treatment of this case with corticosteroids before definitive diagnosis may have worsened the clinical signs.

The severity and unremitting nature of lesions in cases reported by Munson (2004) resulted in the euthanasia of 6/20 individuals.

This response to FHV-1 infection has been reported in domestic cats but is very rare and atypical. The relative prevalence in cheetahs suggests an extreme immune response as is also reported in cheetahs with feline coronavirus and *Helicobacter*. A number of hypotheses exist as to the cause of this immune response (see further reading) but include chronic stress in captivity and a lack of heterogeneity in the major histocompatibility genes.

Further reading

Heeney, J.L., Evermann, J.F., McKeirnan, A.J., et al., 1990. Prevalence and implications of feline coronavirus infections of captive and free-ranging cheetahs (*Acinonyx jubatus*). J. Virol. 64 (5), 1964–1972.

Munson, L., Wack, R., Duncan, M., et al., 2004. Chronic eosinophilic dermatitis associated with persistent feline herpes virus infection in cheetahs (*Acinonyx jubatus*). Vet. Pathol. 41, 170–176.

Munson, L., Terio, K.A., Worley, M., et al., 2005. Extrinsic factors significantly affect patterns of disease in free ranging and captive cheetah (*Acinonyx jubatus*) populations. J. Wildl. Dis. 41, 542–548.

Terio, K.A., Marker, L., Munson, L., 2004. Evidence for chronic stress in captive but not free ranging cheetahs (*Acinonyx jubatus*) based in adrenal morphology and function. J. Wildl. Dis. 40, 259–266.

Case 1.20 *T. A. Bailey*

Clinical history

A 20-month-old male cheetah (*Acinonyx jubatus*) weighing 21 kg, was presented with the following clinical signs of 3 days' duration:

- Inappetence and lethargy
- Loss of condition
- Diarrhoea
- Intermittent regurgitation.

The captive-bred cheetah was part of a breeding programme with 25 other cheetahs. The animal had recently received anthelmintic treatment and was vaccinated against feline panleucopenia, calicivirus and canine distemper.

Clinical examination

Clinical examination and sample collection were performed under general anaesthetic. The cheetah was in poor body condition. Survey radiographs were taken (Fig. 1.51a, b). Blood samples were collected for haematology, blood chemistry and plasma protein electrophoresis analyses. A faecal sample was collected to examine for the presence of endoparasites and for microbiology culture.

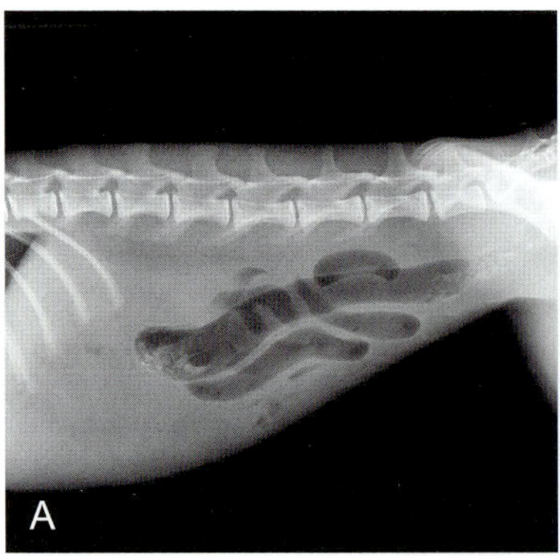

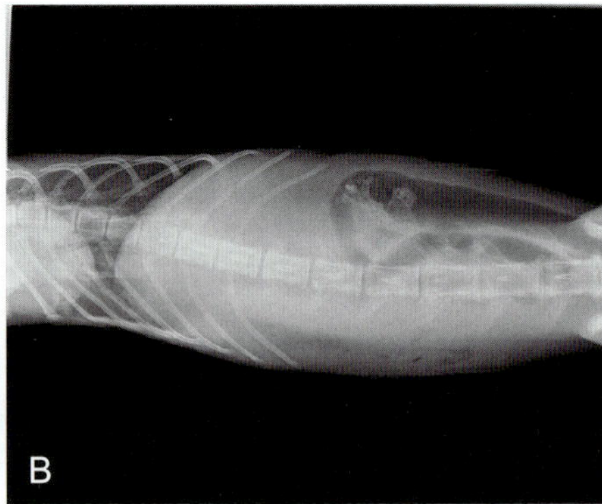

Fig. 1.51 (a) Lateral radiograph of the cheetah abdomen; (b) ventrodorsal radiograph of the abdomen region of the cheetah.

Radiology

1. What is your interpretation of the radiographs in Fig. 1.51a, b?

Radiographic findings included:

- Dilated small intestine and proximal large intestine loops filled with gas
- Small amount of faecal material present in the large intestine
- Loss of abdominal detail (stomach and kidney shadows are not discernible). The ground-glass appearance is suggestive of fluid in the abdominal cavity.

Clinical diagnosis laboratory

The results of the laboratory assays are given in Tables 1.21–1.23.

2. What is your interpretation of the haematology, blood chemistry and protein electrophoresis values shown in Tables 1.21–1.23 and Fig. 1.51a, b?

- ➤ Haematology analysis showed a moderate anaemia with low Hb, PCV, MCH and MCV. The white cells showed a marked leucocytosis with a neutrophilia, lymphopenia. The platelet count is raised
- ➤ Blood chemistry analysis showed elevated TP and globulin levels. BUN levels are mildly elevated

Table 1.21 Haematology values of the cheetah (mean±SD)

Parameters	Results	Reference values
RBC (×10^{12}/l)	6.94	6.84±1.1
Hb (g/dl)	9.5	12.5±1.9
Hct (l/l)	25.1	37.9±5.8
MCV (fl)	36.2	55.6±5.5
MCH (pg)	13.7	18.3±1.7
MCHC (g/dl)	37.8	33.0±2.6
WBC (×10^{12}/l)	24.1	10.35±3.5
Neutrophils (×10^{12}/l)	22.4	6.9±2.7
Lymphocytes (×10^{12}/l)	1.0	2.0±0.9
Monocytes (×10^{12}/l)	0.7	0.3±0.3
Eosinophils (×10^{12}/l)	0	0.8±0.8
Basophils (×10^{12}/l)	0	0.1±0.1
Platelets (×10^{12}/l)	629	349±119

ISIS values are for cheetah.

Table 1.22 Blood chemistry values of the cheetah (colorimetry, mean ± SD)

Analysis	Results	Reference values
Albumin (g/l) (colorimetry)	31	36±4
Total protein (g/l) (colorimetry)	83	67±6
Globulin (g/l) (colorimetry)	52	31±6
Calcium (mmol/l)	2.6	10.6±0.8
Creatinine (μmol/l)	149	212.2±79.6
CK (U/l)	121	296±311
LDH (U/l)	129	92±87
AST (U/l)	60	52±35
Iron (μmol/l)	5	9.3±3.9
Phosphorus (mmol/l)	3.75	1.9±0.6
Total urea (mmol/l)	17.5	12.85±3.2

ISIS values are for cheetah.

Table 1.23 Plasma protein electrophoresis of the cheetah (concentrations g/dl)

Parameters	Results	ISIS normal
Total protein	7.99	6.7±6
Albumin	1.77	3.6±4
Globulin	6.2	3.1±6
Alpha 1 globulins	0.34	0.5±0.2
Alpha 2 globulins	1.91	1.0±0.2
Beta globulins	1.78	0.6±0.3
Gamma globulins	2.19	No data
A:G ratio	0.28	1.2

➤ Plasma protein electrophoresis showed low albumin, raised TP, markedly elevated globulins and low albumin:globulin ratio. Although there are no available published normal values for gamma globulins in normal cheetahs for comparison, the animal appears to have elevated gamma globulins

Results

Other laboratory results included:

- Faecal examination was negative for the presence of endoparasites
- *Salmonella* spp. was isolated from the faecal culture.

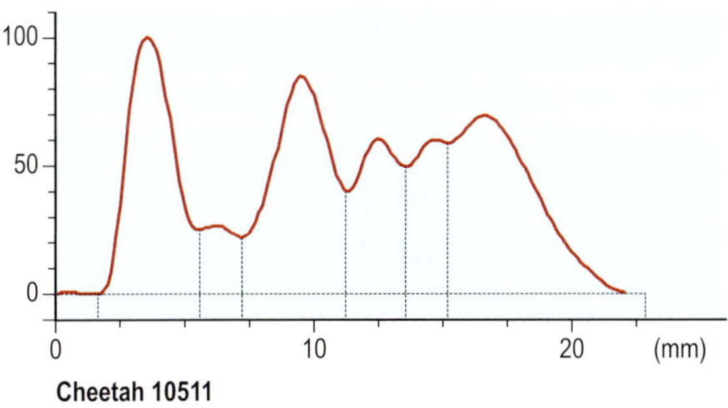

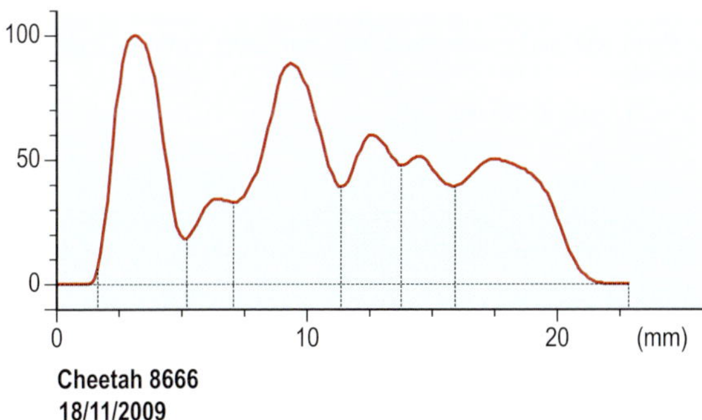

Fig. 1.52 Electrophoresis profile of the cheetah (results in Table 1.23).

Please evaluate the clinical history, Figs 1.51a, b and 1.52, the results of the physical examination and clinical diagnosis laboratory tests.

Q *3. List your differential diagnoses.*

- Feline infectious peritonitis (FIP)
- Salmonellosis
- Peritonitis of other bacterial aetiology
- Pancreatitis
- Rupture of the gallbladder, urinary bladder, or bile duct

Q *4. What additional diagnostic tests would be appropriate to move this case closer to a diagnosis?*

- Ultrasound would be appropriate to identify free fluid within the abdomen and to exclude other conditions, e.g. pancreas or liver abscesses
- Abdominocentesis or diagnostic peritoneal lavage – if abdominal fluid not recovered by paracentesis

- ➤ Culture and sensitivity and cytology of recovered fluid
- ➤ Rivalta's test is useful to differentiate between FIP effusions and effusions caused by other diseases
- ➤ Laparoscopy to observe specific lesions of the peritoneal cavity and to obtain a biopsy sample for histopathology or immunohistochemistry
- ➤ Serum antibody tests – immunoassays detect antibodies against feline coronavirus (FCoV)

Further results

Other laboratory results included:

- A blood sample was tested with a rapid qualitative FCoV immunoassay and was positive
- Cytology of abdominal fluid showed numerous inflammatory cells in a dense granular protein background
- Abdominal fluid was Rivalta's test positive.

Therapy

- ➤ No treatment routinely effective
- ➤ Treatment with immunosuppressive drugs, interferon and antibiotics is tried in domestic cats, but patients with generalized and typical signs almost invariably die
- ➤ In this case, treatment of an individual animal needs to balanced against the risks of continued contact with the remaining animals in the breeding project, especially as treatment is likely to be ineffective

Post-mortem findings

The cheetah was euthanased. On post-mortem, the condition loss was noted along with abdominal distention. A post-mortem examination was performed (Fig. 1.53). Samples from different organs were collected for histopathology.

Q *5. What lesions can you observe in the post-mortem photograph?*

- ➤ Abdominal serous-purulent fluid with adhesions and free-floating pus

Q *6. What further laboratory tests are required to confirm a post-mortem diagnosis?*

Immunohistochemistry assays detect FCoV within specific cells of biopsy samples or histopathologic sections of tissues are excellent for confirming cause of specific lesions, especially inflammatory abdominal disease.

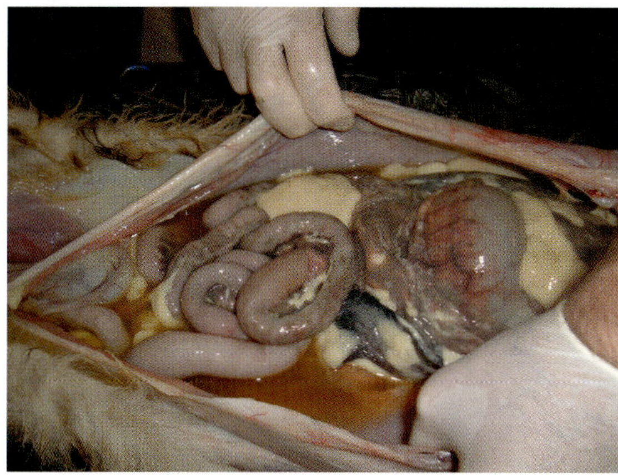

Fig. 1.53 Post-mortem photograph of the cheetah (courtesy of C. Lloyd).

Laboratory findings

- Histology – showed a severe fibrinous polyserositis with histiocyctic vasculitis and perivasculitis of the mesentery, liver, heart, pancreas, spleen, intestine and urinary bladder
- Immunohistochemistry of kidney tissue using antifeline coronavirus monoclonal antibody demonstrated positive staining for feline coronavirus within the pyogranulomatous lesions around the blood vessels in the kidney

Final diagnosis

- Feline infectious peritonitis

Discussion

Feline infectious peritonitis is a fatal viral disease of cats caused by infection with feline coronavirus. In most cases, the virus will cause no clinical signs or only mild transient disease such as self-limiting diarrhoea. Sometimes, infection will result in the development of the progressive fatal manifestation of disease known as FIP.

The diagnosis of FIP described has implications for the cheetah breeding project. Relevant risk factors for developing FIP in cats include: contact with an FCoV antibody-positive cat; breeding catteries or multicat facilities and age (<3 years). In cats, the main method of transmission from mother to offspring is from asymptomatic carrier queens to their kittens at 5–7 weeks of age, after maternally derived immunity wanes. It is recommended to break the cycle of transmission by early weaning at 4–5 weeks of age and isolating the litter from direct contact with other cats, including the mother. Susceptible cats are most likely to be infected following contact with FCoV in faeces from asymptomatic cats. Disposal of faeces and routine disinfection of premises, cages and water/food dishes readily inactivates the virus and reduces transmission. Screening of in-coming cheetahs against FCoV is important so that only FCoV antibody-negative cheetahs from FCoV-free centres are introduced to the facility.

As FIP is a progressive disease, the clinical manifestations will change over time. Reaching a diagnosis in the early stages when clinical signs are vague may be extremely challenging but, in most cases, as time goes by, more classical signs of FIP will develop. However, this does mean that repeat and thorough clinical examinations (and blood tests) may be required in ongoing cases in order to detect the development of these changes.

Results of routine laboratory tests are useful in supporting a presumptive diagnosis of FIP. On routine haematology, the most consistent features are a lymphopenia (low lymphocyte count), a neutrophilic leucocytosis (high neutrophil count) that may be accompanied by a left shift (presence of immature neutrophils), and a mild to moderate non-regenerative anaemia. However, all these are non-specific changes that can occur with other diseases.

Similarly, serum biochemistry changes are non-specific in FIP, with the most common abnormalities being a hyperproteinaemia due to hyperglobulinaemia, often accompanied by low or low to normal serum albumin concentrations.

Interpretation of coronavirus titres requires care. No test is able to distinguish between the different strains of FCoV and a positive result simply shows that a cat has been exposed to a strain of FCoV. The presence and magnitude of the antibody titre cannot distinguish the type of FCoV strain to which a cat has been exposed, whether the infection is current or previous, or whether the cat is susceptible or resistant to the development of FIP.

The analysis of effusions is a valuable routine test for the diagnosis of FIP. The only way of making a definitive diagnosis of FIP is by histopathological examination of affected tissues collected either at post-mortem examination, or collected ante-mortem from appropriate sites. Microscopic examination of tissues affected by FIP yields characteristic signs of inflammation, and additional confirmation can be sought by detecting the presence of FCoV within the lesions using immunohistochemistry.

Acknowledgements

Thanks to Christudas Silvanose and Chris Lloyd (Fig. 1.53) for their contribution to this case.

Further reading

Addie, D., Belák, S., Boucraut-Baralon, C., et al., 2009. Feline infectious peritonitis. ABCD guidelines on prevention and management. J. Feline Med. Surg. 11, 594–604.

Hartmann, K., Ritz, S., 2008. Treatment of cats with feline infectious peritonitis. Vet. Immunol. Immunopathol. 123, 172–175.

Pedersen, N.C., 2009. A review of feline infectious peritonitis virus infection: 1963–2008. J. Feline Med. Surg. 11, 225–258.

The Feline Infectious Peritonitis Website. University of Glasgow, UK. http://www.dr-addie.com/index.htm.

Tilley, L.P., Smith, F.W.K., 2007. In: Blackwell's Five Minute Veterinary Consult: Canine and Feline CD-ROM, fourth ed. Blackwell Publishing. www.blackwellprofessional.com.

Case 1.21 *J-M. Hatt*

Clinical history

A 12-month-old, male African lion (*Panthera leo*) weighing 83 kg, was presented with the clinical signs of ataxia and head tilt for 1 month.

The animal had lived for 5 months with the owner and was kept in an indoor and outdoor enclosure together with a female lion of similar age. The diet consisted mainly of beef to which the owner added a commercial vitamin-mineral mix for carnivores. The lion had originally been hand-reared in a zoo and when received, the current owner noted that growth and body condition were reduced. The animal was regularly dewormed against nematodes, the vaccine status was not known.

Clinical examination

On presentation, the animal was alert and had a body condition of 3/5, however, for its age was of small size. There was a minor head tilt to the left. When walking the animal showed mild to moderate ataxia, especially on the front legs. The clinical examination was made under general anaesthesia, which was induced by ketamine 2.5 mg/kg IM with medetomidine 0.06 mg/kg IM and maintained with isoflurane (1%). Upon palpation and auscultation of the lungs and the heart no abnormal findings were noted. Investigations included a computed tomography evaluation of the head and neck, an ultrasound of the abdomen (for liver biopsy), collection of spinal fluid, conjunctival scraping (for canine distemper analysis) and blood sampling for haematology, blood chemistry, vitamin A and viral analysis (canine distemper, feline leukaemia virus and feline immunodeficiency virus).

Computed tomography

Q *1. What is your interpretation of the CT images in Fig. 1.54a, b?*

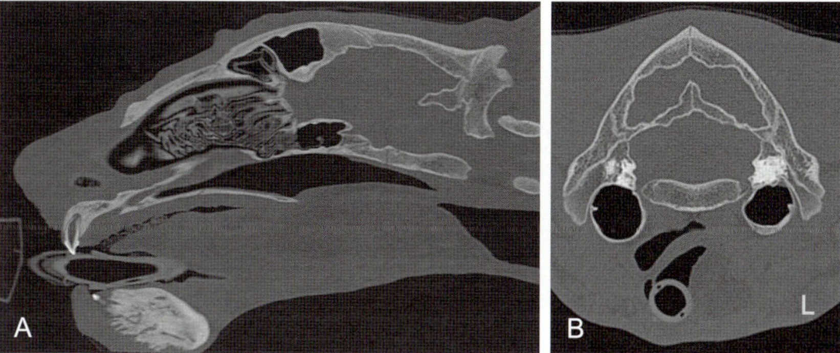

Fig. 1.54 (a) Mid-sagittal computed tomographic image of the skull of the lion; (b) transverse computed tomographic image of the skull at the processus jugularis of the lion, the level of the bullae is visible.

Clinical diagnosis laboratory

The results of the clinical diagnosis laboratory assays are given in Tables 1.24 and 1.25.

RBC and WBC morphology

- Some anisocytosis in the RBC

Viral test results

All test were negative for antigen for canine distemper (PCR and immunofluorescence), feline leukaemia virus (AG ELISA) and feline immunodeficiency virus (Western blot).
- The abdominal ultrasound examination did not reveal any abnormalities.

Q *2. What is your interpretation of the haematology and blood chemistry values shown in Tables 1.24 and 1.25?*

The results of the spinal fluid assays are shown in Table 1.26.

Q *3. What is your interpretation of the spinal fluid values shown in Table 1.26?*

Table 1.24 Haematology values of the lion

Parameters	Results (absolute)	Results (%)	Reference values
Hb (g/dl)	14.3		11.8 ± 2.1
Hct (l/l)	0.42		0.36 ± 0.05
Erythrocytes (×10⁶/μl)	9.12		7.5 ± 1.3
MCHC (g/dl)	29		33.0 ± 3.0
MCH (pg)	16		16.4 ± 1.6
MCV (fl)	46		49.2 ± 5.0
WBC (×10⁹/l)	13.9		12.2 ± 5.0
Unsegmented neutrophils (×10⁹/l)	0.21	1.5	0.19 ± 0.096
Segmented neutrophils (×10⁹/l)	11.8	84	8.5 ± 3.82
Lymphocytes (×10⁹/l)	1.30	9.5	2.3 ± 1.13
Monocytes (×10⁹/l)	0.28	2.0	0.4 ± 0.33
Eosinophils (×10⁹/l)	0.28	2.0	0.3 ± 0.29
Basophils (×10⁹/l)	0.07	0.5	0.1 ± 0.09

Table 1.25 Blood chemistry values of the lion

Analysis	Results	Reference values
Albumin (g/l)	33	34 ± 5
Alkaline phosphatase (U/l)	161	105 ± 57
Amylase (U/l)	1884	160 ± 83
Bilirubin (μmol/l)	1.1	2 ± 2
Calcium (mmol/l)	2.7	2.6 ± 0.18
Chloride (mmol/l)	121	117 ± 4
Cholesterol (mmol/l)	3.7	4.5 ± 1.14
Creatinine (μmol/l)	104	159 ± 53
Glucose (mmol/l)	7.7	7.1 ± 1.72
GPT (U/l)	55	45 ± 13
GOT (U/l)	24	28 ± 10
Lipase (U/l)	7	1.3 ± 1.95
Phosphorus (mmol/l)	2.1	2.2 ± 0.36
Potassium (mmol/l)	3.9	4.5 ± 0.5
Sodium (mmol/l)	159	150 ± 5
Total protein (g/l)	71	67 ± 7
Triglycerides (mmol/l)	0.5	0.5 ± 0.26
Urea (mmol/l)	16.3	10.7 ± 2.14
Vitamin A (Retinol) (μmol/l)	<30	>200

Reference values ISIS Physiological Reference Values, 2002.

Table 1.26 Spinal fluid values of the lion

Analysis	Results	%
Amount (ml)	3	
Transparency	Clear	
Colour	None	
Protein (g/l)	0.2	
Leukocytes/μl	4.3	
Erythrocytes/μl	None	
Neutrophils		27
Monocytes		7
Lymphocytes		66

Results

- Computed tomographic images revealed an enlarged occipital bone and *tentorium osseus cerebelli* and in the left bulla there was sign of fluid accumulation, suggestive of otitis interna
- The mild elevation of RBC, Hct and erythrocytes indicated a mild dehydration; the elevated amylase and lipase may have been related to pancreatic disease, such as inflammation or obstruction, but may also have been due to the general anaesthesia
- The occurrence of neutrophil granulocytes in the spinal fluid suggested a mild inflammatory process
- The low vitamin A serum level suggested hypovitaminosis A

Please evaluate the clinical history, Fig. 1.54a, b, the results of the physical examination and clinical diagnosis laboratory tests.

4. List your most likely diagnosis and the pathophysiology.

Diagnosis

- Hypovitaminosis A, bone malformation (Chiari-like malformation) especially of the skull in the region of the occipital and basisphenoid bone as well as the *tentorium osseus cerebelli* resulting in cerebellar and caudal brainstem compression
- Otitis interna of left side

5. What would be your initial therapy and long-term therapy?

Initial therapy (Table 1.27)

Table 1.27 Initial therapy

Prednisolone	2 mg/kg IV followed by 1 mg/kg PO SID × 2 weeks
Marboflaxacin	2 mg/kg SC followed by 2 g/kg PO SID × 2 weeks
Fluids	Lactated ringer solution 10 ml/kg/h IV
Vitamin A	5000 IU/kg PO SID until adult size is reached
Observe digestion	Look for signs of maldigestion due to pancreatic disease, treat if necessary

Long-term therapy

- Surgical decompression of the caudal fossa through foramen magnum decompression

Final diagnosis

➤ Chronic hypovitaminosis A, bone malformation especially of the skull (Chiari-like malformation)

Discussion

Clinical signs of incoordination, ataxia, opisthotonus, convulsions, head tilt and blindness have been reported in lions worldwide. Several aetiologies have been proposed including infections, neoplasia and deficiency. Vitamin A deficiency has been described several times especially in young animals. It appears likely that vitamin A deficiency results in skull bone malformation. The bones most frequently affected are the *tentorium osseus cerebelli*, occipital and basisphenoid bones and the cranial cervical vertebrae. The thickening of these bones results in compression of the cerebellum and the caudal brainstem, which causes the clinical signs. Initial treatment with prednisolone alleviates the condition, by reducing oedema of the affected central nervous tissue. For long-term improvement, however, it appears that only surgical decompression is effective. The prognosis is good. Untreated cases typically succumb to the disease and conservative treatment with vitamin A alone is not effective once clinical signs are present.

Further reading

Gross-Tsubery, R., Chai, O., Shilo, Y., et al., 2010. Computed tomographic analysis of calvarial hyperostosis in captive lions. Vet. Radiol. Ultrasound 51, 34–38.

McCain, S., Souza, M., Ramsay, E., et al., 2008. Diagnosis and surgical treatment of a Chiari I-like malformation in an African lion (*Panthera leo*). J. Zoo Wildl. Med. 39, 421–427.

Shamir, M.H., Shilo, Y., Fridman, A., et al., 2008. Sub-occipital craniectomy in a lion (*Panthera leo*) with occipital bone malformation and hypovitaminosis A. J. Zoo Wildl. Med. 39, 455–459.

Case 1.22 *C. Lloyd*

Clinical history

Twenty-three dama gazelle (*Gazella dama)* were held in a fenced, sand enclosure with direct contact to a mixed collection of non-domestic ungulates including springbok (*Antidorcas marsupialis)*, fallow deer (*Dama dama*) and nyala (*Tragelaphus angasii*). The enclosure had previously housed domestic goats. The gazelle were fed a commercial browser pellet and mixed browse and hay.

Over a 4-month period, five gazelles from the herd aborted late in their gestation period with no apparent adverse effects to the dam. Fetuses were fully developed with no external signs of illness. Gross post-mortems on all animals revealed no gross abnormalities (Fig. 1.55).

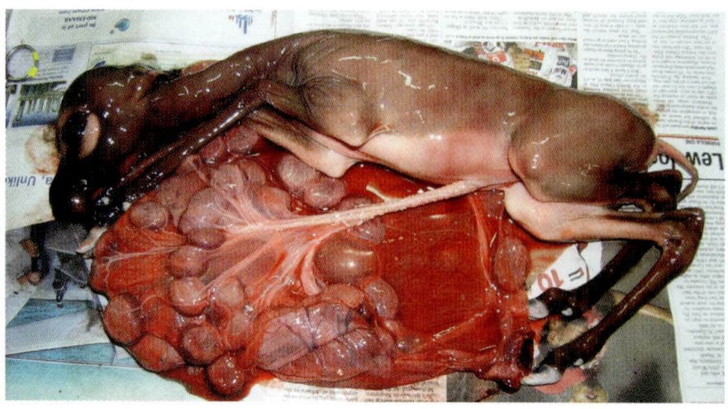

Fig. 1.55 Typical external appearance of aborted dama gazelle fetus.

Q *1. What are your differentials for abortion in this species?*

Differential diagnoses

- *Coxiella burnetii*
- *Brucella abortus*
- *Brucella melitensi*
- *Leptospira* spp.
- *Toxoplasma gondii*
- *Neospora caninum*
- *Ureaplasma diversum*
- *Chlamydophila abortus*
- Bovine viral diarrhoea virus

2. What diagnostic steps would you take to identify the cause of abortion?

- Direct Giemsa stained smears of placental material and vaginal discharge
- Histopathology of fetal liver, lung, spleen and placental material
- Possibly immunohistochemistry
- PCR testing from pooled fetal spleen, lung, liver and placental material
- Viral cultures from fetal spleen, lung, liver and placental material

Results

- Viral cultures were negative
- Histopathological examination of fetal tissues from two cases revealed evidence of meconial aspiration in the lung consistent with fetal distress, otherwise no abnormalities were detected in fetal tissue. Intracytoplasmic aggregations of tiny closely packed basophilic coccoid organisms suggestive of *Coxiella burnetii* were present between the cotyledonary villi. An absence of vasculitis contrasted with the typical appearance of placentitis due to

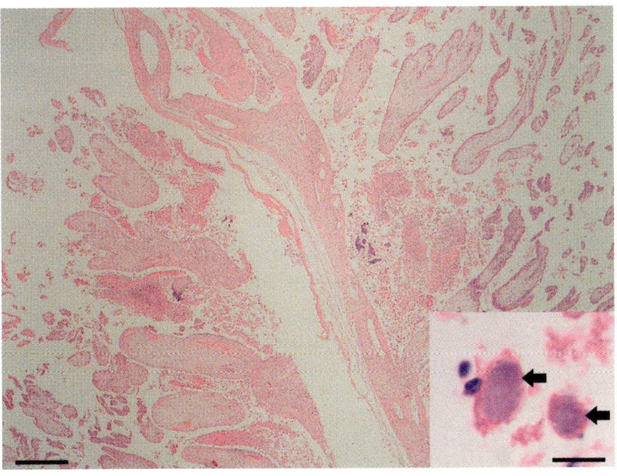

Fig. 1.56 Dama gazelle, placenta. Main image: accumulations of necrotic cellular debris, intermingled with neutrophils, lie between the villi in the cotyledons. Haematoxylin and eosin. Scale bar = 500 μm. Inset: intracytoplasmic aggregations (arrows) of tiny closely packed basophilic coccoid organisms, consistent with *Coxiella burnetti*, within the exudate. Scale bar = 20 μm.

Chlamydophila species, another infectious abortifacient agent generating intracytoplasmic inclusions (Fig. 1.56)

- Immunohistochemistry showed positive labelling for *C. burnetii* organisms
- PCR testing was positive for *C. burnetii*

 *3. What is another name for the disease caused by this pathogen and how is this disease spread?*

C. burnetii is an obligate intracellular, Gram-negative coccobacillus and the cause of the disease Q fever. The organism can infect a large number of animal species with the main clinical manifestation of infection being late-term abortion. The organism is found in large numbers in the placentas of infected animals, but organisms have also been detected in milk, vaginal discharges, semen, urine, amniotic fluid, and faeces. Infection can be vertical or horizontal with the latter being mainly via ingestion or inhalation. *C. burnetii* is extremely resistant to desiccation, probably due to its ability to form spores, and has been found in soil samples for periods of up to 150 days. Reports of the organism being spread on the wind, via tick vectors and on fomites exist. In this case, it is hypothesized that the herd contracted the infection after being moved into a pen that had previously housed infected goats.

 *4: What is the significance of this diagnosis for:*

- *The affected herd*
- *The caregivers.*

Discussion

C. burnetii affects a wide range of animals and has been reported in mammals, birds, reptiles, fish and invertebrates. Infections are mainly asymptomatic but do cause reproductive disease in domestic goats, sheep, non-domestic artiodactyls, perisodactyls and aquatic mammals.

It may be that this herd will have no further issues with reproductive disease, however, there is a high probability that animals within the herd will become carriers and shed the organism at the next parturition.

C. burnetii is a zoonotic pathogen. The disease is highly infectious to humans with a single organism able to cause disease in humans. Humans are usually infected through aerosolized animal products and, while approximately 50% of infections are asymptomatic, clinical disease may occur. Pregnant women, cardiac patients and immunosuppressed people are most at risk. Symptoms include abortion, fever, headache and atypical pneumonia in acute infections and chronic endocarditis develops from approximately 1% of all acute cases. The main sources of human infection depends on the epidemiological context, but animal care workers are at increased risk of exposure. Domestic ungulates, companion animals, zoo animals, and wildlife, as well as their arthropod parasites have been implicated in human outbreaks of disease.

Q *5. What steps could be taken to protect staff and prevent spread of disease?*

- The infected herd should be isolated from direct and indirect contact with other animals
- Staff associated with the infected herd should be minimized and prevented from working on nearby animal facilities. Staff should wear face masks, overalls and gloves when within animal enclosures
- Only essential staff allowed contact with animals and pregnant women banned from the facility
- Separation and isolation of pregnant dams in the herd may be advisable depending on management constraints
- All reproductive material on the farm should be treated as a potential biological hazard
- Effective arthropod control
- Disinfectant foot baths should be placed outside each enclosure and vehicles should be sprayed with disinfectant upon entering and leaving the premises
- Staff could be vaccinated or serologically monitored for exposure to the pathogen
- Herd vaccination: commercial sheep vaccines are reported to reduce both abortion and shedding of the organism
- Treatment of herd: although tetracyclines, enrofloxacin and trimethoprim sulpha have been used in treatment there is no effective regimen. Recent studies in sheep have suggested that oxytetracyline therapy does not prevent the shedding of bacteria or reduce the duration of shedding
- Serological identification of carrier animals: there are limitations to serological testing of individual non-domestic and domestic ungulates. ELISA testing in a sheep herd showed 50% of the sheep that were PCR positive from vaginal mucus remained serologically negative. It is hypothesized that, in some animals, infection may be localized to the placenta or uterus without stimulating an antibody response
- Cases of abortion in a zoological collection should always be investigated. Sporadic abortion in a small herd may be considered uneconomical to investigate fully and incorrectly attributed to non-infectious causes. Causes of abortion in ruminants should be dealt with carefully and clinicians should be aware of the significant number of zoonotic diseases that may be implicated

Further reading

Berri, M., Souriau, A., Crosby, M., et al., 2001. Relationship between the shedding of *Coxiella burnetii*, clinical signs and serological responses of 34 sheep. Vet. Rec. 148, 502–505.

European Association of Zoo and Wildlife Veterinarians Transmissible disease fact sheets 2009. Coxiellosis or Q fever.

Lloyd, C., Stidworthy, M.F., Wernery, U., 2010. *Coxiella burnetii* abortion in dama gazelle (*Gazella dama*) in the United Arab Emirates. J. Zoo Wildl. Med. 41 (1), 82–88.

Maurin, M., Raoult, D., 1999. Q-fever. Clin. Microbiol. Rev. 12, 518–553.

Case 1.23 *J. Samour, J. Naldo*

Clinical history

A sub-adult female and a juvenile male common Arabian gazelle (*Gazella gazella*) were taken to the veterinary clinic for examination. The gazelles were part of a herd of 25 individuals housed in a paddock measuring 500 m × 500 m planted with trees to provide natural shade. The gazelles were maintained at a private zoological collection. Several other groups of gazelles and other antelopes were housed in the same collection, but no further cases had been reported.

On examination at a distance using binoculars, the gazelles exhibited numerous growths on the face and neck (Fig. 1.57a, b). The gazelles were bright and alert and showed normal flight response when approached, characteristic of the species. The gazelles were lured with fresh food into a smaller enclosure and were sedated with a combination of xylazine hydrochloride (1 mg/kg) and ketamine hydrochloride (2 mg/kg) IM at a ratio of 2:1 using a remote injecting system.

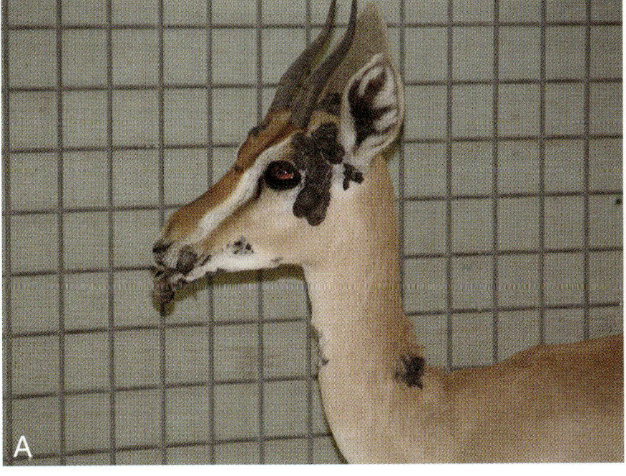

Fig. 1.57 (a) Lateral and (b) frontal view of the face and neck on the sub-adult female common Arabian gazelle showing multiple skin growths.

Continued

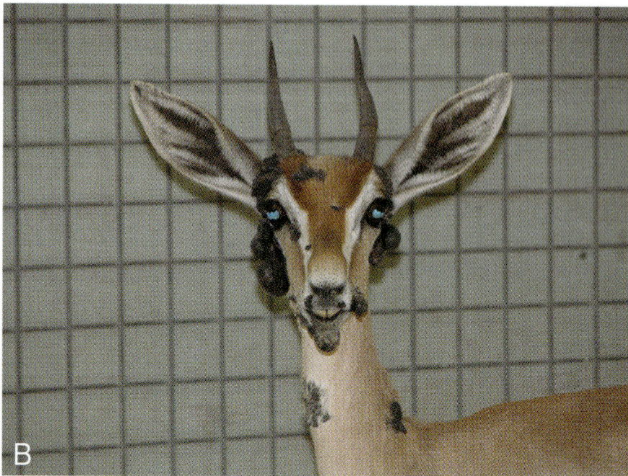

Fig. 1.57—cont'd

Physical examination

The juvenile male was anaesthetized for physical examination with a mixture of isoflurane and oxygen delivered via a face mask. On examination, the gazelle presented multiple firm, round, nodular, large to small fibrous growths, dark brown to black in colour and firmly attached to the skin (Fig. 1.58). Nothing else abnormal was detected.

Q *1. Can you suggest a presumptive diagnosis from studying the images of the gazelles?*

Q *2. What samples would you examine in order to confirm your diagnosis?*

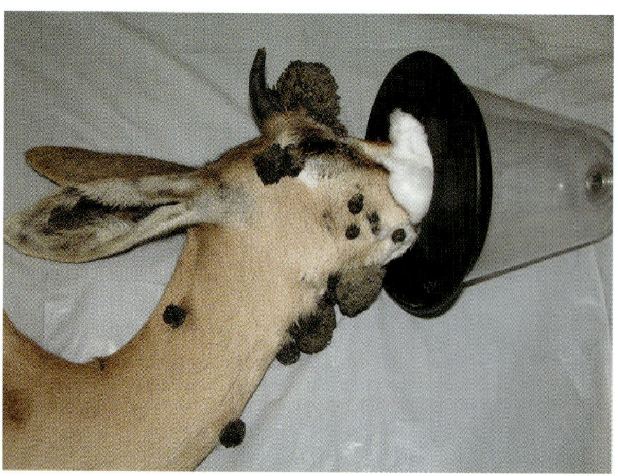

Fig. 1.58 Juvenile male common Arabian gazelle showing the multiple skin growths on the face and neck under isoflurane anaesthesia.

Clinical diagnosis laboratory examination

Biopsies of the growths were obtained, fixed in buffered formalin solution and then sent to the laboratory for histopathological examination.

 *3. Can you offer a list of differential diagnoses?*

Differential diagnoses

- ➤ Sarcoptic mange
- ➤ Squamous cell carcinoma
- ➤ Dermatophytosis
- ➤ Pox
- ➤ Papillomatosis

Histopathology findings

The histopathology report read as follows:

- Skin growth: thickened epidermis with prominent epithelial pegs extending into massive dermal proliferation of fibroblasts in whorls and herringbone pattern.

Final diagnosis

- ➤ Dermal papillomatosis or fibromatosis

Q *4. What would be your suggested therapeutic management of this case?*

Therapy

Since these were isolated cases in the collection affecting only two individuals, the veterinarian in charge opted for euthanasia in order to prevent spreading of the condition to other individuals in the same or other herds.

Q *5. Can the keeping staff become infected with papillomatosis from the gazelles?*

Q *6. What aetiological agent is responsible for papillomas in gazelles?*

Q *7. How is papillomatosis transmitted from animal to animal?*

Discussion

Skin papillomas or cutaneous fibromas have been reported in the domestic cow, horses, camels, cotton-tailed rabbits (*Sylvilagus floridanus*), moose (*Alces alces*), caribou (*Rangifer caribou*), chamois (*Rupicapra rupicapra*), serow (*Capricornis crispis*), impala (*Aepyceros melampus*), giraffe (*Giraffa camelopardis*), opossum (*Didelphis marsupialis*), coyote (*Canis latrans*) and several species of deer and primates.

The causative agent is bovine papillomavirus (BPV), a group of DNA viruses of the family *Papillomaviridae*. The virus causes papillomas and fibropapillomas of the skin, digestive and reproductive tracts. Six types of the virus have been characterized, subdivided into three large groups:

- *Deltapapillomavirus or fibropapillomaviruses*: BPV-1, BPV-2, cause benign fibropapillomas involving the epithelium and the underlying dermis, affect mainly the paragenital areas, urinary bladder, udder, teats, digestive system and skin
- *Xipapillomavirus or epitheliotropic*: BPV-3, BPV-4 and BPV-6, may cause pure papillomas, affect the skin, upper digestive system, the udder and teats
- *Epsilonpapillomavirus*: BPV-5, may cause pure papillomas and fibropapillomas, affects mainly the udder and teats.

BPV type 1 and 2 appear to be associated with the pathogenesis of equine sarcoid producing locally aggressive, skin fibroblastic benign tumours in horses, donkeys, mules and zebras.

In deer, skin papillomas tend to occur more often in individuals less than 2 years old with a higher incidence reported in bucks. It had been suggested that papillomas are transmitted from individual to individual by direct contact through open skin growths or fomites that have been in contact with infected individuals. Mosquitoes, biting flies and other insects have also been suspected to be involved with the transmission. The virus is species specific and is not known to occur or to affect humans.

Treatment is generally not recommended as the papillomas and fibropapillomas appear to regress spontaneously over a period of time. Surgical removal is sometimes indicated if occurring as a single growth affecting the nose, mouth, prepuce or vulva, but excision has been known to lead to recurrence. Adequate disinfection of animal quarters and fomites could help prevent transmission to other animals in the herd. Vaccination using virus-killed papilloma tissue suspension is useful for long-term protection against the same BPV type but it is ineffectual against existing papillomas.

Further reading

Chambers, G., Ellsmore, V.A., O'Brien, P.M., et al., 2003. Association of bovine papillomavirus with the equine sarcoid. J. Gen. Virol. 84, 1055–1062.

Karstad, L., Kaminjolo, J.S., 1978. Skin papillomas in an impala (*Aepyceros melampus*) and a giraffe (*Girafa camelopardalis*). J. Wildl. Dis. 14, 309–313.

Sundberg, J.P., Nielsen, S.W., 1981. Deer fibroma: a review. Can. Vet. J. 22, 385–388.

Case 1.24 *P. Zucca*

Clinical history

At the end of the summer, several free-ranging alpine chamois (*Rupicapra rupicapra*) living in the same alpine valley of a natural reserve (Fig. 1.59) have been exhibiting abnormal changes in behaviour with reduced mobility, circling movements, decreased feeding activity, poor general body condition and increased fearful reactions to environmental stimuli. The "flight" responses to a stimulus were characterized by incoordination, high stepping falls and self-injuries due to collisions with rocks, trees and other objects. A closer observation of sick chamois by means of a telescope revealed an increased ocular lacrimation and ocular lesions.

Inside the natural reserve there were no domestic animal farms or breeding centres, although a sheep herd of about 200 individuals was translocated on an alpine meadow one month before the disease outbreak. An adult chamois severely affected by this pathological condition was captured by hand without any chemical restraint and hospitalized at the local wildlife rescue centre.

1. Do you think domestic sheep could play a role in the epizoology of this pathological condition?

Physical examination

A complete physical examination revealed a poor general body condition score and a corneal and conjunctival inflammation with mucoserous effusions as shown in Fig. 1.60. The adult chamois was lethargic, hypothermic, dehydrated and it was not able to keep its normal quadrupedal position (Fig. 1.61).

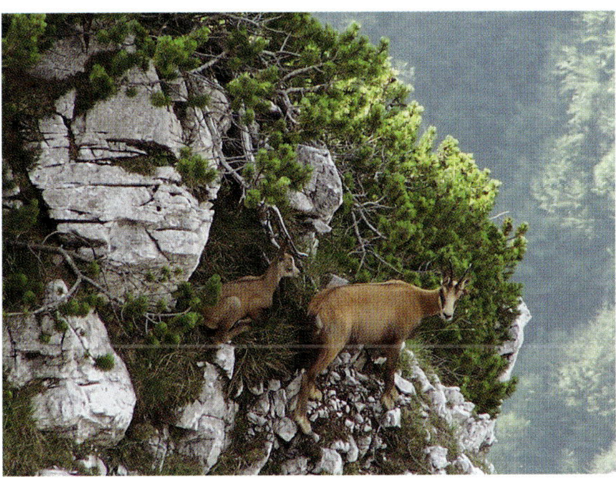

Fig. 1.59 Mortality caused by this disease is higher in females and juveniles (courtesy of V. Coradazzi).

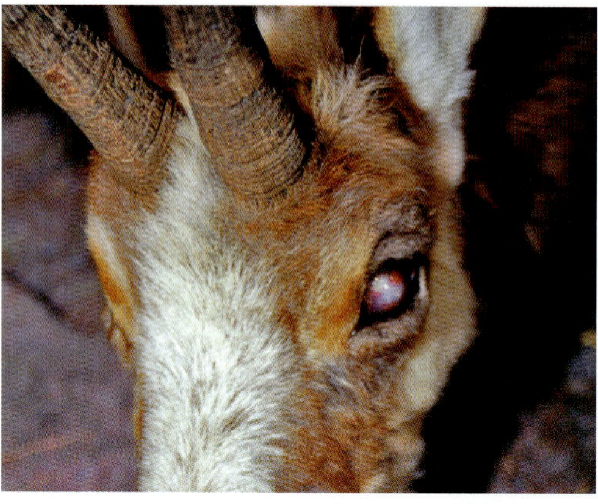

Fig. 1.60 Detail of the left eye, please note the wide corneal neovascularization.

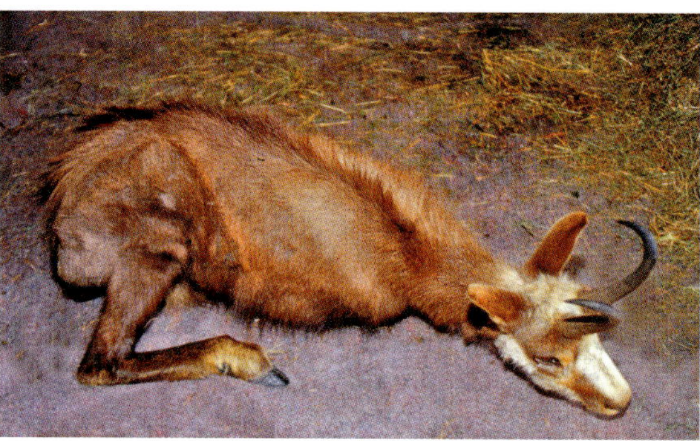

Fig. 1.61 The chamois was not able to stand up on its own and was starving.

Clinical diagnosis examination

The examination of the eyes and periocular structures revealed that the chamois was blind. The left eye showed a hyperaemic conjunctiva with seromucous effusions and corneal ulcerations were neovascularized all over the ulcerations, as shown in Fig. 1.62, while the right eye was severely affected and its cornea was perforated (Fig. 1.63). Several alopecic areas were identified along the trunk, abdomen and forelimb (see Fig. 1.61). However, the skin was not thickened or encrusted.

2. Do you think that the ocular lesion depicted in Fig. 1.63 is reversible?

Clinical diagnosis laboratory examination

Swabs were collected from both eyes and using a transport medium were processed for isolation of the organisms by culture. Swabs were positive for *Mycoplasma conjunctivae* and *Streptococcus* spp. Deep skin scrapings from several alopecic locations were examined in 10% potassium hydroxide (KOH).

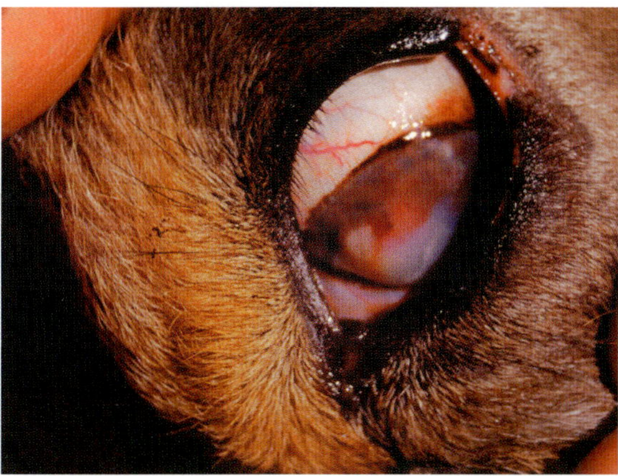

Fig. 1.62 The left eye showed a hyperaemic conjunctiva with seromucous effusions and the corneal ulcerations showed extensive neovascularization.

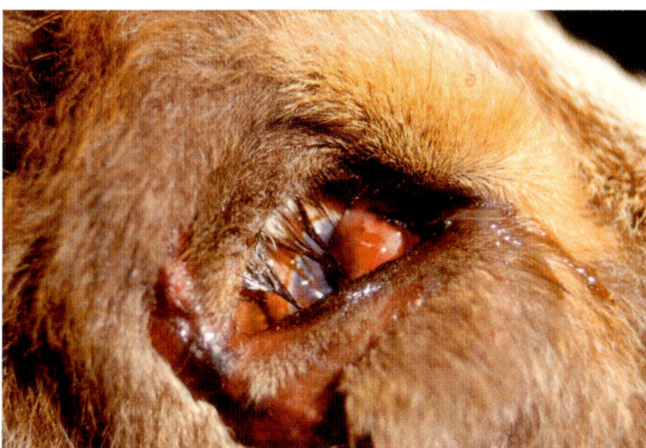

Fig. 1.63 Right eye, corneal perforation.

3. Do you think that direct culture is the best method for proving the presence of M. conjunctivae in the chamois eye?

Summary of diagnostic results

- Abnormal changes in behaviour of free-ranging chamois
- Self-injuries related to "flight" behavioural patterns
- Poor general conditions that could lead to starvation
- Alopecia along the trunk, abdomen and limbs
- Increased lacrimation and bilateral conjunctival and corneal lesions
- Corneal perforation on the right eye
- Isolation of *M. conjunctivae* and streptococci from the eyes
- Photophobia

 *4. List your differential diagnoses.*

Q *5. List your therapeutic strategy.*

Differential diagnoses

- Infectious or parasitic diseases that cause central nervous system clinical signs
- Bacterial infection of the eyes due to heterogeneous flora (mixed infection)
- Sarcoptic mange

Therapy

The hospitalized chamois was euthanized on humane grounds. It was an adult subject with a severe general illness and an irreversible lesion to the right eye. Free-ranging chamois affected by the same ocular disease have not been treated and a small number of individuals with similar condition have been shot by the local wildlife services on humane grounds.

Post-mortem examination

The main post-mortem findings were related to starvation and to the ocular infections. The left eye was affected by keratitis with oedema and neovascularization while the right cornea was necrotic and perforated. The eye chambers collapsed and secondary bacterial infections were found in the orbital area. The brain and the central nervous system were not affected. Deep skin scraping and histopathology from several alopecic locations were negative for sarcoptic mites.

 *6. What is your provisional post-mortem diagnosis?*

Summary of post-mortem examination findings

- Poor general body condition
- Bilateral keratitis and conjunctivitis
- Corneal perforation of the right eye
- Negative skin scraping for sarcoptic mites from alopecic locations

Provisional post-mortem diagnosis

- *Chlamydophila* spp.
- Infectious keratoconjunctivitis caused by *Mycoplasma conjunctivae*
- Mixed infection due to heterogeneous flora like *Staphylococcus aureus*, streptococci, *Haemophilus* spp., *Corynebacterium pyogenes* and other bacteria

Post-mortem laboratory findings

- Microbiology: cultural isolation from the eye and the periorbital area of *M. conjunctivae* and heterogeneous flora like *S. aureus*, streptococci, *Haemophilus* spp.
- Histology: eye: mononuclear inflammatory cell infiltrations of conjunctiva and neutrophil infiltration in the corneal ulceration of the right eye. The other organs and apparatus were not affected by any significant pathological alterations that could be related to the ocular disease. Alopecic locations along the body and forelimbs: histopathology confirmed the skin scraping diagnosis and it was negative for sarcoptic mange

Final diagnosis

- Infectious keratoconjuctivitis of chamois (IKC) due to *Mycoplasma conjunctivae* infection

Discussion

Mycoplasma conjunctivae is the pathogenic agent of infectious keratoconjunctivitis of chamois (IKC). This pathological condition is a non-generalized, specific and highly contagious ocular disease that can affect chamois, ibex (*Capra ibex*) and several domestic ruminants like goats and sheep. These two domestic species play a major role as reservoirs for the infection of wild *Caprinae* because it has been proved that *M. conjunctivae* is not self-maintained in free-ranging chamois populations. Transmission occurs through direct contact or by means of eye-frequenting insects. Lacrimation attracts flies that, moving from one pasture to another, transmit the infection from domestic herds to wild *Caprinae*. Outbreaks of infectious keratoconjunctivitis in chamois can cause up to 30% mortality, although average mortality is usually lower than 5% of the population. In fact, most sick chamois usually completely recover after a while. Abnormal behavioural patterns shown by affected animals are related to a visual deficit and this pathological condition can be initially confused with diseases that affect the central nervous system (CNS). However, changes in behaviours are not a consequence of a CNS lesion but they are related to blindness and the stress that this pathological condition causes to wild animals. Therefore, only starving subjects with non-reversible eye lesions like corneal perforations should be euthanized on humane grounds. Great efforts should be taken to reduce direct contact with infected domestic herds and disturbance to sick chamois in affected areas. Domestic sheep and goats that move to summer meadows should be evaluated for ocular diseases and topical or systemic treatments should be administered to symptomatic subjects. Pharmacological treatment of free-ranging chamois is not suggested at all.

Further reading

Giacometti, M., Janovsky, M., Belloy, L., et al., 2002. Infectious keratoconjunctivitis of ibex, chamois and other Caprinae. Rev. Sci. Tech. 21 (2), 335–345.

Giacometti, M., Janovsky, M., Jenny, H., et al., 2002. Mycoplasma conjunctivae infection is not maintained in alpine chamois in eastern Switzerland. J. Wildl. Dis. 38 (2), 297–304.
Mayer, D., Degiorgis, M.P., Meier, W., et al., 1997. Lesions associated with infectious keratoconjunctivitis in alpine ibex. J. Wildl. Dis. 33 (3), 413–419.

Case 1.25 *P. Zucca*

Clinical history

A Risso's dolphin (*Grampus griseus*) was swimming actively close to the shore "patrolling" a limited area. It was sighted in the early morning but started to show signs of tiredness during the late morning and it stranded toward a sandy shallow during the evening. The main abnormal behavioural patterns observed before stranding were:

- "Circular" swimming pattern close to the shore
- Incoordination and rolling during active swimming
- Increasing frequency of "rest at surface" behaviour with short periods of active mobility.

Physical examination

The dolphin was an adult mature 310 kg male, 3 metres long. Like every adult Risso's dolphin it had several linear scars covering almost all its body as observed in Fig. 1.64. These lines are the consequence of superficial wounds caused by conspecific teeth and they should not be confused with a clinical sign of illness. The general body condition of the dolphin was very poor but no other clinical signs were detected.

1. Is it easy to judge the health condition of a stranded cetacean only by its outward appearance?

Clinical diagnosis examination

A preliminary inspection of the mouth did not reveal any hook in the first tract of the oral cavity; breath frequency and heart rate were quite stable.

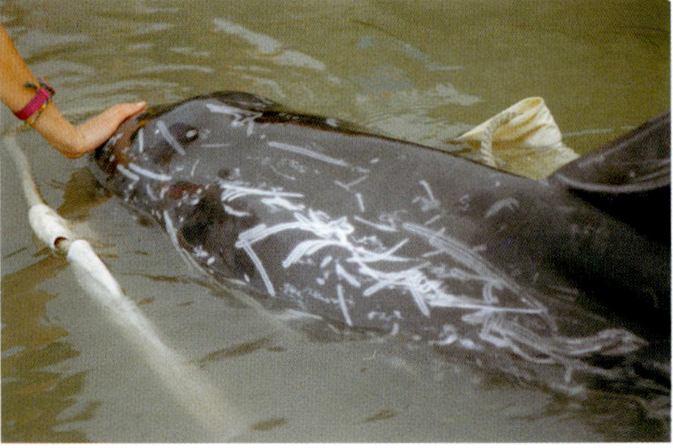

Fig. 1.64 The stranded Risso's dolphin was alert and responsive to environmental stimuli (noise and touch).

Clinical diagnosis laboratory examination

Blood samples were collected for haematological and blood chemistry analyses (Fig. 1.65). Although there are no available haematological and biochemical reference intervals for Risso's dolphins, hepatic enzyme values were several times higher than the 95th percentile of serum biochemical reference intervals for free-ranging common bottlenose dolphins (*Tursiops truncatus*) suggesting an ongoing hepatic damage.

Summary of diagnostic results

- Abnormal pre-stranding behavioural patterns
- Poor general body condition
- Alert and responsive to environmental stimulation
- Stable breathing frequency and heart rate
- Ongoing hepatic damage

Q *2. List your differential diagnoses.*

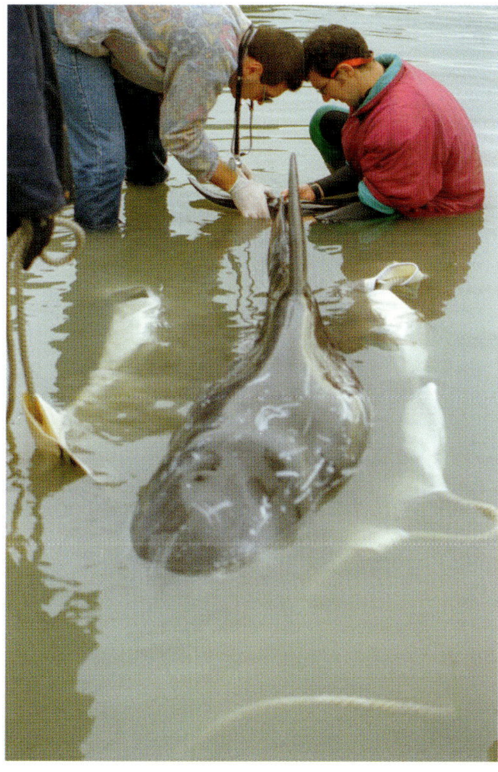

Fig. 1.65 Blood samples were collected for haematological and blood chemistry analyses.

Differential diagnoses

- Ingestion of plastic debris and gastrointestinal obstruction
- Xenobiotic contamination
- Toxoplasmosis
- Morbillivirus

Therapy

The first aid on the beach was focused on preventing further injuries and on reducing the dolphin's stress by means of:

- Providing shade
- Keeping moist
- Digging holes for flippers (allowing them to stay in a natural position).

During the short hospitalization time in a local temporary facility the dolphin was monitored continuously. It suddenly died without showing any specific clinical sign and without eating anything.

Post-mortem examination

Post-mortem examination of the body and the internal organs did not show any pathognomonic lesion related to a specific disease or condition that could explain the stranding and the death. The body condition was very poor and the stomach and intestine were empty, suggesting that it had not eaten for some time. The animal had a multiple spleen and the liver showed signs of degeneration with several necrotic foci. Samples for microbiology, histopathology and toxicology were collected from all the organs as suggested by marine mammal necropsy standard protocol. Due to the fact that Risso's dolphins are frequently affected by endoparasites of the nasal and pterygoid sinuses, a computed axial tomography (CAT) scan of the head was performed in order to evaluate the presence of such parasites inside the head of the dolphin before carrying out a gross necropsy.

The main macroscopical lesions suggested by the CT scan (Figs 1.66 and 1.67) and confirmed by the necropsy were related to a heavy nematode infection of the nasal and pterygoid sinuses, as well as infection close to the periauricular air spaces and the tympanic *bullae*.

3. What is your provisional post-mortem diagnosis?

Summary of post-mortem examination findings

- Nasal and pterygoid sinuses, periauricular air space, tympanic *bullae*: high burden of thin elongated nematodes and several concretions of parasitic origin
- Liver: several necrotic degeneration areas
- Empty stomach and intestine

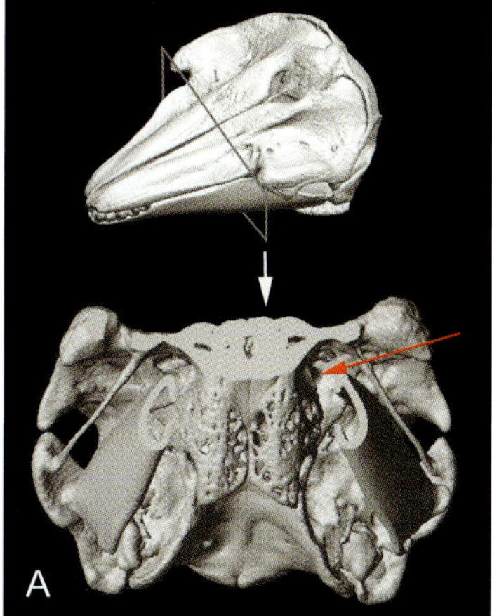

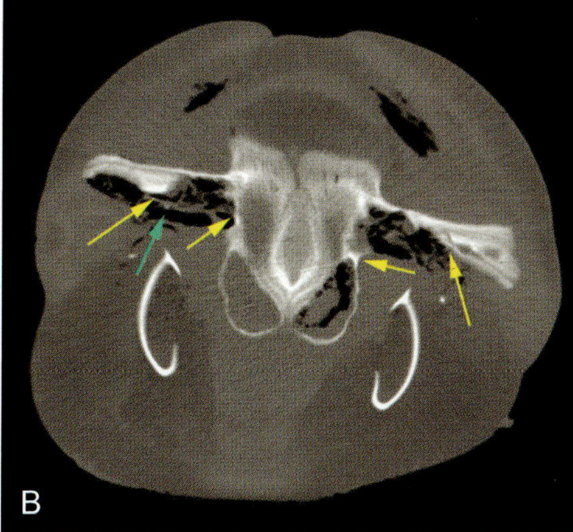

Fig. 1.66 (b) CT scan transverse section at about red arrow level of Fig. 1.66a, yellow arrows show a bony reaction due to the inflammatory action of parasites while the cyan arrow shows a small concretion of parasitic origin.

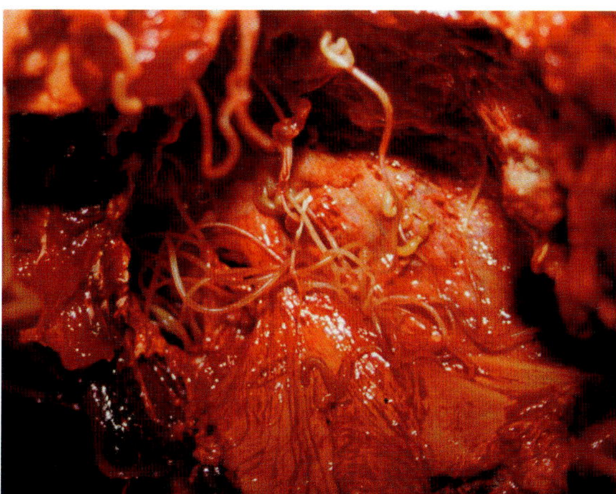

Fig. 1.67 Left lateral view (red arrow of Fig. 1.66a) of the parasitic infection of the sinuses. The large number of worms and the inflammation of the mucosa are clearly visible.

Provisional post-mortem diagnosis

- *Crassicauda grampicola* infection
- Xenobiotic contamination

Post-mortem laboratory findings

- Microbiology: nothing significant was isolated
- Histology: liver shows chronic circulatory disturbances, with evidence of degenerative and necrotic changes affecting several hepatocytes; severe

inflammatory lesions with multiple and extensive necrotic foci associated with haemorrhage at submucosal location of the nasal and pterygoid sinuses and the timpanic *bullae* surrounding area

- Toxicology: high levels of mercury in the liver (498 mg/kg ww)

Final diagnosis

- *Crassicauda grampicola* infection

Discussion

Whenever a live dolphin strands on the shore it is important to evaluate as soon as possible what are the survival chances of the subject for medical, logistic and ethical reasons. In fact, there are three different intervention options: release, hospitalize or euthanize the dolphin according to the severity of the pathological condition. Unfortunately, it is quite difficult to judge the health condition of a stranded cetacean only by a preliminary physical and clinical examination on the shore and usually other parameters like species, season, individual or group stranding are taken into account for a general assessment of the stranding severity. The general condition of this dolphin was very poor and a social deep-water cetacean like the Risso's usually strand individually when it is affected by a severe illness condition. However, its responsiveness to environmental stimuli was very good and therefore it was decided temporarily to hospitalize it for a better assessment of the health condition. It died after a couple of days due to a fatal infection by *Crassicauda grampicola*. Several authors consider this nematode a primary parasitic pathogen and an important regulatory factor of marine mammal and especially of Risso's dolphin populations. However, the immune-suppressive action of mercury levels may have contributed to the occurrence of the liver damage and may have compromised the immune response, making the Risso's dolphin more vulnerable to parasitic infection.

Further reading

Geraci, J.R., Lounsbury, V.J., 1993. Marine Mammals Ashore: A Field Guide for Strandings. Texas A&M Sea Grant Publication, Galveston.

Raga, J.A., Balbuena, J.A., Aznar, J., et al., 1997. The impact of parasites on marine mammals: a review. Parassitologia 39, 293–296.

Zucca, P., Di Guardo, G., Pozzi-Mucelli, R., et al., 2004. Use of computer tomography for imaging of *Crassicauda grampicola* in a Risso's dolphin (*Grampus griseus*). J. Zoo Wildl. Med. 35, 391–394.

Zucca, P., Di Guardo, G., Francese, M., et al., 2005. Causes of stranding in four Risso's dolphins (*Grampus griseus*) found beached along the North Adriatic Sea Coast. Vet. Res. Commun. 29 (Suppl. 2), 261–264.

CHAPTER

Birds 2

Case 2.1 *R. J. Doneley*

Clinical history

A 2-year-old female ostrich (*Struthio camelus*) was examined to assess a weight loss of several months' duration.

The bird was housed in a large outdoor grassed pen with another hen and a cock. The farm was in a high-rainfall coastal area on sandy soil, and held over 300 birds in numerous pens. The birds were fed a daily diet of a commercial ostrich maintenance pellet and grain. Water was supplied via polypropylene pipes. There were several dams on the property, attracting large numbers of ibis and egrets to the farm.

The bird had been purchased 18 months previously but had not yet bred. Its appetite was poor.

Clinical examination

On presentation, the bird was weak and in very poor body condition, with a prominent spine and pelvic bones. There was no evidence of dyspnoea or increased respiratory effort. Skin tone was reduced and urine production was scant. The bird's faeces were small and pelletized. Abdominal palpation and auscultation of the cardiorespiratory system were normal. Cloacal examination revealed multiple nodules on the cloacal mucosa.

Blood was collected for haematology and biochemistry analysis, and a cloacal mucosal nodule was biopsied. Faeces were collected for parasitological examination.

Clinical diagnosis laboratory

The results of the clinical diagnosis laboratory assays are shown in Tables 2.1 and 2.2.

RBC, WBC and thrombocyte morphology

➤ Cellular morphology was normal

1. What is your interpretation of the haematology and blood chemistry values shown in Tables 2.1 and 2.2?

Table 2.1 Haematology values of the ostrich

Parameters	Results	Reference values
RBC ($\times 10^3/\mu l$)	1.9	1.7–2.17
Hb (g/dl)	16.1	14–17.2
Hct (l/l)	45	41–57
MCV (fl)	211	205–218
MCH (pg)	79.8	76.4–88.4
MCHC (g/dl)	37.3	34.7–41.2
WBC ($\times 10^9/l$)	60	10–24
Heterophils (%)	33	58–89
Lymphocytes (%)	40	12–41
Monocytes (%)	27	0–1
Eosinophils (%)	0	0–4
Basophils (%)	0	0–1

Table 2.2 Blood chemistry values of the ostrich

Analysis	Results	Reference values
AST (U/l)	781	226–547
Bile acids (μmol/l)	102	2–30
CK (U/l)	12 412	800–6508
Uric acid (μmol/l)	950	59.5–892.2
Urea nitrogen (mmol/l)	4	0–1
Total protein (g/l)	22	24–53
Calcium (mmol/l)	2.2	2.0–3.39
Glucose (mmol/l)	7.8	9.1–18.3

Results

- Faecal examination was negative for the presence of endoparasites
- Haematology analysis showed an elevated WBC with marked monocytosis
- Blood chemistry analysis showed elevated levels of aspartate aminotransferase (AST), creatine kinase (CK), bile acids, uric acid, and urea nitrogen
- The cloacal biopsy revealed a granulomatous lesion associated with numerous acid-fast bacilli

Please evaluate the clinical history, the results of the physical examination and clinical diagnosis laboratory tests.

2. List your differential diagnoses.

Differential diagnoses

- Aspergillosis
- Proventricular impaction
- Mycobacteriosis
- Chronic disease of unknown origin

Outcome

A presumptive diagnosis of avian mycobacteriosis was made. In light of the bird's physical condition and clinical pathology findings, the owner opted for euthanasia.

Post-mortem findings

The cloacal nodule biopsy revealed a granulomatous reaction associated with numerous acid-fast bacilli. A thorough post-mortem examination was performed. Samples from different organs were collected for histopathology, culture and polymerase chain reaction (PCR).

On necropsy, the bird was emaciated with bright yellow subcutaneous and internal body fat. The liver was enlarged with multifocal, densely packed, small white nodules (>5 mm in diameter) on the surface and throughout the parenchyma (Fig. 2.1a, b). Similar nodules of various sizes (2–35 mm) were scattered over the serosa and mucosa of the intestinal tract, protruding into the lumen. Both caecae were covered with a yellow fissured membrane and the lumen contained a clear gelatinous material in which some flocculent material was suspended.

The heart, lungs, air sacs, kidneys and spleen appeared normal.

Summary of post-mortem examination findings

- Liver: enlarged with multifocal, densely packed, small white nodules (>5 mm in diameter) on the surface and throughout the parenchyma
- Intestines: similar nodules of various sizes scattered over the serosa and mucosa
- Caecae: covered with a yellow fissured membrane and the lumen contained a clear gelatinous material in which some flocculent material was suspended
- Other internal organs: normal

Q *3. What is your provisional post-mortem diagnosis?*

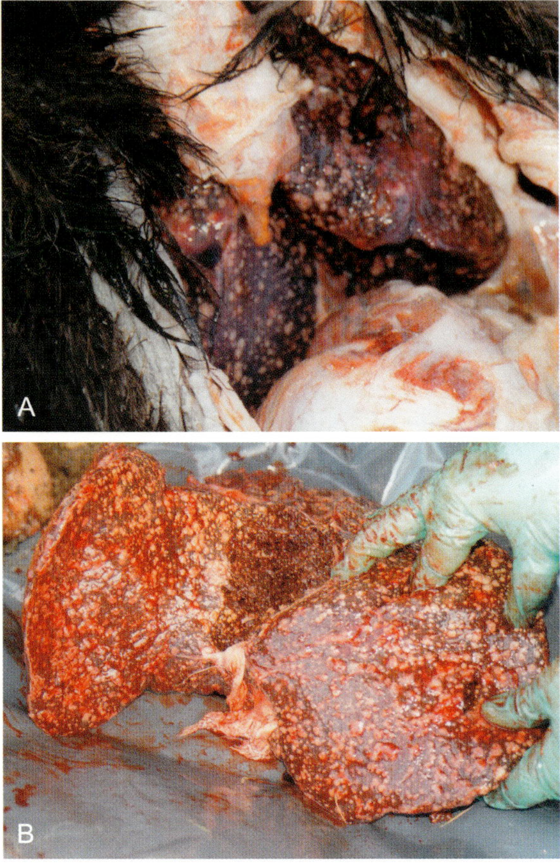

Fig. 2.1 (a) Post-mortem examination of the ostrich showing necrotic foci in the liver (courtesy of Kaye and Marcus Holdsworth); (b) section of the liver showing small and large necrotic foci on the surface and throughout the parenchyma of the liver (courtesy of Kaye and Marcus Holdsworth).

Provisional post-mortem diagnosis

- Avian mycobacteriosis

Laboratory findings

- Microbiology: mycobacterial cultures of eight tissue samples (liver, cloaca, caecum and intestine) failed to grow mycobacteria
- Histology: multiple granulomas were present in the liver, spleen and intestine. Most of the granulomas had a central area of coagulative necrosis surrounded

by giant cells, epithelioid macrophages, plasma cells and occasional heterophils. Ziel-Neelsen stains of these lesions revealed masses of slender acid-fast bacilli in the necrotic centres of the granulomas and in the surrounding giant cells and macrophages. No lesions were observed in other tissues
- PCR: a multiplex PCR was performed; the results were consistent with *Mycobacterium avium*

Final diagnosis

- Mycobacterial hepatitis, enteritis and splenitis due to *M. avium*

4. What advice would you give the owner of this bird regarding the infectious and zoonotic potential of this disease?

Discussion

Avian mycobacteriosis is an uncommonly reported disease of ratites, although reports in other avian species are widespread.

M. avium is an opportunistic pathogen in birds and mammals, including humans. It can cause disease in most, if not all, avian species and is characterized by its chronic nature, its persistence in a flock once established, and its tendency to cause wasting and finally death. It can be found in soil, feed and water, particularly where faecal contamination by infected birds can occur, and it can persist in soil for several years. On an ostrich farm, contamination of soil and water could be expected to be due to infected ostriches or wild birds, or by mechanical transmission on clothing, vehicles and equipment.

Infection is believed to be due to ingestion and, as ostriches are noted for their soil-eating behaviour, it is likely that this was the source of infection in this case. The disease is primarily gastrointestinal in presentation; lymphatic drainage of the gastrointestinal tract then spreads the infection to other organs in the body, especially the liver.

Although *M. avium* can be associated with disease in humans – an Australian study showed that, between mid-1985 and late 1988, 17.3% of people with AIDS had concomitant *M. avium* infections – birds are not thought to be the direct source of infection. Rather, it is the contamination of food and water that is thought to lead to human infection. Nevertheless, the zoonotic potential of this disease is present and owners of infected birds should be advised of this.

In the poultry industry, avian mycobacteriosis is not considered to be a major production threat because of the early slaughter age for chickens. In ostriches, however, where the slaughter age is much older (8–12 months), it is possible that mycobacterial infection in a flock could pose a threat to production.

Ante-mortem diagnosis of avian mycobacteriosis is difficult. Intradermal tuberculin sensitivity testing is not considered reliable in an individual bird and, in fact, a strong response could indicate a highly resistant bird rather than an infected bird. The potential use of intradermal testing may be to determine if a flock, rather than an individual, is infected with mycobacteria. Its use in ostriches has yet to be fully evaluated.

Further reading

Dawson, D.J., 1990. Infection with *Mycobacterium avium* complex in Australian patients with AIDS. Med. J. Aust. 15 (153), 466–468.

Doneley, R.J.T., Gibson, J.A., Thorne, D., et al., 1999. Mycobacterial infection in an ostrich. Aust. Vet. J. 77 (6), 368–370.

Phalen, D., 1998. Avian mycobacteriosis. In: Proceedings of the Association of Avian Veterinarians Conference Australian Committee. pp. 71–73.

Reece, R.L., Beddome, V.D., Barr, D.A., et al., 1992. Common necropsy findings in captive birds in Victoria, Australia, 1978–1987. J. Zoo Wildl. Med. 23, 301–312.

Sanford, S.E., Rehymulla, A.J., Josephson, G.K.A., 1994. Tuberculosis in farmed rhea (*Rhea americana*). Avian Dis. 193–196.

Shane, S.M., Camus, A., Strain, M.G., et al., 1993. Tuberculosis in commercial emus (*Dromaius novaehollandiae*). Avian Dis. 1172–1176.

Thorel, M.F., Huchzermeyer, H., Weiss, R., et al., 1997. *Mycobacterium avium* infections in animals. Literature review. Vet. Res. 28, 439–447.

Case 2.2 *T. A. Bailey*

Clinical history

An adult female African fish eagle (*Haliaeetus vocifer*) weighing 1800 g, was presented with the following clinical signs of three days' duration:

- Steadily decreasing appetite and vomiting
- Lethargy
- Progressive weight loss
- Green-coloured urates
- Dyspnoea.

The bird had recently been imported from Africa into Dubai as a display bird for a falconry show, but was not being trained.

Clinical examination

On presentation, the bird was thin with marked loss of pectoral muscle condition and pale mucous membranes. Parasitology crop swabs for wet preparation and faecal samples for direct smear and flotation were performed. Survey radiographs were taken while the bird was under anaesthesia (Fig. 2.2a, b). Blood samples were collected for haematology analysis. Endoscopy examination of the caudal thoracic air sacs and upper digestive tract and trachea was also performed.

Radiology

1. What is your interpretation of the radiographs in Fig. 2.2a, b?

➤ Radiographic findings included a generalized increased radio-opacity of the lung fields and air spaces causing loss of detail over the heart and liver on VD view. Focal radiodensities are apparent in the lung fields and are particularly evident

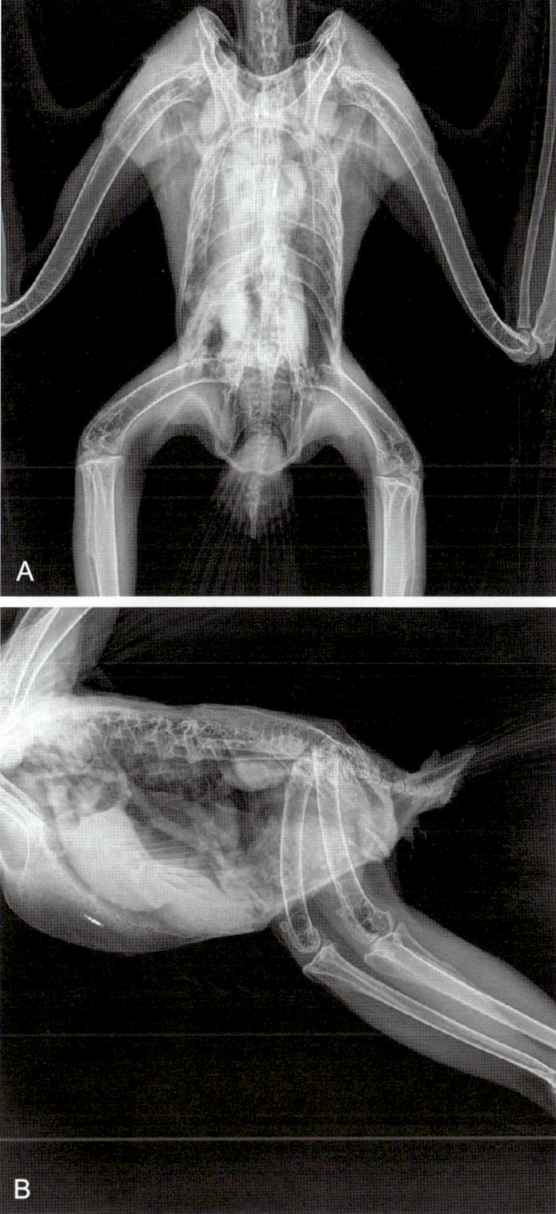

Fig. 2.2 (a) Ventrodorsal survey radiograph of the African fish eagle; (b) lateral survey radiograph of the African fish eagle.

in the right air space adjacent to the liver on the VD view. The proventriculus wall appears thickened and air is evident in the lumen of the proventriculus. The gizzard is small and empty and the spleen is enlarged. The lateral view also reveals increased radio-opacity of the kidneys which are also enlarged.

Endoscopy

- Endoscopy examination of the upper gastrointestinal tract and trachea revealed no abnormal findings. Endoscopy of the caudal thoracic air sacs was conducted (Fig. 2.3). A swab was collected from the caudal thoracic air sacs and submitted for microbiological and cytology investigations (Fig. 2.4).

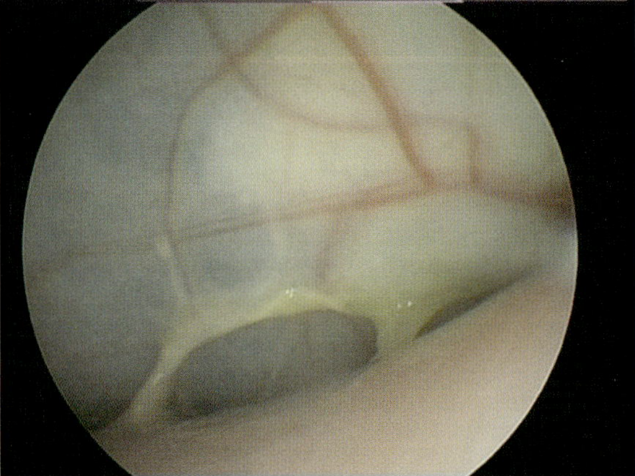

Fig. 2.3 Endoscopic view inside the caudal thoracic air sac of the African fish eagle.

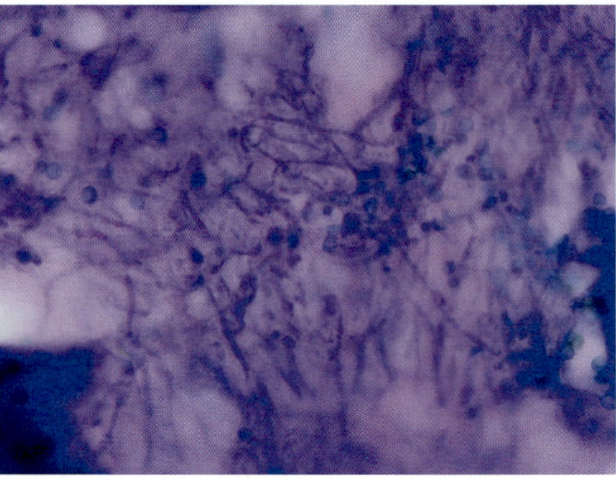

Fig. 2.4 Photomicrograph of cytology preparation from a swab of the caudal thoracic air sacs of the African fish eagle. Note the smear was negative for acid-fast bodies.

Cytology

An endoscopic image and photomicrograph of the cytology preparation collected during endoscopy are shown in Figs 2.3 and 2.4.

2. What is your interpretation of the endoscopic findings shown in Fig. 2.3? What is your interpretation of the cytology preparation from the air sac?

- The air sac is opaque and vascularized. Thick yellow fluid is present in the margin of the air sac along with the edge of a yellow plaque
- The impression smear from the swab collected from the air sac reveals numerous fungal hyphae and spores

These observations along with the radiography findings would be consistent with a diagnosis of a mycotic airsacculitis.

3. List your differential diagnoses based on the clinical, radiography and endoscopy findings.

Causes of lower respiratory tract disease to be considered include pneumonia/airsacculitis caused by bacterial, viral, fungal, mycobacterial or parasitic infestation (*Serratospiculum* spp.).

Clinical diagnosis laboratory

The results of the clinical diagnosis laboratory assays are shown in Table 2.3 and the blood film in Fig. 2.5.

Table 2.3 Haematology values of the African fish eagle

Parameters	Results	Reference values*
RBC (×10^{12}/l)	2.1	2.3±0.2
Hb (g/dl)	3.6	12.2±1.1
Hct (l/l)	10	42±4
MCV (fl)	47.62	182.5±19.3
MCH (pg)	17.1	50±1
MCHC (g/l)	36	29.7±0.8
WBC (×10^9/l)	3.4	14.5±6.8
Heterophils (×10^9/l)	2.2	10.5±6
Lymphocytes (×10^9/l)	1.1	2.3±1.4
Monocytes (×10^9/l)	0.1	0.6±0.6
Eosinophils (×10^9/l)	0	0.8±0.6
Basophils (×10^9/l)	0	0.2±0.1

**ISIS values are for African fish eagles (n 2–11).*

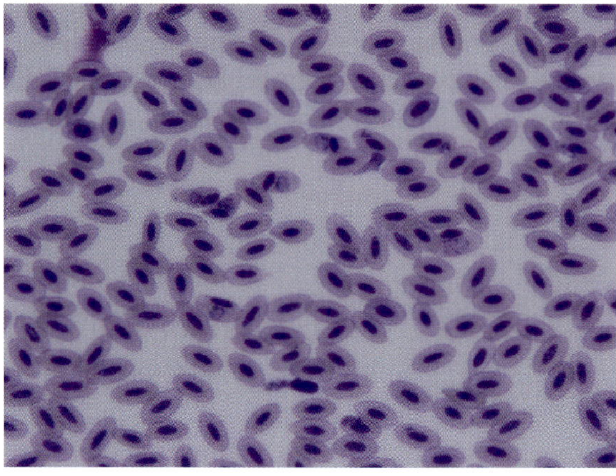

Fig. 2.5 Photomicrograph of blood film from the African fish eagle.

Q *4. What is your interpretation of the haematology values shown in Table 2.3? What is your interpretation of the blood film in Fig. 2.5?*

- Haematology analyses showed low RBC, Hb, Hct and WBC
- The blood film shows gametocyte, trophozoite and shizont stages of malaria
- The gold standard for diagnosis of *Plasmodium* is a Giemsa-stained thin blood smear

Other laboratory results

- Faecal examination was negative for the presence of endoparasites
- Examination of saline crop swabs was negative for the presence of parasites
- *Aspergillus fumigatus* was cultured from the swab of the air sac

Please evaluate the clinical history, Figs 2.2–2.5, the results of the radiography and endoscopic examinations and clinical diagnosis laboratory tests.

Q *5. List your final diagnosis.*

Clearly, there are two pathological processes contributing to the morbidity of this bird.

- Aspergillosis
- Avian malaria

Q *6. List your therapeutic strategy.*

Therapy

Treatment for malaria comprises giving chloroquine at a dose of 25 mg/kg PO and 1.3 mg/kg primaquine PO initially. Twelve hours after the initial combination, 15 mg/kg chloroquine is given and 24 hours after the initial combination dose 15 mg/kg PO of chloroquine is repeated; 48 hours after the initial combination dose the final 15 mg/kg chloroquine is given.

The profound anaemia of this bird should also be addressed. Homologous blood transfusions have been shown to be beneficial for birds with severe anaemia (PCV <20%) and are feasible where there is a donor bird of the same species available. The haemoglobin-based oxygen carrier, Oxyglobin (Biopure, USA) is becoming more widely used in avian medicine. This product is indicated during resuscitation when increased oxygen delivery to the tissues is desired. Intravenous colloids with replacement fluids (isotonic crystalloids) are indicated if neither Oxyglobin nor a homologous blood transfusion are possible.

If the disease is diagnosed in the early stages, aspergillosis can be successfully treated with oral itraconazole or voriconazole and nebulization with amphotericin B or F10 (Table 2.4). One caution in such a profoundly anaemic bird would be to deal with the malaria first because sometimes the azole antifungal agents can cause anorexia, particularly in debilitated birds.

Supportive therapy including fluids (IV, SC, IO), tube feeding, antibiotics, antiemetic drugs, immune stimulants and vitamin A supplementation should be given according to the needs of the case. Vitamin B complex and iron injection are both recommended initially for anaemic birds.

Discussion

One criticism of the workup in this case was the diagnostic workup that involved a lengthy anaesthesia to enable radiography and endoscopy examinations. However, in this case, the radiographic findings resulted in the endoscopy investigation to establish the cause of the radiographic lesions. The blood findings were only apparent some hours later when the results were released from the laboratory.

In general, the pathogenicity of blood parasites in most birds of prey is relatively low, but *Plasmodium* spp. has been linked with deaths in gyr falcons and snowy owls.

Plasmodium spp. use mosquitoes as vectors. *Plasmodium* spp. has been reported in free-living African fish eagles in Africa. In a dual aspergillosis–malaria infection such as this case, it is possible that the bird developed aspergillosis as a result of the stress of being shipped between countries and may have precipitated the recrudescence of the *Plasmodium* infection.

One important consideration hampers the diagnostic procedure for malaria. Stress resulting from manual restraint to collect blood samples has caused death in gyr falcons with malaria. Isoflurane anaesthesia of the patient to minimize stress before diagnostic sampling and treatment is recommended.

In countries where there is a high prevalence of malaria, prevention is important. Prevention is based on two approaches. First, vector exclusion through mosquito control and prophylactic treatment. Prophylactic treatment consists of a once weekly

Table 2.4 Dosage protocols of some antifungal agents in birds

Drug	Route	Dose
Itraconazole	PO	Treatment or prevention – 20 mg/kg q24h or 10–15 mg/kg q12h for 30–60 days
Voriconazole	PO	12.5 mg/kg q12h for 30–60 days

single treatment with chloroquine–primaquine combination commencing 1 month before and finishing 1 month after the mosquito season.

Prophylactic itraconazole is recommended for captive-held birds undergoing a change in management to reduce the chances of mycotic pneumonia occurring, especially high risk species and during times of stress such as transportation between countries.

Further reading

Atkinson, C., 2008. Avian malaria. In: Atkinson, C.T., Thomas, N.J., Hunter, D.B. (Eds.), Parasitic Diseases of Wild Birds. Wiley-Blackwell Publishing, Ames, pp. 35–53.

Dorrestein, G.M., 1997. Metabolism, pharmacology and therapy. In: Altman, R.B., Clubb, S.L., Dorrestein, G.M., et al. (Eds.), Avian Medicine and Surgery. WB Saunders Company, Philadelphia, pp. 661–670.

Greiner, E.C., 1994. Parasites. In: Ritchie, B., Harrison, G., Harrison, L. (Eds.), Avian Medicine: Principles and Application. Wingers Publishing, Lake Worth, pp. 1008–1029.

Hollamby, S., Afema-Azikuru, J., Sikarskie, J.G., et al., 2004. Clinical pathology and morphometrics of African fish eagles in Uganda. J. Wildl. Dis. 40 (3), 523–532.

Krone, O., Cooper, J., 2002. Parasitic diseases. In: Cooper, J. (Ed.), Birds of Prey Health and Disease. Blackwell Science, Oxford, pp. 105–120.

Lichtenberger, M., 2005. Shock, fluid therapy and CPCR for the avian patient. In: Proceedings of the 8th European Conference of the Association of Avian Veterinarians. Arles, France, pp. 374–387.

Remple, D., 2004. Intracellular hematozoa of raptors: a review and update. J. Avian Med. Surg. 18 (2), 75–88.

Williams, R.B., 2005. Avian malaria: clinical and chemical pathology of *Plasmodium gallinaceum* in the domesticated fowl *Gallus gallus*. Avian Pathol. 34 (1), 29–47.

Case 2.3 *J. Chitty*

Clinical history

A 15-year-old female Harris' hawk (*Parabuteo unicinctus*) weighing 910 g was presented as a referral with thickening and ulceration of the skin on the neck. The bird was reportedly irritated by the lesion. The referring veterinarian had not performed any diagnostics. However, the bird had not responded to two courses of antibiosis (enrofloxacin) or to topical fusidic acid, but had responded to a fusidic acid/corticosteroid topical gel preparation. During this time the lesion had regressed partially. However, when the gel was discontinued, the lesion returned. At the time of examination the bird had been on no therapy for 2 weeks.

Physical examination

The bird was in good body condition. No abnormality was detected other than a large ulcerated, thickened skin lesion of the ventral neck (Figs 2.6 and 2.7).

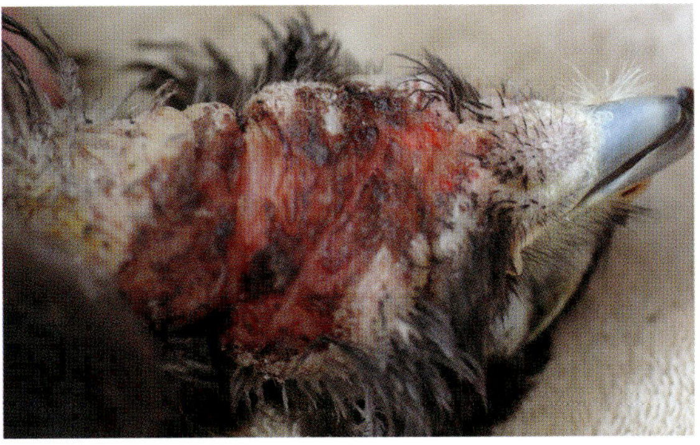

Fig. 2.6 Ventral view of the neck of the Harris' hawk clearly showing the lesion.

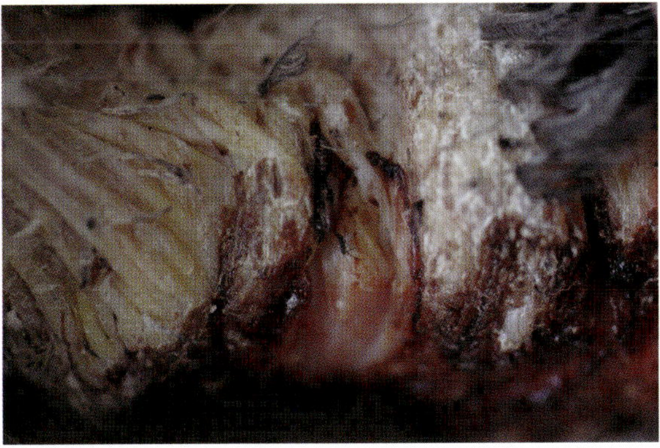

Fig. 2.7 Close-up view of the lesion on the ventral neck.

 *1. What are your differential diagnoses?*

- Infection – bacterial/yeast
- Ectoparasites – especially epidermoptid mites
- Chronic irritation/allergy
- Tumour – especially squamous cell carcinoma
- Idiopathic mutilation
- Oral/pharyngeal lesion causing irritation resulting in self-trauma

The bird was anaesthetized using isoflurane.

Q *2. What clinical investigations would you perform?*

Clinical diagnosis examination

Endoscopy examination was carried out of the upper gastrointestinal tract.

Clinical diagnosis laboratory examination

Blood samples were collected for haematology, blood chemistry and protein electrophoresis (Fig. 2.8) analyses (Tables 2.5–2.7). In addition, cytology smears, skin biopsies and bacteriology swabs were collected from the lesion.

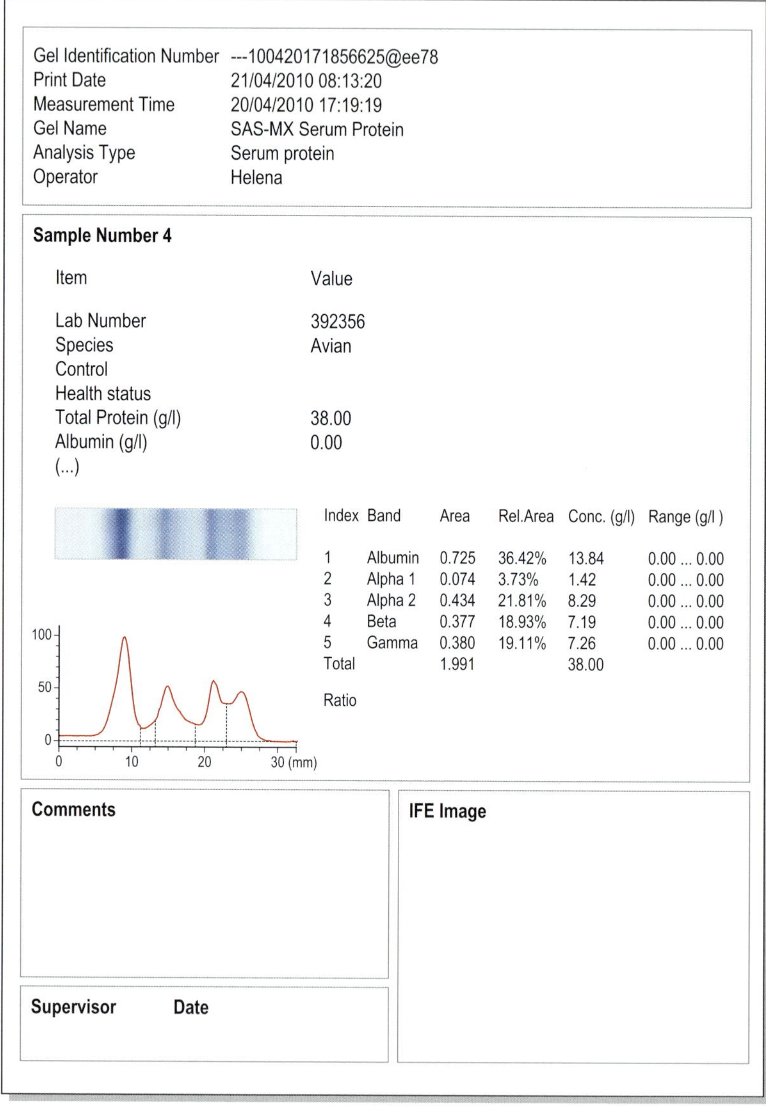

Gel Identification Number	---100420171856625@ee78
Print Date	21/04/2010 08:13:20
Measurement Time	20/04/2010 17:19:19
Gel Name	SAS-MX Serum Protein
Analysis Type	Serum protein
Operator	Helena

Sample Number 4

Item	Value
Lab Number	392356
Species	Avian
Control	
Health status	
Total Protein (g/l)	38.00
Albumin (g/l)	0.00
(...)	

Index	Band	Area	Rel.Area	Conc. (g/l)	Range (g/l)
1	Albumin	0.725	36.42%	13.84	0.00 ... 0.00
2	Alpha 1	0.074	3.73%	1.42	0.00 ... 0.00
3	Alpha 2	0.434	21.81%	8.29	0.00 ... 0.00
4	Beta	0.377	18.93%	7.19	0.00 ... 0.00
5	Gamma	0.380	19.11%	7.26	0.00 ... 0.00
Total		1.991		38.00	

Ratio

Comments

Supervisor **Date**

IFE Image

Fig. 2.8 Plasma protein electrophoresis graph in the Harris' hawk.

Table 2.5 Results of the biochemistry analyses in the Harris' hawk

Analysis	Results	Reference ranges
Total protein (g/l)	38	22–40
Albumin (g/l)	13	9–26
Globulin (g/l)	25	12–29
Albumin:globulin ratio	0.5	
Total calcium (mmol/l)	2.55	1.78–2.95
Phosphate (mmol/l)	1.5	0.39–3.65
Uric acid (μmol/l)	348	143–980
AST (U/l)	171	118–723
Gamma GT (U/l)	8	1–20
CK (U/l)	549	240–1500

Table 2.6 Results of the haematology analyses in the Harris' hawk

Analysis	Results (absolute)	Results	Reference range
RBC ($\times10^{12}$/l)	2.13		1.46–3.46
Hb (g/dl)	11.9		5–15
HCT (%)		37	35–50
WBC ($\times10^{9}$/l)	8.5		3–12
Heterophils ($\times10^{9}$/l)	4.76	56%	1.8–7.4
Lymphocytes ($\times10^{9}$/l)	0.94	11%	0.6–2.36
Monocytes ($\times10^{9}$/l)	1.62	19%	0–2.1
Eosinophils ($\times10^{9}$/l)	0.85	10%	0–6.3
Basophils ($\times10^{9}$/l)	0.34	4%	0.0–0.8

Blood film examination

Two fresh blood smears and a film made from the submitted heparin were examined. Red cells appear normocytic and normochromic showing no evidence of increase in polychromasia. No abnormal white cells seen. Thrombocyte count and morphology appear normal on smear evaluation.

Table 2.7 Results of the plasma protein electrophoresis analysis in the Harris' hawk

Fraction	Results (g/l)
Total protein	38.0
Pre-albumin	
Albumin	13.84
Alpha 1 globulin	1.42
Alpha 2 globulin	8.29
Beta globulin	7.19
Gamma globulin	7.26

Summary of diagnostic results

- Endoscopy of the oral cavity and oesophagus showed no abnormalities
- Impression smears of the lesion showed mixed bacteria and a heterophilic response
- A bacteriological swab from the lesion grew a pure growth of non-haemolytic *Escherichia coli* sensitive to all routine antibiotics

Q *3. What is your interpretation of the blood analyses?*

The albumen:globulin (A:G) ratio suggests inflammatory disease and this is borne out by the electrophoresis. A prominent alpha 2 fraction suggests an acute phase inflammatory reaction while a polyclonal gammopathy indicates a chronic component. Otherwise there are no significant findings.

Q *4. What do you think of the significance of the bacterial isolate?*

This was clearly a contaminant or opportunistic invader. Had it been a primary cause there would have been a more significant response to previous antibiosis.

Histopathology confirmed the presence of squamous cell carcinoma with a secondary bacterial pyoderma.

Final diagnosis

- Squamous cell carcinoma

Q *5. What will be your course of action?*

Squamous cell carcinoma is common in older Harris' hawks. While radical excision and phototherapy may be appropriate in some cases, this was clearly not possible in this situation. Given the previous beneficial response to topical corticosteroid/

fusidic acid gel, it was decided to resume using this. While topical corticosteroids are normally contraindicated, this case had a hopeless prognosis so therapy was deemed palliative at best. Euthanasia was offered but declined by the owner at that time as the bird appeared well. The bird did well on topical therapy for over six months before euthanasia.

Further reading

Chitty, J., 2008. Raptors: feather and skin diseases. In: Chitty, J., Lierz, M. (Eds.), BSAVA Manual of Raptors, Pigeons & Passerine Birds. British Small Animal Veterinary Association, Gloucester, pp. 270–277.

Forbes, N.A., Cooper, J.E., Higgins, R.J., 2000. Neoplasms of birds of prey. In: Lumeij, S., Remple, D., Redig, P., et al. (Eds.), Raptor Biomedicine. Zoological Education Network, Lake Worth, pp. 127–147.

Lightfoot, T., Garner, M., 2006. Overview of tumors. In: Harrison, G., Lightfoot, T. (Eds.), Clinical Avian Medicine. Spix Publishing, Palm Beach, pp. 559–572.

Case 2.4 *N. A. Forbes*

Clinical history

A 13-year-old female Harris' hawk (*Parabuteo unicinctus*) was presented for examination. The bird had only been in the owner's possession for 2 years, but there was no history of ever having previously been bred from. The owner ran a falconry experience company and took clients out flying with his birds. However, he was unable to fly this bird with guests as it was aggressive towards all humans except the falconer himself. In the past month, the bird had been increasingly vocal and had built a nest in her aviary. The falconer had observed that the bird had laid an egg 3 days previously and now had a red soft tissue structure protruding from her vent.

Clinical history summary

- Laid first egg ever (in absence of a mate) 3 days previously
- Was aggressive to all humans apart from the falconer
- Inflamed soft tissue mass protruding from the cloaca on the day of presentation
- Otherwise bright and vocal

Physical examination

On examination, the hawk was found to be in good body condition, with a well-developed ventral brood patch and a cloacal prolapse as shown in Fig. 2.9.

Clinical diagnosis examination

1. What are the structures which could be found prolapsed from a cloaca of a female bird?

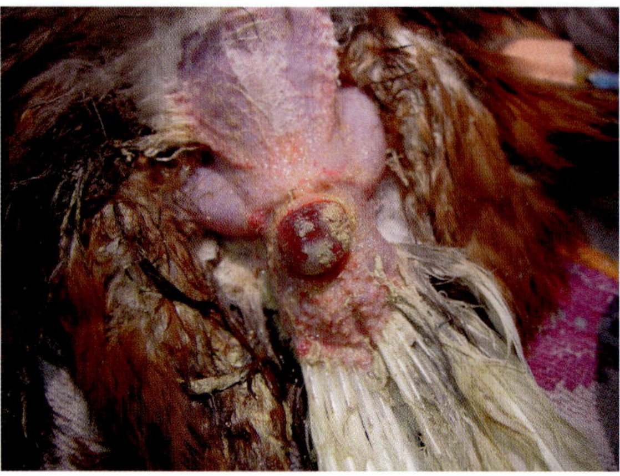

Fig. 2.9 Cloacal prolapse in the Harris' hawk. The bird had laid an egg 3 days previously.

Q *2. What are the possible causes of cloacal prolapse?*

Q *3. What structure is prolapsed in this case?*

Q *4. What tests should be performed to elicit the cause of prolapse in this case?*

A1. Cloaca, oviduct, colon.

A2. Any cause of tenesmus (e.g. oviductitis, egg peritonitis, cloacitis, cloacolith, hypersexuality resulting in masturbation and physical trauma, egg laying-related trauma, trauma subsequent to mating or artificial insemination, bacterial, yeast or parasitic enteritis, gut or oviduct obstruction), relaxed cloacal sphincter (typically secondary to egg laying or hypersexuality) with secondary cloacal exposure or trauma.

A3. Cloaca.

A4. Cloacal cytology, faecal cytology for parasites or infection, radiography and coelioscopy (endoscopic visualization of internal viscera), clinical examination of the cloaca and cloacal sphincter.

Summary of diagnosis results

- Haematology and biochemistry parameters were all normal, with the exception of an elevated total calcium level (a common feature in egg laying or pre-egg laying female birds)
- Radiography normal
- Coelioscopy normal – no indication of peritonitis, further egg progression, enteritis, or cloacitis
- Faecal cytology normal, no abnormal bacteria, yeasts or parasites
- Cloacal cytology normal
- Clinical examination: the cloacal sphincter is dilated and floppy. The oviductal entrance to the cloaca is inflamed and apparently traumatized

Q *5. List your differential diagnoses.*

Q *6. List your therapeutic strategy.*

Differential diagnoses

- Cloacitis secondary to trauma at egg laying
- Cloacal sphincter trauma following first egg laying at an advanced age
- Cloacal sphincter stretching secondary to hypersexuality
- The aggression noted towards other humans and egg laying in absence of a mate tends to indicate that the bird has a desired breeding relationship with the owner. Such an abnormal relationship will often result in abnormal egg laying, cloacal sphincter stretching and secondary cloacitis.

Therapy

- Reduction of cloacal prolapse
- Topical treatment for cloacitis
- Cloacopexy – i.e. after reduction of the cloacal prolapse, placing a cotton bud into the cloaca and pushing as craniad as possible, then fixation either percutaneous or via an abdominal incision, to the ventral abdominal wall, or if possible bilaterally to the last (8th) rib
- Cloacoplasty – i.e. reduction of the internal circumference of the cloacal sphincter, by bilateral removal of mucosa and placement of sutures from the external skin surface, through the skin, muscle and mucosa and back to the skin, in order to reduce the cloacal circumference
- Antibiosis and analgesia
- On recovery, maintaining the bird in a darkened environment, without exposure to the falconer

Response to therapy

- The bird's condition settled, no further straining was observed

Discussion

This problem appears to have arisen due to an inappropriate desired breeding relationship between the bird and the keeper. The same desired relationship is also likely to be the cause of the bird's aggression towards other humans when out flying. Both repeated attempted breeding and territorial or mate, hormonally-derived behaviour can be effectively controlled by the subcutaneous insertion of a gonadotrophin-releasing (GnRH) implant (Suprelorin, Virbac Animal Health). This bird received an implant one week after the prolapse episode. She did not attempt to lay eggs again over the subsequent 12 months and became a friendly bird capable of being flown with guests. Implants remain efficacious for approximately 12 months in birds.

Further reading

Forbes, N.A., 2008. Soft tissue surgery. In: Samour, J. (Ed.), Avian Medicine, second ed. Mosby Elsevier Ltd., Oxford, pp. 163–164.

Forbes, N.A., 2009. The use of GnRH implants in the treatment of sexually derived behavioural abnormalities in birds. In: Proceedings of the European Association of Avian Veterinarians. Antwerp, pp. 119–122.

Case 2.5 *L. Crosta*

Clinical history

During a standard consultation at a breeding facility with a mixed psittacine and birds of prey population, a 5-year-old male snowy owl (*Bubo*{*Nyctea*} *scandiacus*) was presented with the following clinical signs of several weeks:

- Inability to fly
- Progressive weight loss
- Mild diarrhoea.

The bird was housed in a breeding aviary measuring around 4×4 m and 2.5 m height. The owner reported that the bird had been involved in an accident a few months before when he accidentally lost his balance, and to avoid falling down, he put all his weight on the bird's back. He suspected he damaged the bird's spine and that as a consequence, the bird could not fly since then.

Clinical diagnosis examination

On presentation, the bird had a reduced body condition of 2/5. Survey radiographs were taken while the bird was under anaesthesia (Fig. 2.10a, b).

Radiology

1. What is your interpretation of the radiographs in Fig. 2.10a, b?

The radiographs did not show any skeleton abnormality, but several undefined radiodense masses were detected within the coelomic cavity.

Clinical diagnosis laboratory examination

Blood samples were collected for haematology, but the client declined blood chemistry. The results of the haematology analysis are shown in Table 2.8.

Film comments

- Moderate leucocytosis
- Heterophilia
- Heterophil toxicity

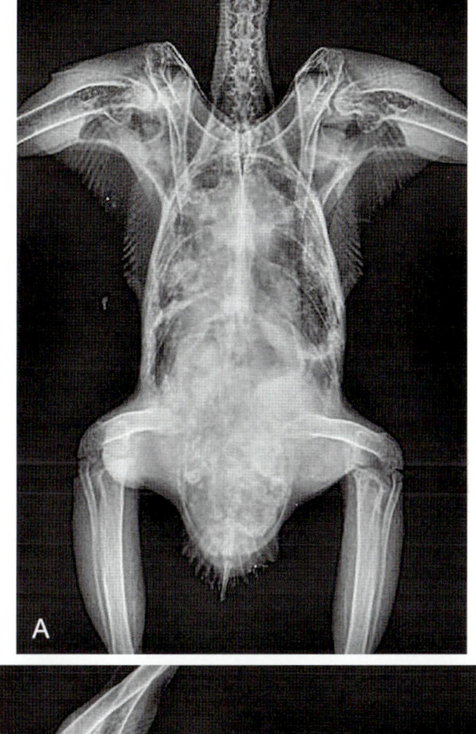

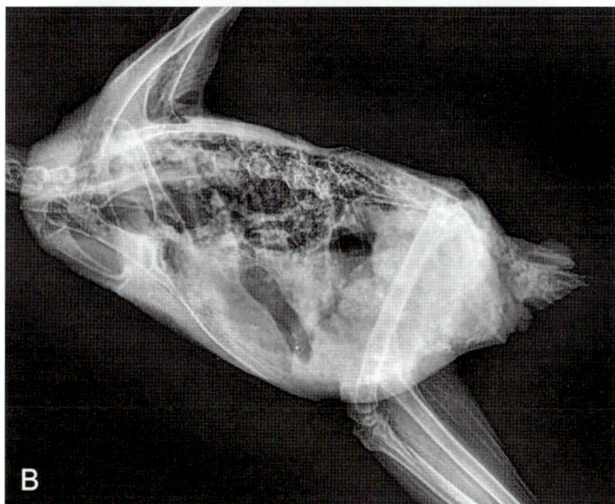

Fig. 2.10 (a) Ventrodorsal survey radiograph of a 5-year-old male snowy owl; (b) lateral survey radiograph of the snowy owl.

Table 2.8 Haematology values of the snowy owl

Parameters	Results (absolute)	Results (%)	Reference values
RBC (×10^12/l)	2.91		2.0–3.7
Hb (g/dl)	20.1		12.3–16.2
Hct (l/l)	0.48		33–52
MCV (fl)	166		118–212
MCH (pg)	67.1		38.4–67.5
MCHC (g/dl)	41.6		28.2–31.8
WBC (×10^9/l)	29.55		8.0–28.7
Heterophils (×10^9/l)	26	88	1.16–18.3
Lymphocytes (×10^9/l)	2.364	8	0.47–15.2
Monocytes (×10^9/l)	0	0	0.063–2.14
Eosinophils (×10^9/l)	591	2	0.021–1.36
Basophils (×10^9/l)	0	0	0.08–1.56
Thrombocytes (×10^9/l)	70.7		n-d

Q *2. What is your interpretation of the haematology values shown in Table 2.8?*

After having explained the results, the owner agreed to a coelioscopy, to investigate the abdominal radiodense masses as observed in the survey radiographs (Fig. 2.11a, b).

The endoscopy examination showed disseminated whitish masses within the coelomic cavity. During the procedure samples were taken for cytology and microbiology.

Cytology

- Cytology: high number of cells, monomorphic population of large foamy cells, with marked anisocytosis/anisokaryosis. Furthermore, large atypical fibroblasts and very few heterophils were observed. No microorganisms were observed

Microbiology

- No bacteria or fungi were cultured from the swabs collected from the coelomic cavity

Summary of clinical diagnosis laboratory results

- Haematology revealed a moderate leucocytosis, a moderate to high heterophilia and heterophil toxicity
- Both Gram staining and cytology confirmed the absence of microorganisms
- Furthermore, cytology detected large foamy cells with marked anisocytosis and anisokaryosis, and large atypical fibroblasts

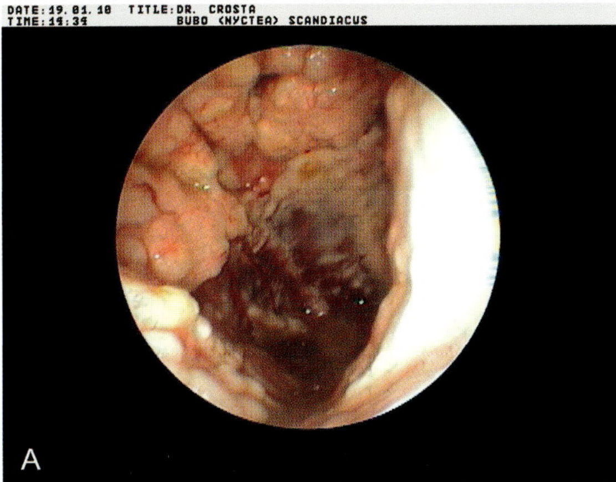

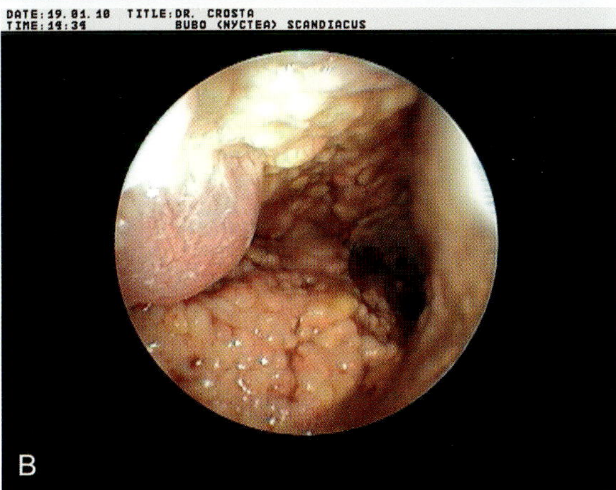

Fig. 2.11 (a,b) Endoscopic view of the coelomic cavity of the snowy owl.

Please evaluate the clinical history, Figs 2.10a, b, 2.11a, b, the results of the physical examination and clinical diagnosis laboratory tests.

Q *3. List your differential diagnoses.*

Q *4. List your therapeutic strategy.*

Differential diagnoses

- Granulomatous disease (mycobacteriosis, aspergillosis)
- Disseminated neoplasm (adenocarcinoma, liposarcoma)

Therapy (Table 2.9)

Unfortunately, after 2 days of treatment and no obvious improvement, the owner opted for euthanasia.

Table 2.9 Therapy

Ceftriaxone	100 mg/kg IM BID × 1 week
Vitamin ADE	Vitamin A 20 000 IU/kg IM once
Fluids/vitamin B complex	Ringer's lactate 20 ml/kg with 30 mg/kg thiamine SC BID
Itraconazole	10 mg/kg PO BID

Post-mortem findings

A thorough post-mortem examination was performed (Fig. 2.12a–d). Samples from different organs were collected for histopathology.

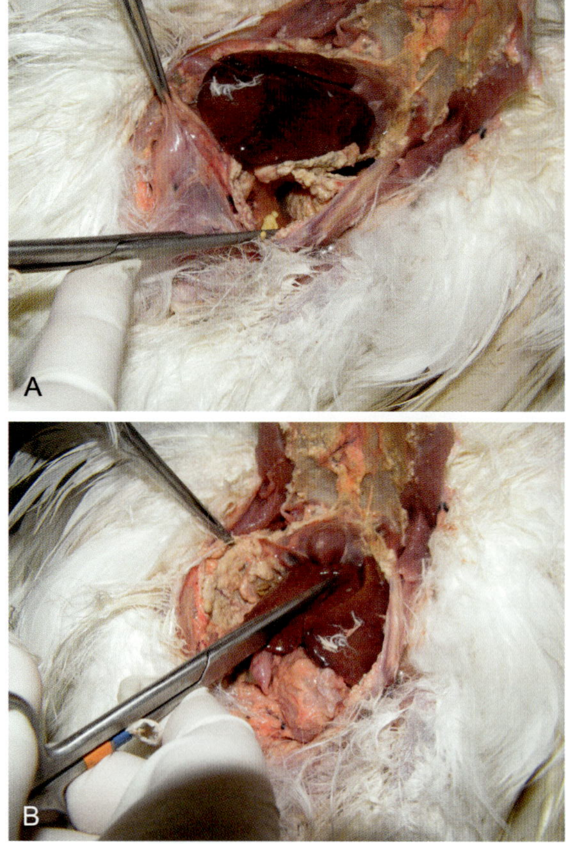

Fig. 2.12 (a–d) Post-mortem photographs of the snowy owl.

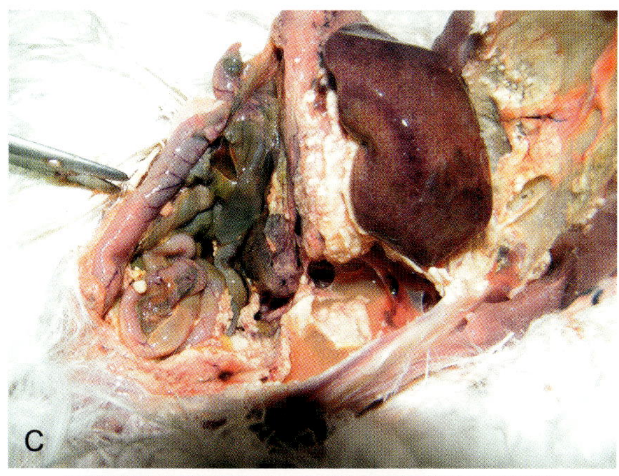

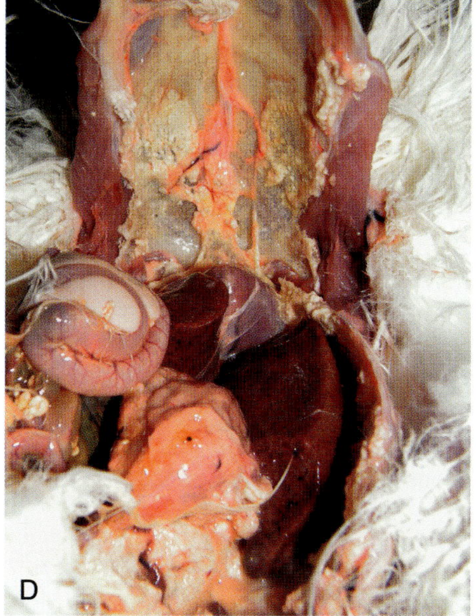

Fig. 2.12—cont'd

Q *5. What lesions can you observe in the post-mortem photographs?*

Q *6. What is your provisional post-mortem diagnosis?*

Summary of post-mortem examination findings

- Almost every organ looked "rotten" inside the bird
- Liver: marbled, but without specific focal foci

- Coelomic cavity: presence of multiple small, caseous masses, possibly granulomatous in origin, infiltrating several organs and serosa
- Intestine: no gross changes, apparently only involved mechanically

During the examination, it was suspected that the pathology had started from the kidney region. The kidneys could not be located and had been "replaced" by a large whitish mass.

Provisional post-mortem diagnosis

- Disseminated tumour (to be defined histologically)
- Tuberculosis
- Coligranulomatosis (unlikely because no bacteria were detected)
- Aspergillosis (unlikely because no fungi were detected)

Laboratory findings

Histology

- Spongy tissue with trabecula that often looked necrotic. In the spaces between the mesh large macrophages and granulocytes, but in many of these "chambers" basophilic crystal-like cigar to round structures that were small (diameter 2–3 μm) and irregular
- In other places it looked more like a xanthoma, including cholesterol clefts
- Intestines no changes
- Liver reactive with mixed cellular periportal and sinusoidal infiltrates
- In the lungs locally parabronchi filled with the large spongy macrophages seen in the tumour and also basophilic changes (metastasis or inhalation?)

Final diagnosis

- Disseminated tumour, most likely xanthoma

Discussion

The owner suspected trauma as the cause of the bird's inability to fly. Radiographs revealed the presence of disseminated masses that could not be related to trauma. Haematology pointed to a possible infection (leucocytosis, heterophilia and heterophil toxicity), but this was not supported by the microbiology samples collected during endoscopy. The endoscopy examination showed several small masses filling almost every space of the air sacs. This was a very unusual endoscopy finding. The bird was euthanased as there was little that could have been done to save the bird. This became obvious at post-mortem examination. The perception of the owners could very often lead to a wrong diagnosis, but a professional approach to the case often leads, if not to save a bird, at least to provide a definite diagnosis. Unfortunately, it was not possible to carry out histopathology examination. The most important aspect of the case for the owner was that the bird was not undergoing an infectious process that could have threatened the rest of the birds in the breeding facility.

Further reading

Cooper, J.E., 2002. Miscellaneous and emerging diseases. In: Birds of Prey: Health and Disease. third ed. Blackwell Publishing, Oxford, pp. 200–201.

Forbes, N.A., 2000. Raptor medicine. Seminars in Avian and Exotic Pet Medicine 9, 197–203.

Forbes, N.A., Cooper, J.E., Higgins, R.J., 2000. Neoplasm of birds of prey. In: Lumeij, J.T., Remple, J.D., Redig, P.T., et al. (Eds.), Raptor Biomedicine III. Zoological Education Network, Lake Worth, FL, pp. 127–146.

Garner, R.R., 2006. Overview of tumors: section II – a retrospective study of case submissions to a specialty diagnostic service. In: Harrison, G.J., Lightfoot, T. (Eds.), Clinical Avian Medicine. Spix Publishing, Inc., Palm Beach, pp. 5665–5671.

Latimer, S.K., 1994. Oncology. In: Ritchie, B.W., Harrison, G.J., Harrison, L.R. (Eds.), Avian Medicine: Principle and Application. Wingers Publishing, Inc., Lake Worth, pp. 640–672.

Lightfoot, T.L., 2006. Overview of tumors: section I – clinical avian neoplasia and oncology. In: Harrison, G.J., Lightfoot, T. (Eds.), Clinical Avian Medicine. Spix Publishing, Inc., Palm Beach, pp. 560–565.

Raynor, P.L., Kollias, G.V., Krook, L., 1999. Periosseous xanthogranulomatosis in a fledgling great horned owl (*Bubo virginianus*). J. Avian Med. Surg. 13 (4), 269–274.

Rettenmund, C., Sladky, K.K., Rodriguez, D., et al., 2010. Pulmonary carcinoma in a great horned owl (*Bubo virginianus*). J. Zoo Wildl. Med. 41 (1), 77–82.

Ridgway, R.L., 1977. Oral xanthoma in a budgerigar (*Melopsittacus undulatus*): a case report. Vet. Med. Small Anim. Clin. 72 (2), 266–267.

Schmidt, R.E., Reavill, D.R., Phalen, D.N., 2008. Pathology of Pet and Aviary Birds. Blackwell Publishing, Ames.

Case 2.6 *J. Samour, J. Naldo*

Clinical history

A 6-month-old female gyr falcon (*Falco rusticolus*) was presented for examination. The captive-bred bird was used in the sport of falconry and it was in the early stages of training. One afternoon the falcon owner noticed the falcon drooling saliva and repeatedly making a clacking noise after feeding. He inspected the oro-pharynx and palpated the neck thinking of a bone caught at the entrance of the crop, but could not find anything abnormal. The following day, the falcon was normal so he ignored the symptoms observed the previous day. Two days later, the bird began passing green-coloured urates and did not look well, therefore he decided to take it to a veterinarian for consultation. The falcon was presented for examination with the following clinical signs observed in the past 2 days:

- Inappetence
- Progressive weight loss
- Pastel green-coloured urates
- Reduced interactive activity.

Physical examination

On examination, the falcon was found relatively alert and responsive. The bodyweight was 1156g with a body condition of 3/5 and was mildly dehydrated. The bird was weak and had to be assisted back to the glove after a failed attempt to carry out an endurance test.

Clinical diagnosis examination

Survey radiographs were taken while the bird was under anaesthesia (Fig. 2.13a, b). Endoscopy examination of the upper digestive tract and trachea was also performed.

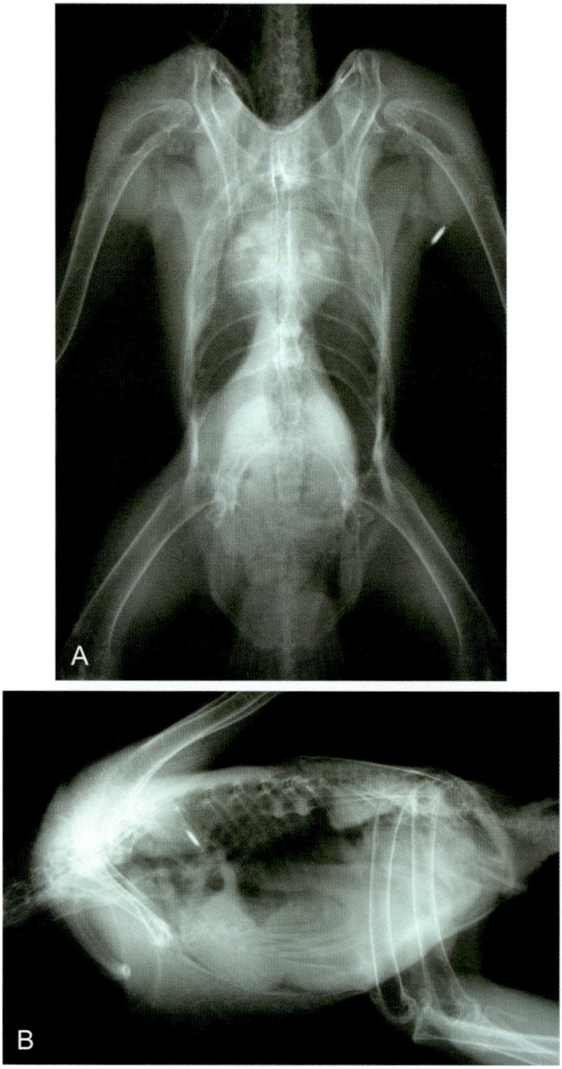

Fig. 2.13 (a) Ventrodorsal survey radiograph of a 6-month-old female gyr falcon; (b) lateral survey radiograph of the gyr falcon.

Radiology

1. What is your interpretation of the radiographs in Fig. 2.13a, b?

Clinical diagnosis laboratory examination

Blood samples were collected for haematology, blood chemistry and plasma protein electrophoresis analyses. A faecal sample was collected to examine for the presence of endoparasites.

The results of the clinical diagnosis laboratory assays are shown in Tables 2.10–2.12.

Table 2.10 Haematology values of the gyr falcon

Parameters	Results (absolute)	Results (%)	Reference values
RBC ($\times 10^{12}$/l)	2.13		3.91±0.14 (3.1–5.12)
Hb (g/dl)	14.3		18.85±0.23 (16.0–21.2)
Hct (l/l)	0.39		0.51±0.09 (0.44–0.59)
MCV (fl)	183		135.83±3.59 (106.18–162.36)
MCH (pg)	67.1		49.44±1.32 (39.17–59.67)
MCHC (g/dl)	36.6		36.41±0.16 (35.47–37.84)
WBC ($\times 10^9$/l)	11.9		7.3±0.38 (4.2–10.8)
Heterophils ($\times 10^9$/l)	2.7	23	4.67±0.34 (2.31–8.85)
Lymphocytes ($\times 10^9$/l)	8.8	74	1.43±0.10 (0.48–2.36)
Monocytes ($\times 10^9$/l)	0.119	1	0.42±0.05 (0.03–0.9)
Eosinophils ($\times 10^9$/l)	0	0	0.27±0.04 (0.0–0.68)
Basophils ($\times 10^9$/l)	0.238	2	0.05±0.02 (0.0–0.29)
Thrombocytes ($\times 10^9$/l)	12.6		22.57±1.04 (12.67–29.93)
Fibrinogen (g/l)	4.0		3.61±0.21 (1.72–5.63)

Table 2.11 Blood chemistry values of the gyr falcon

Analysis	Results	Reference values
Albumin (g/l)	12.4	11.8 (1.7)
ALKP (U/l)	97.54	-
Amylase (U/l)	60.1	86 (116)
Bile acids (μmol/l)	460	-
Bilirubin (μmol/l)	17.44	4.6 (1.7)
Calcium (mmol/l)	2.13	2.3 (0.27)
Cholesterol (mmol/l)	2.15	5.44 (1.03)
Creatinine (μmol/l)	116.69	38 (14)
CK (U/l)	1066.4	-
GGT (U/l)	5.73	-
AST (U/l)	418.4	149 (110)
ALT (U/l)	221.6	135 (125)
Glucose (mmol/l)	16.21	20.4 (1.7)
Iron (μmol/l)	12.27	-
LDH (U/l)	7335.5	1917 (879)
Phosphorus (mmol/l)	1.70	1.52 (0.40)
Total protein (g/l)	32.0	25.0 (8.7)
Total urea (mmol/l)	1.73	3.6 (2.2)
Uric acid (μmol/l)	1225	370 (170)

Table 2.12 Plasma protein electrophoresis of the gyr falcon

Parameters	Fractions (%)	Concentrations (g/l)
Total protein		32.0
Albumin	12.7	4.06
Alpha 1 globulins	8.0	2.56
Alpha 2 globulins	22.0	7.04
Beta globulins	36.0	11.52
Gamma globulins	21.3	6.82
A:G ratio		0.15

RBC, WBC and thrombocyte morphology

➤ Nothing abnormal detected

2. What is your interpretation of the haematology, blood chemistry and protein electrophoresis values shown in Tables 2.10–2.12?

 *3. In view of the early nervous clinical signs, would you request any other laboratory diagnosis test?*

Summary of diagnostic results

- Radiographic findings included mainly an enlarged liver shadow and a slightly distended gizzard
- Endoscopy examination of the upper gastrointestinal tract and trachea revealed no abnormal findings
- Faecal examination showed negative result for the presence of endoparasites
- Haematology analysis showed low RBC, low Hb and low Hct. The WBC was slightly elevated with marked lymphocytosis
- Blood chemistry analysis showed elevated levels of bile acids, CK, glutamic oxaloacetic transaminase (GOT), glutamic pyruvic transaminase (GPT), lactate dehydrogenase (LDH) and uric acid
- Plasma protein electrophoresis showed low albumin, elevated globulins and low albumin:globulin ratio

Please evaluate the clinical history, Fig. 2.13a, b, the results of the physical examination and clinical and laboratory diagnostic tests.

 *4. List your differential diagnoses.*

 *5. List your therapeutic strategy.*

Differential diagnoses

- Visceral gout
- Hepatopathy
- Renal disease

Therapy

The falcon was placed on the therapeutic management shown in Table 2.13.

Table 2.13 Therapy

Marbofloxacin 10%	15 mg/kg IM SID × 1 week
Vitamin ADEC	To provide Vitamin A 20 000 IU/kg IM, once
Vitamin B complex	To provide thiamine 30 mg/kg IM, once
Fluids	Ringer's lactate 20 ml/kg SC BID
Forced feeding	Mixture of ground whole quail, ground quail liver, Spark liquid concentrate™ and water, 30–40 ml TID

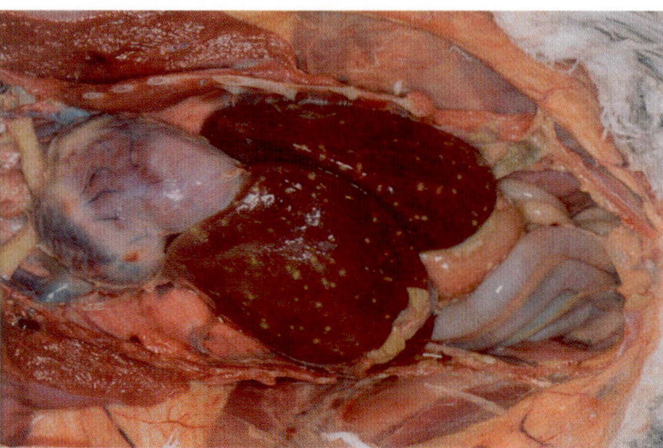

Fig. 2.14 Post-mortem photograph of the gyr falcon.

Post-mortem examination

The falcon continued deteriorating despite support therapy and died on the fourth day of admission. A thorough post-mortem examination was performed (Fig. 2.14). Samples from different organs were collected for microbiology, histopathology and virus isolation.

 *6. What lesions can you observe in the post-mortem photograph?*

 *7. What is your provisional post-mortem diagnosis?*

Summary of post-mortem examination findings

- Liver: enlarged with numerous focal necrotic foci
- Intestines: inflamed mucosa with mild haemorrhages
- Spleen and kidneys: enlarged, congested, with a few necrotic foci
- Lungs: bilateral mild congestion
- Trachea: congested blood vessels

Provisional post-mortem diagnosis

- Herpesvirus hepatitis
- *Escherichia coli* septicaemia
- Salmonellosis

Post-mortem laboratory findings

- Microbiology: nothing significant was cultured
- Histology:
  - Liver: recent necrotic foci with some surrounding cells containing eosinophilic intranuclear inclusions

- Pancreas, spleen: few small necrotic foci
- Other tissues: no lesions observed

➤ Virology: herpesvirus isolated

Final diagnosis

➤ Herpesvirus hepatitis

Discussion

There are three different herpesvirus producing hepatitis in birds of prey. The causal agent in falcons is falconid HV1 (FHV1). Inclusion body hepatitis of falcons is an infectious viral disease commonly transmitted through direct contact with infected pigeons. Transmission is believed to be accomplished through viral particles entering the ocular route. The infection usually follows a super-acute (0–48 hours), acute (48–72 hours) to chronic (>78 hours) course. In some cases, sudden death is observed. The presence of multiple caseous necrotic foci in the liver and spleen are characteristic of the infection. Transmission was very likely through close contact with pigeons used in the training process. This report includes the occurrence of nervous signs at the beginning of the infection. This is certainly unusual and was the first time the authors ever observed nervous clinical signs associated with this disease. Subsequently, similar clinical signs were observed in an outbreak involving nine individuals affected by the same infection. It is difficult to ascertain as to whether the unusual clinical signs may have been caused by a particular virulent strain of the virus.

Further reading

Samour, J., 2006. Management of raptors. In: Harrison, G.J., Lightfoot, T.L. (Eds.), Clinical Avian Medicine. Spix Publishing, Inc., Palm Beach, pp. 915–956.

Stanford, M., 2008. Raptors: infectious diseases. In: Chitty, J., Lierz, M. (Eds.), BSAVA Manual of Raptors, Pigeons and Passerine Birds. British Small Animal Veterinary Association, Gloucester, pp. 212–222.

Wernery, U., 2008. Viral diseases. In: Samour, J. (Ed.), Avian Medicine, second ed. Mosby Elsevier, Oxford, pp. 358–373.

Case 2.7 *J. Samour, J. Naldo*

Clinical history

An adult, female, saker falcon (*Falco cherrug*) was taken to a local veterinary hospital for clinical examination. The falcon was used as part of an avian pest control programme around monuments and historical buildings. The falconer reported the following clinical symptoms:

- Severe depression
- General weakness
- Absence of preening and interactive activities
- Shredding and flicking of food
- Regurgitation
- Foetid diarrhoea
- Anorexia of 48 h.

Physical examination

On examination, the falcon displayed almond-shaped eyes, it showed mild dehydration, and was unable to stand or to maintain its balance on the glove when handled.

Clinical diagnosis examination

The falcon was anaesthetized to obtain radiographs (Fig. 2.15a, b) and to perform exploratory endoscopy of the upper digestive tract (Fig. 2.16).

Radiology

1. Can you observe any radiological abnormality in Fig. 2.15a, b?

Endoscopy

2. Is the endoscopic view of the ventriculus of the saker falcon normal?

3. If not, what is the most important finding in the endoscopic view of the ventriculus?

Clinical diagnosis laboratory examination

Blood samples were collected for haematology (Table 2.14) and blood chemistry analyses. A direct faecal examination was conducted to determine the presence of internal gastrointestinal parasites.

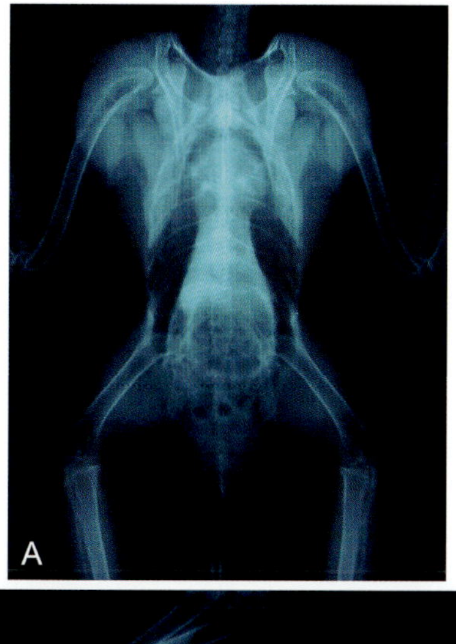

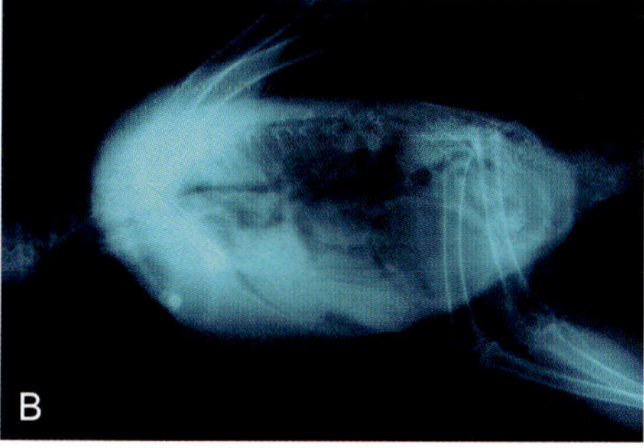

Fig. 2.15 (a) Ventrodorsal radiographic view of the saker falcon; (b) latero-lateral radiographic view of the saker falcon.

Blood chemistry

Nothing abnormal was observed in the results of the blood chemistry values in the saker falcon with the exception of a mild increment in bile acids (18 µmol/l, normal range 1.7–14.4 µmol/l).

White blood cell morphological characteristics

Approximately 50% of the heterophils showed slightly basophilic cytoplasm, loss of granulation and loss of lobulation (left-shift), while a smaller percentage of lymphocytes (15%) showed intracytoplasmic azurophilic granules. Approximately 5% of the thrombocytes could be classified as megathrombocytes due to their large size.

4. What is the interpretation of the haematology and blood chemistry results?

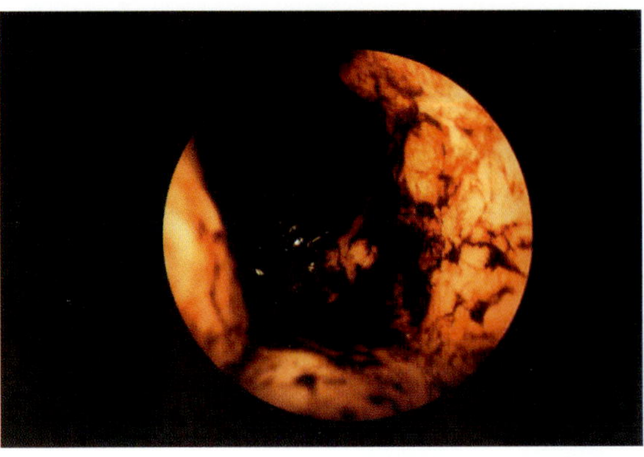

Fig. 2.16 Endoscopic view of the ventriculus of the saker falcon under anaesthesia.

Table 2.14 Relevant results of the haematology analysis on the saker falcon

Parameter	Absolute value	Normal range	Percentage value	Normal range
WBC ($\times 10^9$/l)	11.2	5.7±0.31 (3.8–11.5)	16.3	5.7±0.31 (3.8–11.5)
Heterophils ($\times 10^9$/l)	8.95	4.14±0.24 (2.6–5.85)	84.2	65–70
Eosinophils ($\times 10^9$/l)	0.3	0–0.2	1.7	0–2
Basophils ($\times 10^9$/l)	0.03	0.08±0.01 (0–0.45)	0.2	0–2
Lymphocytes ($\times 10^9$/l)	0.9	1.33±0.09 (0.8–4.25)	7.3	20–30
Monocytes ($\times 10^9$/l)	0.8	0.21±0.03 (0.0–0.8)	7.0	2–5

5. How important is it to provide haematology results in both absolute and percentage values?

Summary of diagnostic results

- Faecal examination was negative for the presence of gastrointestinal parasites
- Survey radiographs obtained showed mainly a severely distended ventriculus together with a distinct thickening of the ventricular wall
- Endoscopy examination of the ventriculus showed the presence of partially digested blood due to extensive petechial haemorrhages across the ventricular wall
- Haematology analysis revealed a mild elevated WBC count. Absolute heterophilia (>80%). Toxic changes observed in the heterophils and lymphocytes. Mild monocytosis
- Mild increment of bile acids

 *6. Based on clinical history, clinical examination and clinical diagnostic and laboratory findings, could you propose differential diagnoses?*

Differential diagnoses

- Gastroenteritis
- *Escherichia coli* septicaemia
- Toxicosis
- Newcastle disease

 *7. Can you list your proposed therapeutic management of the case?*

Therapy

The falcon was prescribed 100 mg/kg piperacillin IM BID for 7 days and was given 20 ml Ringer's lactate IV before recovering from anaesthesia and prescribed force feeding 30–40 ml ground whole quail TID or BID as indicated.

Post-mortem examination

The falcon died overnight and a post-mortem examination was carried out the following morning (Fig. 2.17a–c). Samples were collected from all major organs including brain, heart, lung, spleen, liver and kidneys for virus isolation and histopathology. Bacteriological swabs were also collected from intestinal content, liver and spleen.

 *8. What gross post-mortem changes can be observed in Fig. 2.17a?*

 *9. Can you describe the pathological findings in Fig. 2.17b and c?*

Summary of post-mortem examination findings

Severely distended proventriculus; moderate to severe petechial haemorrhages were observed on the mucosal membrane around the isthmus of the proventriculus and across the ventricular wall. Severe petechial and ecchymotic haemorrhages along the entire intestinal tract. Slightly enlarged spleen.

Provisional post-mortem diagnosis

- Gastroenteritis
- Newcastle disease

Post-mortem laboratory findings

- Microbiology: no significant growth was observed on the samples cultured
- Histopathology: nothing abnormal was observed in the histopathology examinations
- Virus isolation: paramyxovirus isolated

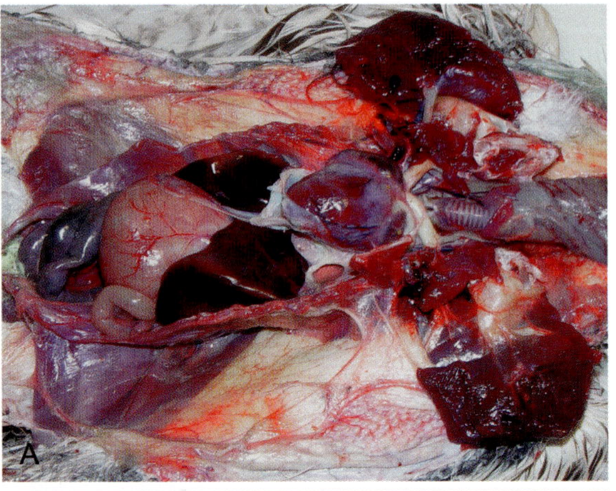

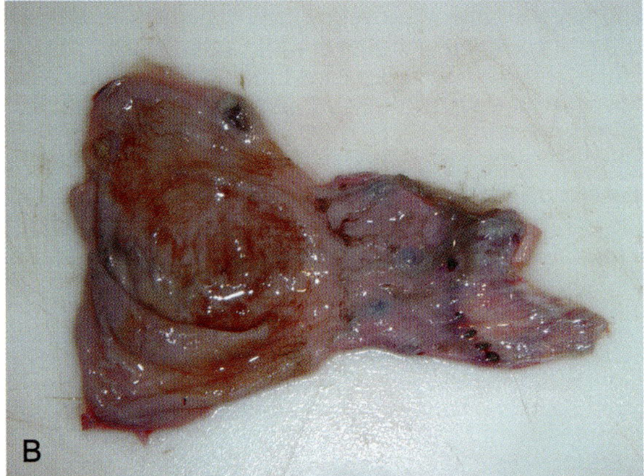

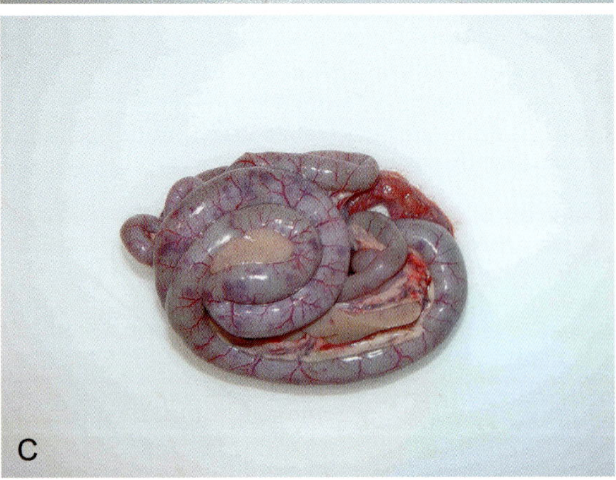

Fig. 2.17 (a–c) Post-mortem findings.

Final diagnosis

➤ Newcastle disease viscerotropic form

Discussion

The falcon was affected with the viscerotropic form of Newcastle disease. The infection was probably contracted due to close contact with pigeons commonly found in urban areas. The clinical symptoms associated with the viscerotropic form of Newcastle disease may not be easily recognized by veterinarians and could represent a challenge in establishing a diagnosis. The haematology findings are of particular interest and highlight the importance of expressing the results of the differential white cell count in both absolute and percentage values. In this case, the absolute heterophil count was within established normal ranges. However, absolute heterophilia was only detected when the percentage of heterophils in the blood films was taken into consideration. The toxic changes observed in the heterophils were considered typical of the acute phase of the Newcastle disease infection. The radiographic observations of ventricular dilatation and thickening of the proventricular wall were also of particular interest. These findings have never been reported in the literature. The occurrence of petechial haemorrhages in the ventriculus is a common finding in poultry affected with Newcastle disease, however, this has not been mentioned in the literature in falcons. Vaccination programmes using commercially available inactive vaccines are vital to ensure that falcons are adequately protected against this relatively common and fatal disease.

Further reading

Samour, J., 2006. Management of raptors. In: Harrison, G.J., Lightfoot, T.L. (Eds.), Clinical Avian Medicine. Spix Publishing Inc., Palm Beach, pp. 915–956.

Samour, J., Naldo, J.L., 2003. The use of serum bile acids in the assessment of hepatobiliary function in saker falcons in Saudi Arabia. In: European Association of Avian Veterinarians Conference. Tenerife, pp. 292–296.

Stanford, M., 2008. Raptors: infectious diseases. In: Chitty, J., Lierz, M. (Eds.), BSAVA Manual of Raptors, Pigeons and Passerine Birds. British Small Animal Veterinary Association, Gloucester, pp. 212–222.

Wernery, U., 2008. Viral diseases. In: Samour, J. (Ed.), Avian Medicine, second ed. Mosby Elsevier Ltd., Oxford, pp. 358–373.

Case 2.8 *J. Samour, J. Naldo*

Clinical history

An imprinted adult female peregrine falcon (*Falco peregrinus*) used in a captive breeding programme was presented to a veterinary hospital with the following history:

- Progressive weight loss
- Shredding and flicking of food
- Delay emptying the crop
- Regurgitation
- Decreased appetite.

Physical examination

On examination, the bird was found alert and responsive. The bodyweight was 805 g with a body condition score of 3/5. The bird was alert and responsive.

Clinical diagnosis examination

The falcon was anaesthetized to undergo full clinical diagnosis examination including survey radiographs, endoscopy of the upper respiratory (Fig. 2.18) and digestive tract.

Endoscopy

 ***1. What abnormality can you observe in this endoscopic view of the crop?***

 ***2. What additional sample would you collect to aid in the diagnosis?***

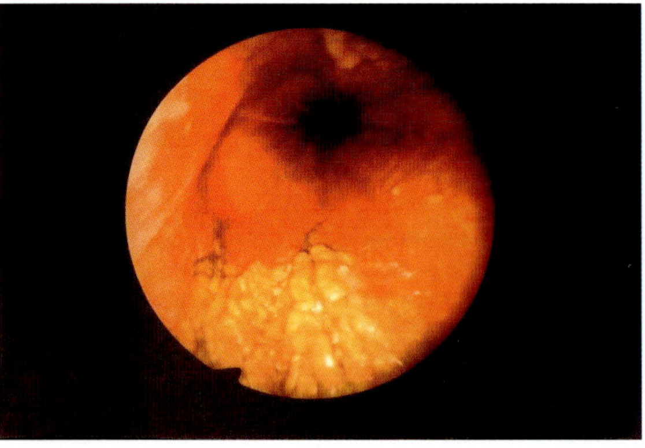

Fig. 2.18 Endoscopic view of the crop of the peregrine falcon.

Clinical diagnosis laboratory examination

A faecal sample was collected for parasitology analysis and blood samples were obtained for routine haematology and blood chemistry analyses. In addition to these, a swab was collected from the crop to make cytology preparations. Impression smears were made on microscope slides. These were stained with methylene blue stain and examined under 1000× oil immersion using a light microscope.

Summary of diagnostic results

Nothing abnormal could be detected in the haematology or blood chemistry analyses. Similarly, the radiographs obtained did not show any abnormality. Faecal sample examination was negative for the presence of endoparasites. Fig. 2.19 was obtained from an impression smear from the crop.

Cytology

Q *3. Is this an artefact within the preparation?*

Q *4. If not, can you describe the findings on this preparation?*

Q *5. Please revise the clinical history and clinical pathology findings and formulate differential diagnoses.*

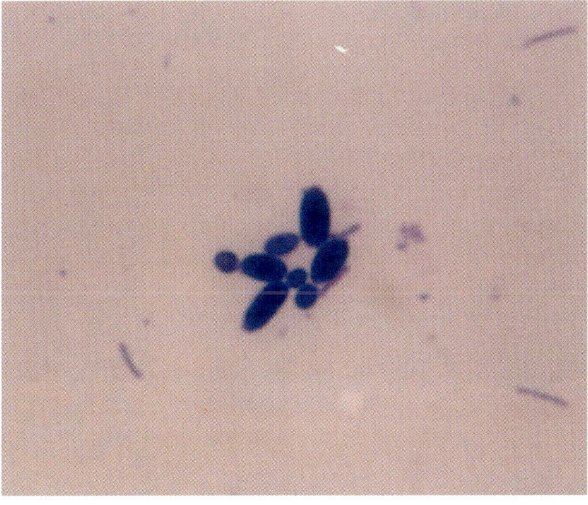

Fig. 2.19 Cytology finding in the impression smear made from the swab taken from the crop of the peregrine falcon.

Differential diagnoses

- Vitamin A deficiency
- Capillariasis
- Candidiasis
- Foreign body

 *6. Based on the findings can you establish a diagnosis?*

 *7. Can you formulate a therapeutic plan?*

Final diagnosis

- Candidiasis

Discussion

The cytology preparation in Fig. 2.19 clearly shows typical budding yeast cells characteristic of *C. albicans*. The falcon was affected with candidiasis. This is a fungal disease very commonly linked in birds to prolonged use of antibiotics and poor husbandry. The bird in this particular case had just finished moulting and the owner was eager to increase the bodyweight fast. In this respect, the falcon was allowed to take a full crop for several days. In a clinically normal falcon, a full crop should empty within 2 to 3 hours with a maximum of 4 hours. This bird used to take between 6 to 8 hours to empty the crop. The repeated retention of food in the crop is very dangerous for a bird of prey leading to candidiasis and, in worse cases, to "sour crop" and death.

Several pharmaceutical compounds have been used successfully for the treatment of candidiasis in avian species. These include nystatin, ketoconazole, itraconazole and fluconazole. Miconazole in gel form (Daktarin®) topically BID for 3 to 5 days has been used with great success in falcons affected with candidiasis. Force feeding should be considered for the duration of the treatment if the bird is not eating well and if the bodyweight continues to decrease. The administration of 15 000 to 25 000 IU Vitamin A IM per week for 2 to 3 weeks should also be considered.

Further reading

Lloyd, C., 2008. Raptors: gastrointestinal tract diseases. In: Chitty, J., Lierz, M. (Eds.), BSAVA Manual of Raptors, Pigeons and Passerine Birds. British Small Animal Veterinary Association, Gloucester, pp. 260–269.

Samour, J., 2006. Management of raptors. In: Harrison, G.J., Lightfoot, T.L. (Eds.), Clinical Avian Medicine. Spix Publishing, Inc., Palm Beach, pp. 915–956.

Samour, J.H., Naldo, J.L., 2002. Diagnosis and therapeutic management of candidiasis in falcons in Saudi Arabia. J. Avian Med. Surg. 16 (2), 129–132.

Silvanose, C., 2008. Fungal diseases – candidiasis. In: Samour, J. (Ed.), Avian Medicine, second ed. Mosby Elsevier Ltd., Oxford, pp. 388–390.

Case 2.9 *M. Lierz, D. Fischer*

Clinical history

Three, 9–12-day-old gyr falcon chicks (*Falco rusticolus*), weighing 220–300 g, were presented with the following clinical signs:

- Empty crop
- Respiratory distress
- Weakness.

The falcon chicks came from a commercial falcon breeder, who kept a couple of breeding pairs and imprinted falcons for artificial insemination. The birds were hatched in an incubator after the eggs had been removed from the parental nest on the 10th day of natural incubation. After hatching in the artificial incubator the falcons were reared by hand for 6–7 days before placing them back with an imprinted brooding female for rearing. During the first 7 days the chicks received baby rats as feed. The mother and other breeding pairs were fed with freshly slaughtered 4-week-old cockerels and thawed young laboratory rats. Cockerels were raised separately by the falcon breeder using commercial poultry feed. Three days after placing the chicks back with the imprinted mother, the breeder observed that their crops were empty, although the rearing-experienced female attempted to feed them several times.

Physical examination

On presentation, all birds were weak and showed severe respiratory symptoms, such as acute tachypnoea and dyspnoea with open-mouthed respiration and double pump respiration. One chick died on the day of admission and was sent for post-mortem examination. From the remaining two chicks tracheal swabs were taken for microbiological examination.

1. List your differential diagnoses for respiratory symptoms.

Differential diagnoses for tachypnoea and dyspnoea in falcons

- Foreign body aspiration
- Inhaled respiratory toxins (e.g. fumes)
- Anaemia
- Aspiration pneumonia
- Pulmonary congestion following trauma
- Fungal infection (e.g. *Aspergillus* spp., *Mucor* spp., *Penicillium* spp., *Histoplasma* spp.)
- Bacterial infection (e.g. *Pseudomonas aeruginosa, Pasteurella* spp., *Proteus mirabilis, Escherichia coli, Klebsiella* spp., *Staphylococcus aureus, Chlamydophila* spp., and *Mycoplasma* spp.)
- Viral infection (avian influenza virus and paramyxovirus-1)
- Parasitic infection (*Syngamus trachea, Capillaria* spp., *Serratospiculum* spp., *Cryptosporidium* spp.)
- Oral lesions (e.g. granuloma, trichomoniasis, avipox, bacterial stomatitis, candidiasis, capillariasis)
- Space-occupying masses (e.g. granuloma, neoplasm, hepatomegaly, egg binding) or including fluid (ascites, haemorrhage, egg-related peritonitis) in the coelomic cavity

Post-mortem findings

One chick died on the day of admission. A thorough post-mortem examination was performed (Fig. 2.20). Samples from different organs (heart blood, lungs, liver and air sacs) were collected for microbiology and histopathology analyses.

Q *2. What lesions can you observe in the post-mortem photographs?*

Q *3. What is your provisional post-mortem diagnosis?*

Summary of post-mortem examination findings

- Liver: enlarged
- Air sacs: filled with serofibrinous exudates

Provisional post-mortem diagnosis

- Hepatomegaly
- Airsacculitis

Q *4. Please evaluate the clinical history, Fig. 2.20 and the results of the post-mortem examination.*

Q *5. List your therapeutic strategy.*

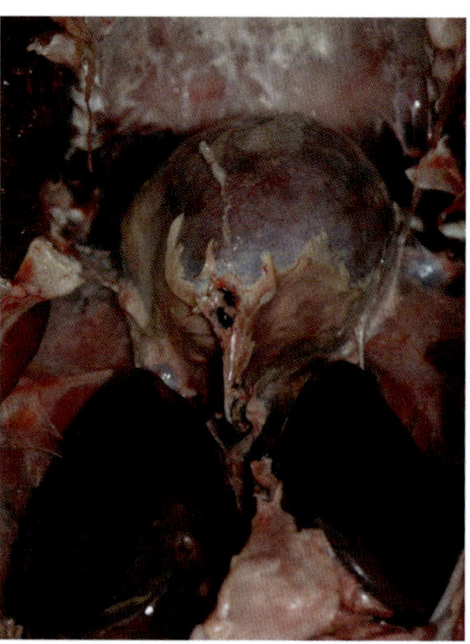

Fig. 2.20 Pericarditis and airsacculitis induced by *Ornithobacterium rhinotracheale* in a hybrid falcon chick.

Therapy (Table 2.15)

Table 2.15 Therapy

Long-acting tetracycline (Doxycycline-SF®)	100 mg/kg IM twice in an interval of 3 days
Fluids	Ringer's lactate and glucose solution 5% mixed to equal parts 20 ml/kg SC BID × 3 days
Vitamin B complex	Thiamine 30 mg/kg SC in the infusion SID × 3 days
Nebulization	5 ml of an inhalant mix (=1% enilconazole solution with saline) for 30 min SID × 6 days
Hand feeding	Mixture of ground whole quail, ground quail liver, Spark liquid concentrate™ and water, 30–40 ml TID
Keeping warm	Infrared light

Laboratory findings

- Microbiology:
  - In samples from lungs and air sacs, fine, circular, greyish, non-haemolytic colonies of *Ornithobacterium rhinotracheale* (ORT) were cultured on blood agar with 10% sheep blood. On Gassner agar there was no growth detectable. The samples were incubated for 48 hours at 37 °C under microaerobic conditions. A biochemical identification was done using a commercial biochemical test kit
  - Gram stain: Gram-negative cocci and pleomorphic, short, plump rods were visible in a tracheal smear
  - Serological typing by heat-stable antigen with known antisera in an agar gel precipitation test showed the isolate to belong to ORT serotype A
  - Antimicrobial sensitivity of the ORT isolate using a disc diffusion test showed the isolate sensitive to amoxicillin, ampicillin, penicillin, tetracycline and enrofloxacin, but resistant to colistin, erythromycin, gentamicin, neomycin, spectinomycin and sulphamethoxol–trimethoprim
  - A culture of lung and air sac for mycoplasma and *Mycoplasma*-genus specific PCR showed negative results for the presence of *Mycoplasma* spp.
  - No *Salmonella* spp. were isolated or detected by PCR from liver and intestines
- Histology:
  - Air sac: severe acute fibrinous airsacculitis
  - Lung: visceral pleuritis
  - Spleen: focal necrosis foci with lymphocytic depletion
  - Other tissues (liver, heart, trachea, kidney and intestines): no lesions observed

Final diagnosis

- Ornithobacteriosis

Discussion

Depression and a decrease in food intake are common findings in poultry chicks associated with an ORT infection. Also in the falcons the food intake was disturbed. Food deprivation affects the development of young falcons. Chicks should receive around five meals daily, without requiring food at night. Between the meals the crop should empty within 3–4 hours. However, when raised by their parents the crop is usually never empty, except early in the morning before first feeding. Weakness of chicks has to be treated as an emergency case with direct support by fluids.

Respiratory problems are common findings in falcons. There is a great variety of possible causative agents of upper and lower respiratory tract disorders. Although some of the listed differentials, e.g. neoplasm or egg binding, are extremely unlikely in young animals, chicks in general are not fully immunocompetent. Therefore they are susceptible to infections, such as respiratory infections, with several bacteria. Also, in this case, the young falcon chicks suffered from a clinically apparent ORT infection, whereas the adults were clinically inapparent. ORT infections are commonly known from chickens and turkeys. In these animals, clinical disease usually appears in animals older than 14 days (turkeys) or 21 days (chickens), although infection might take place earlier. In falcons, previous studies indicated an inapparent infection in adult birds with persisting infections for more than 12 months.

ORT is suspected as a contributing causative agent in respiratory disease complexes in poultry. Concomitant infections with other respiratory pathogens are described regularly. Beside poultry (turkey, chicken, quail) and waterfowl (duck, goose), ORT has been isolated from the respiratory tracts of many different avian species (chukar partridge, guinea fowl, pheasant, partridge, ostrich, rock, gull) and recently from falcons as well. The bacterium is known to be transmitted horizontally by direct and indirect contact, whereby wild birds might act as the source of an infection in poultry. It is susceptible to warm temperatures, but remains viable in a cold environment for a long time (>40 days at 4 °C, >150 days at −12 °C). Consequently, this may be a reason for the higher incidence of ORT infection in poultry during the winter months. Tracheitis, sinusitis, pericarditis, airsacculitis and pneumonia are associated clinical signs of an ornithobacteriosis.

In falcons, the young individuals seem to be more susceptible than older ones. In a previous report, only 10–14-day-old chicks were affected by ORT while older ones and especially adults were inapparent. However, in this report, poor weather conditions might have affected the younger birds, weakening them for disease, whereas the older birds were already more resistant to the cold weather.

As a potential source of the ORT infection, cockerels were identified by ORT-specific PCR, while the baby rats were tested negative for ORT DNA. Additionally, the ORT serotype A, which was isolated from the falcon chicks, is very common in chickens, so that might indicate its origin too. Parallel to this highly contagious infectious agent, a period of cold and rainy weather is likely to contribute to the clinical disease.

Therapy should be based on the results of antibiotic sensitivity tests, as the susceptibility of ORT stains varies distinctly. Amoxicillin and chlortetracycline are probably a good initial choice. Successful vaccination with inactivated vaccines and live vaccines was done solely in poultry but might be an option in falcons as well.

Further reading

Bailey, T., 2008. Raptors: respiratory problems. In: Chitty, J., Lierz, M. (Eds.), BSAVA Manual of Raptors, Pigeons and Passerine Birds. British Small Animal Veterinary Association, Gloucester, pp. 223–234.

Chin, R.P., Van Empel, P.C.M., Hafez, H.M., 2003. *Ornithobacterium rhinotracheale* infection. In: Saif, Y.M. (Ed.), Diseases of Poultry, eleventh ed. Iowa State University Press, Ames, pp. 683–690.
Hafez, H.M., Lierz, M., 2010. *Ornithobacterium rhinotracheale* in nestling falcons. Avian Dis. 54, 161–163.
Lierz, M., 2008. Raptors: reproductive disease, incubation and artificial insemination. In: Chitty, J., Lierz, M. (Eds.), BSAVA Manual of Raptors, Pigeons and Passerine Birds. British Small Animal Veterinary Association, Gloucester, pp. 235–249.
Lierz, M., Hagen, N., Hafez, H.M., 2008. Occurrence of mycoplasmas in free-ranging birds of prey in Germany. J. Wildl. Dis. 44 (4), 845–850.

Case 2.10 *J. Chitty*

Clinical history

A 6-year-old male white-naped raven (*Corvus albicollis*) was presented (Fig. 2.21) as a referral with intermittent appetite and lesions in the mouth. No diagnostics or therapy had been attempted by the referring veterinarian.

Physical examination

The bird was thin, weighing 790 g. There were no obvious clinical signs on examination.

1. How would you examine the bird's mouth?

Ravens have large powerful beaks with sharp edges for tearing. Opening the beak with bare hands is not recommended and with gloves it is hard to control the head adequately. Metal mouth gags may be used though there is a risk of iatrogenic damage to the beak with these (the raven beak being less hard than that of parrots). It was therefore decided to examine the oropharyngeal cavity under isoflurane anaesthesia.

The mouth contained multiple nodules over the pharynx, tongue and oropharyngeal mucosa (Fig. 2.22a, b).

2. What are your differential diagnoses?

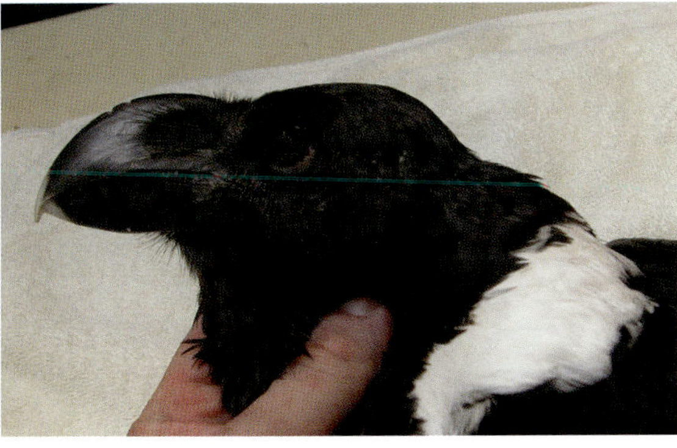

Fig. 2.21 Photograph of the white-naped raven presented for examination.

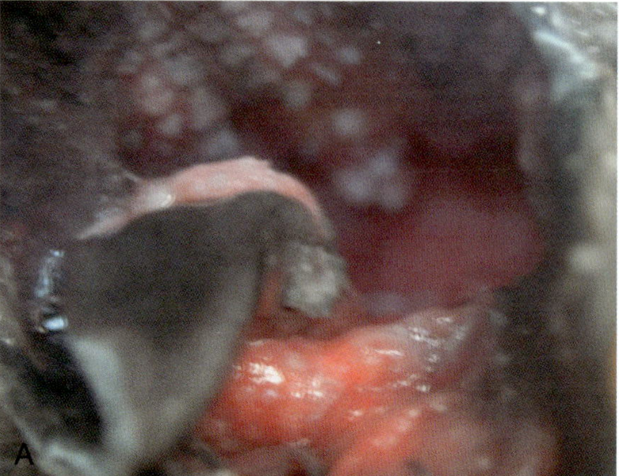

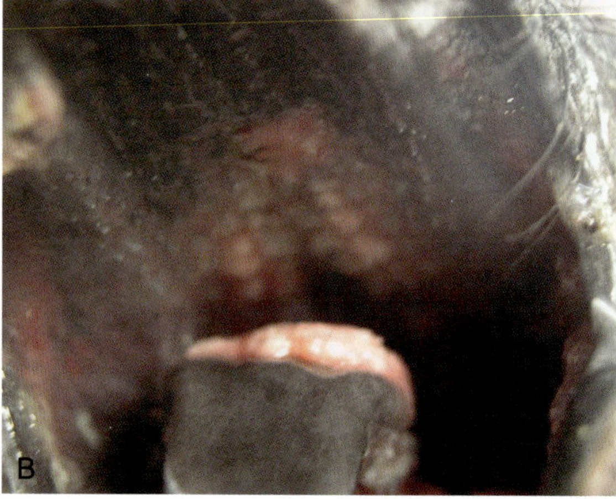

Fig. 2.22 (a) Photograph from the oropharyngeal cavity of the white-naped raven; (b) close-up photograph from the oropharyngeal cavity of the white-naped raven.

Differential diagnoses

- Infection
  - Bacterial (possibly secondary to trauma)
  - Fungal (especially *Candida* spp.)
  - Parasitic (especially *Trichomonas* spp. and *Capillaria* spp.)
- Neoplasia
- Irritant reaction
- Hypovitaminosis A and squamous metaplasia

Q *3. How would you investigate these lesions?*

- Blood
- Faecal examination

- Pharyngeal/crop endoscopy
- Biopsy

Clinical diagnosis laboratory examination

Given financial constraints, the owner elected for faecal examination and biopsy only. Biopsies were taken as pinch specimens using 5FR endoscopic grabs.

- Faecal examination revealed eggs of *Capillaria* nematodes
- Biopsy confirmed capillariasis with no secondary infection

 ***4. How would you treat this bird?***

Therapy

Fenbendazole was given at a rate of 20 mg/kg SID for 5 days. A second faecal sample was checked a few days after this and found to be clear for the presence of ova. The oral lesions largely resolved within 3 months though there was some residual scarring.

 ***5. Would you start any long-term prophylaxis?***

Discussion

Given the feeding habits of ravens and their inquisitive nature, they are always prone to parasitic infection in captivity as they will eat invertebrates or small mammals that enter the aviary.

The owner was unwilling to concrete over or to cover the natural flooring of the aviary. Therefore a system of 3–6 monthly faecal checks was instigated with deworming based on the results of these tests.

This case illustrates the effects of a bird's feeding habits on the infections they are likely to pick up. This is especially worth considering with particularly exotic species such as this. Aviary design and prophylactic regimens should reflect this.

Capillariasis is common and can be life threatening. Avermectins appear not to be effective nor are single high doses of benzimidazoles. Fenbendazole given at low dose over several days appears effective in most cases though some may require a second course.

Further reading

Gelis, S., 2006. Evaluating and treating the gastrointestinal system. In: Harrison, G., Lightfoot, T. (Eds.), Clinical Avian Medicine. Spix Publishing, Palm Beach, pp. 411–440.

Yabsley, M., 2008. Capillarid nematodes. In: Atkinson, C.T., Thomas, N.J., Hunter, D.B. (Eds.), Parasitic Diseases of Wild Birds. Wiley-Blackwell, Ames, pp. 463–500.

Zucca, P., Delogu, M., 2008. Helminths. In: Samour, J. (Ed.), Avian Medicine, second ed. Mosby Elsevier, Oxford, pp. 325–336.

Case 2.11 *L. Crosta*

Clinical history

An adult female Canada goose (*Branta canadensis*), hosted in a zoological garden, was presented because of the presence of a mass in the lower eyelid/conjunctival sac for the past 2 months (Fig. 2.23). Although the bird was apparently behaving normally, it was often blinking and was separated from the flock.

Clinical examination

On presentation, the bird was in good physical conditions (4/5). The lesion was localized and apparently did not affect the bird other than local distress. Blood was collected to run haematology and blood chemistry testing. In addition, a faecal sample was taken to screen for the presence of endoparasites.

1. What is your interpretation of the lesion in Fig. 2.23?

Clinical diagnosis laboratory

The results of the clinical diagnosis laboratory assays are shown in Tables 2.16 and 2.17.

RBC, WBC and thrombocyte morphology

- Nothing abnormal detected

2. What is your interpretation of the haematology and blood chemistry values shown in Tables 2.16 and 2.17?

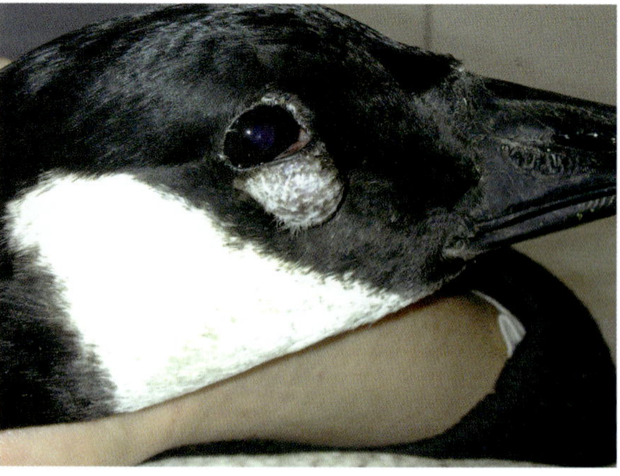

Fig. 2.23 The mass on the lower eyelid of the Canada goose female.

Table 2.16 Haematology values of the Canada goose

Parameters	Results (absolute)	Results (%)	Reference values
Hct (l/l)	0.46		0.47±0.07 (0.40–0.54)
WBC (×10⁹/l)	30.9		9.47±3.68 (13.15–15.79)
Heterophils (×10⁹/l)	24.1	78	5.77±3.2 (2.57–8.97)
Lymphocytes (×10⁹/l)	6.79	22	3.07±3.0 (0.07–6.07)
Monocytes (×10⁹/l)		0	0.42±0.05 (0.03–0.9)
Eosinophils (×10⁹/l)		0	0.27±0.04 (0.0–0.68)
Basophils (×10⁹/l)		0	0.05±0.02 (0.0–0.29)

Table 2.17 Blood chemistry values of the Canada goose

Analysis	Results	Reference values
Albumin (g/dl)	2.0	1.6±0.2
Bile acids (µmol/l)	86	<100
Calcium (mmol/l)	9.5	10.3±0.7
CK (U/l)	780	779±562
GOT (U/l)	58	45±20
Globulin (g/dl)	3.8	2.1±0.4
Glucose (mg/dl)	254	195±86
LDH (U/l)	403	367±207
Phosphorus (mg/dl)	3.4	2.0±0.9
Total protein (g/dl)	5.8	4.1±0.7
Uric acid (mg/dl)	7.0	5.5±2.4

Results

- No parasites were observed in the faecal examination
- Haematology analysis showed elevated WBC with heterophilia
- The blood chemistry analysis showed an elevated globulin level

Please evaluate the clinical history, Fig. 2.23, the results of the physical examination and clinical diagnosis laboratory tests.

Q *3. List your differential diagnoses.*

Q *4. List your therapeutic strategy.*

Differential diagnoses

- Abscess
- Tuberculosis
- Neoplasm

Therapy

The primary treatment selected was the surgical removal of the lesion and submission for histopathology and microbiology.

Laboratory findings

- Microbiology: no bacteria or fungi were isolated from the lesion
- Histology: abscess with centrally caseous necrotic material surrounded by active cellular mass with regularly large multinuclear reactive cells. The whole process is encapsulated in a fibrous capsule
- Acid-fast staining: negative

Final diagnosis

- Sterile abscess

Discussion

Canada geese are among the most common waterfowl species kept in captivity. Although avian tuberculosis is not believed to be very common in wild Canada geese, it is reported more frequently in captive waterfowl. Avian tuberculosis is predominantly a chronic and wasting disease, but localized forms, such as when the eye is involved, may have only local symptoms. This is why avian TB must always be taken into consideration when dealing with wasting diseases in captive waterfowl, but also in the presence of isolated masses. The very high WBC and the relative heterophilia are indicative of a serious inflammatory process. Furthermore, the bird was kept in a bird park and it may have been in contact with visitors. All these facts must be taken into consideration when dealing with zoo animals. Euthanasia is always an option when there is a serious problem with public health. In this case, the zoo premises allowed for a strict isolation of the bird until the lesion was excised and analysed. To date, the gold standard for the diagnosis of mycobacterial infection is culture, since acid-fast staining is not able to differentiate between different *Mycobacterium* species. Nevertheless, negative histopathology coupled with negative Ziehl-Neelsen staining was enough to exclude avian TB.

Further reading

Converse, K.A., 2007. Avian tuberculosis. In: Thomas, N.J., Hunter, B.D., Atkinson, C.T. (Eds.), Infectious Diseases of Wild Birds. Blackwell Publishing, Ames, pp. 289–302.

Flinchum, G.B., 2006. Waterfowl. In: Harrison, G.J., Lightfoot, T. (Eds.), Clinical Avian Medicine. Spix Publishing Inc., Palm Beach, pp. 831–848.

Forbes, N.A., Cromie, R.L., Brown, M.J., et al., 1993. Diagnosis of avian tuberculosis in waterfowl. In: Proceedings of the Annual Conference of the Association of Avian Veterinarians. pp. 182–186.

Olsen, J.H., 1994. Anseriformes. In: Ritchie, B.W., Harrison, G.J., Harrison, L.R. (Eds.), Avian Medicine: Principle and Application. Wingers Publishing, Inc., Lake Worth, pp. 1237–1275.

Tell, L.A., Woods, L., Cromie, R.L., 2001. Mycobacteriosis in birds. Rev. Sci. Tech. 20, 180–203.

Tell, L.A., Foley, J., Needham, M.L., et al., 2003. Diagnosis of avian mycobacteriosis: comparison of culture, acid-fast stains, and polymerase chain reaction for the identification of *Mycobacterium avium* in experimentally inoculated Japanese quail (*Coturnix coturnix japonica*). Avian Dis. 47, 444–452.

Case 2.12 *M. Lierz, D. Fischer*

Clinical history

A 2-year-old Toulouse gander (*Anser anser dom.*) weighing 7200 g (Fig. 2.24) was presented with the following clinical signs:

- Reduced to somnolent behaviour
- Inappetence
- Progressive weight loss
- Slight enophthalmus
- Slightly flushed conjunctivas
- Dehydration.

The gander was kept outside together with 40 other geese as companion animals, not destined for food production. The feed consisted of grass from the field, supplemented with corn and other cereals.

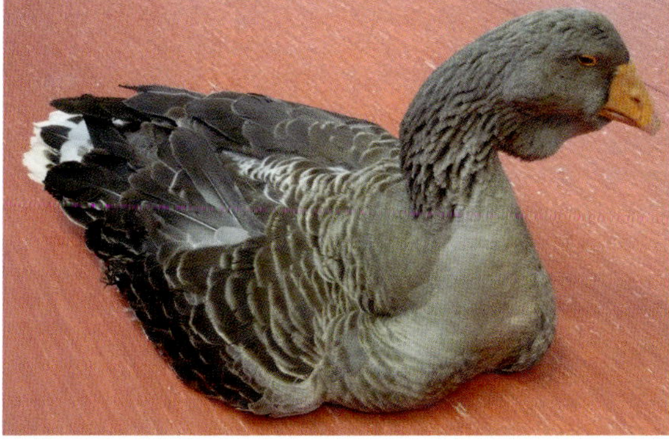

Fig. 2.24 Toulouse gander (*Anser anser dom.*) unable to stand as presented for examination.

Physical examination

At presentation, the gander had a moderate to reduced body condition (body condition score of 2.5/5). It was unable to stand or to walk on its own, but able to stand and to extend the wings when it was supported by the owner. The gander demonstrated swallowing behaviour and regurgitation parallel to a slight tremor. The mucous membranes of the oropharynx were pale rose. Inspection and palpation of neck, abdomen and both legs revealed no abnormal findings or injuries.

Clinical diagnosis examination

Radiographs were taken in the ventrodorsal and latero-lateral views (Fig. 2.25a, b). Blood samples were collected for haematocrit analysis, blood chemistry and examination for the presence of lead or zinc. A faecal sample was collected to examine as fresh smear and following the flotation process.

Radiology (see Fig. 2.25)

1. What is your interpretation of the radiographs in Fig. 2.25a, b?

Clinical diagnosis laboratory examination

The results of the clinical diagnosis laboratory assays are shown in Tables 2.18 and 2.19.

2. What is your interpretation of the blood chemistry and haematocrit values shown in Table 2.18?

Results

- Radiographic findings included numerous radiopaque particles in the proventriculus and ventriculus. Some of the particles were longish, narrow and pointed, while other particles were circular shaped. Air sacs, kidneys and the liver appeared normal. The great vessels in the cardiac region were distinctly visible. No injuries of bones or joints were detectable
- The faecal examination revealed a few flagellates in the fresh smear. Following the flotation process (9 g NaCl/l *aqua destillata*) a high amount of nematode eggs of the genus *Amidostomum* and a moderate amount of *Capillaria* eggs were demonstrated
- Blood chemistry analysis showed low values of total protein, albumin, AST and potassium
- Haematocrit analysis showed low PCV/Hct
- A marked heterophilia was present
- The blood examination for the presence of heavy metals showed no evidence of zinc or lead toxicity

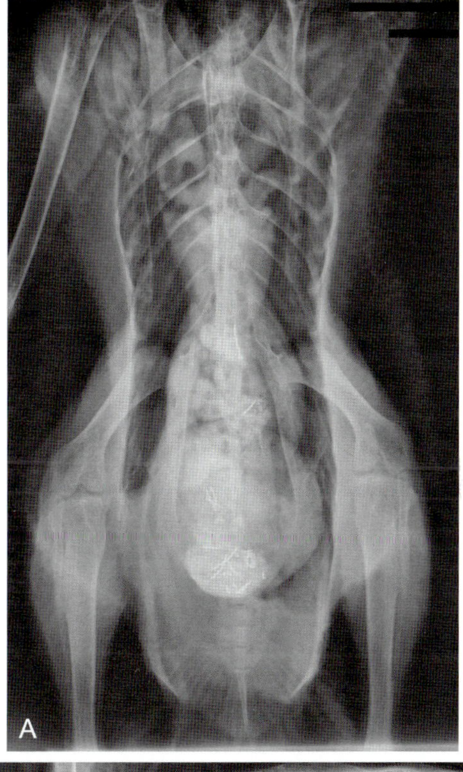

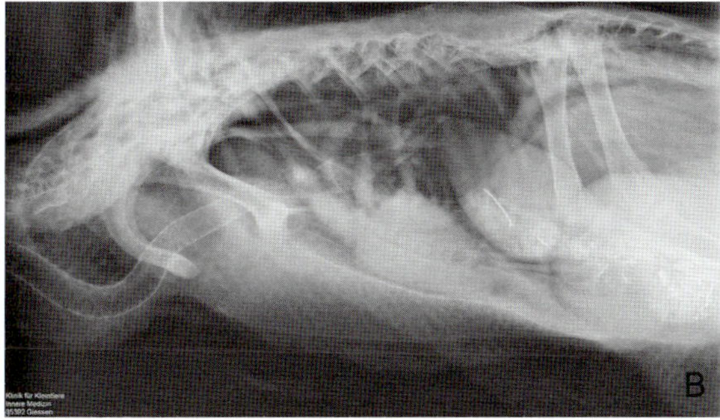

Fig. 2.25 (a) Radiography of the Toulose gander in ventrodorsal and (b) latero-lateral views. Radiodense material is clearly visible in the proventriculus and ventriculus.

Please evaluate the clinical history, Fig. 2.25a, b, the results of the physical examination and clinical diagnosis laboratory tests.

Q *3. List your differential diagnoses for reduced motility, for nervous and central nervous abnormalities and for inappetence and weight loss.*

Q *4. List your therapeutic strategy.*

Table 2.18 Blood chemistry and haematological values of the Toulouse gander

Analysis	Results	Reference values[1]
Albumin (g/dl)	<1.0	1.5±0.2
Bile acids (μmol/l)	35	—
CK (U/l)	1146	—
AST (U/l)	40	125±82
Glucose (mg/dl)	202	230±31
Total protein (g/dl)	2.5	4.4±0.7
Phosphorus (mg/dl)	3.1	3.3±1.3
Calcium (mmol/l)	9.3	10.1±0.6
Ca/P	3/1	—
Sodium (mmol/l)	141	140
Potassium (mmol/l)	2.6	3.1
Uric acid (mg/dl)	5	7.5±1.9
	Results	**Reference values[2]**
PCV (%)	33	38±3
Heterophils (%)	80	47.4
Eosinophils (%)	1	3.3
Basophils (%)	0	< 1
Lymphocytes (%)	15	38.7
Monocytes (%)	4	6.7
Thrombocytes	15.4 giga/l	—

[1]*Reference values = values for male Embden goose as there are none available for Toulouse or grey geese (*Anser anser*); published in: Ritchie BW, Harrison GJ, Harrison LR (1994) Avian Medicine – Principles and Application. Wingers Publishing, Lake Worth, p. 1344.*

[2]*Lucas and Jamroz (1961) Atlas of Avian Hematology. Agriculture Monograph 25, United States Department of Agriculture, Washington.*

Table 2.19 Lead and zinc levels of the Toulouse gander

	Results	Toxic limit value
Zinc (μg/l/ppm)	1680/1.68 ppm	>2000/>3
Lead (μg/l/ppm)	8/l/0.08 ppm	/>0.4

Differential diagnoses for reduced motility

- Orthopaedic reasons – inflammatory, degenerative and traumatic lesions of the musculoskeletal system (skin, soft tissue, bones, joints, tendons, tendon sheets)
- Lesions to the spinal cord/other parts of the central nervous system of various geneses
- Nephropathy of various geneses, e.g. parasitic (coccidia), viral (polyomavirus), bacterial, toxic (heavy metals, pesticides, mycotoxins), drugs (aminoglycosides) or neoplastic
- Abdominal pain of various geneses, e.g. parasitic (flagellates)

Differential diagnoses for nervous and central nervous abnormalities

- Viral (e.g. Newcastle disease virus, avian influenza virus, West Nile virus)
- Bacterial (e.g. *Salmonella* spp., *Chlamydophila* spp., *Mycobacterium* spp., *Listeria* spp.)
- Fungal (e.g. *Aspergillus* spp.)
- Parasitic (e.g. *Toxoplasma gondii)*
- Toxic (e.g. botulinum toxin, heavy metals, carbamates, organic phosphates, mycotoxins)
- Vitamin B1 (thiamine) deficiency
- Vitamin E (alpha-tocopherol) and/or selenium deficiency
- Metabolic (e.g. hypocalcaemia, hypoglycaemia, hypernatraemia)
- Excretory disorders (e.g. uricaemia)
- Hepatic encephalopathy (hyperammonaemia)

Differential diagnoses for inappetence and weight loss

- Lesions of the oropharynx and the gastrointestinal tract of various geneses (e.g. traumatic, inflammatory, neoplastic)
- Lesions of mucous membranes due to hypovitaminosis A
- Parasitic (e.g. different endoparasites, trichomonads)
- Fungal (e.g. *Macrorhabdus ornithogaster*)
- Bacterial

Final diagnosis

- Foreign body uptake
- Capillariosis, amidostomumosis
- Anaemia

Surgery and aftercare

As an endoscopic removal of the numerous, splinter-like and sharp foreign bodies was predicted impossible, surgery was performed under isoflurane inhalation anaesthesia. Previous to surgery the patient was given premedication (Table 2.20).

Table 2.20 Premedication

Carprofen	5 mg/kg IM once
Marbofloxacin 1%	10 mg/kg IM once
Fluids	Ringer's lactate mixed with 5% glucose solution to same parts 20 ml/kg SC

The goose was positioned in dorsal recumbency with lifted upper body and extended legs. A continuous infusion with Ringer's lactate was given via intravenous catheter in the left basilic vein. As a surgical approach, a T-shaped approach in the ventral midline was chosen. After opening the coelomic cavity, the ventriculus and proventriculus were positioned to the surgical wound and fixed with stay sutures. Proventriculotomy was performed on the ventral aspect of the organ to remove the inner foreign bodies. It was possible to access the ventriculus through the proventriculotomy incision. Using a magnetic bar, 22 splinter-like metallic pieces, two nails and one ring washer, were removed from the ventriculus (Fig. 2.26). Endoscopic exploration of the gastric organs and control radiographs confirmed the successful removal of all foreign bodies, so that the proventriculotomy incision was sutured. After coelomic lavage with saline solution, the incisions in muscles and skin were stitched. Local disinfection and covering of the suture with bandage was performed. The bird recovered well from anaesthesia and received post-surgical care (Table 2.21).

On the fourth day post-surgery the gander was able to eat on its own. Two weeks post-surgery it was successfully released from the veterinary clinic.

Discussion

The combination of foreign body-induced pain and the negative impact of endoparasites might have caused the clinical symptoms in the Toulouse gander. *Amidostomum anseris* is reported with clinical symptoms such as inappetence, weakness, diarrhoea, weight loss, anaemia, protein loss and death. These findings are common in 3–8-week-old chicks, while adults are mostly asymptomatic carriers. Capillariosis may cause similar symptoms in young geese after the epithelial cells of crop, oesophagus, small intestine and caecum are destroyed by the parasites.

The uptake of foreign bodies is common in birds, especially in parrots, ratites and water fowl. Fishhooks, plastics, wood, stones and nails are frequently swallowed by water fowl. *Anseriformes* in particular seem to be predisposed to foreign body uptake because of their unselective way of grazing. Fortunately, in most cases, the *corpus alienum* is not related to clinical symptoms or afflictions, so that a surgical removal is not indicated.

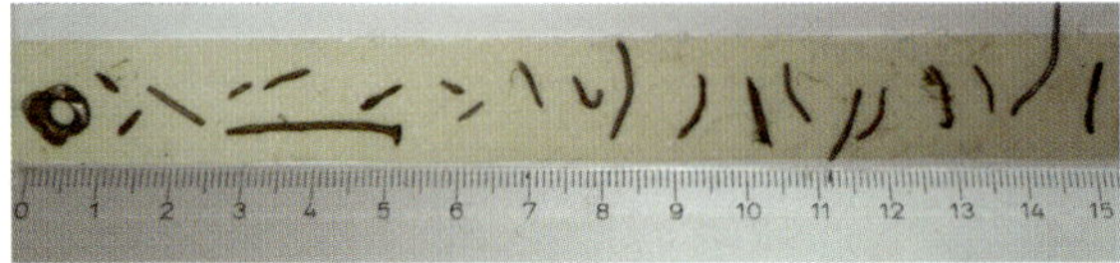

Fig. 2.26 Foreign bodies surgically removed from the proventriculus and ventriculus of the Toulouse gander.

Table 2.21 Post-surgical care

Marbofloxacin 1%	10 mg/kg IM SID × 10 days
Itraconazole	10 mg/kg PO SID 10 days prophylactic
Fluids	Ringer's lactate mixed with 5% glucose solution to same parts 20 ml/kg SC TID × 3 days
Meloxicam 0.5%	0.4 mg/kg IM × 5 days past surgery
Vitamin E	30 g alpha tocopherol/kg IM once
Ca-EDTA	Initial 200 mg/kg IM, from second day on 40 mg/kg IM × 3 days (prophylactic, until the negative results for zinc and lead became known)
Forced feeding with a plastic tube	Mixture of Harrison's Bird Food Recovery Formulary™, Herbi Care Plus® and water, 40–60 ml BID one day after surgery and TID on the following 3 days
Fenbendazole 10%	25 mg/kg PO × 3 days
Physiotherapy	Starting on 4th day post-surgery

In some cases, the incorporated material, e.g. lead or zinc, leads to a clinical manifestation of intoxication. In suspected cases, blood tests are required as a diagnostic measure to confirm a started therapy with antidotes. In the described case, Ca-EDTA was given prophylactically after the removal of potentially zinc-coated nails, until the lab results negated the presence of zinc or lead poisoning.

If foreign bodies cause clinical symptoms, an endoscopic removal should be preferred to a surgical removal. In this case, a proventriculotomy was chosen because of the numerous and hard to reach foreign bodies. The successfully used surgical approach in the ventral midline was reported in ratites previously as an approach for proventriculotomy. In other bird species, a lateral approach on the left vent was used alternatively. A proventriculotomy was preferred to a ventriculotomy in this case, because the latter was estimated as more difficult due to strong muscle layers and a potent blood supply of the ventriculus. However, a gastrotomy by incising the saccus caudalis ventriculi has been described in ducks as a practical method with low risk too. The use of a flexible bar magnet benefitted in the removal of the metallic particles, whereas it would have been of no advantage in the removal of non-magnetic foreign bodies.

Further reading

Bowles, H.L., Odberg, E., Harrison, G.J., et al., 2006. Surgical resolutions of soft tissue disorders. In: Harrison, G.J., Lightfoot, T.L. (Eds.), Clinical Avian Medicine. Spix Publishing, Palm Beach, pp. 806.

Fischer, D., Kraut, S., Hampel, M.R., et al., 2010. Surgical removal of foreign bodies in a gander by using a bar magnet. Tierärztl. Prax. 38 (K), 172–177.

Forbes, N.A., 2002. Avian gastrointestinal surgery. Seminars in Avian and Exotic Pet Medicine 11 (4), 196–207.

Lloyd, M., 1992. Heavy metal ingestion: medical management and gastroscopic foreign body removal. J. Assoc. of Avian Vet. 6 (1), 25–29.

McCluggage, D., 1992. Proventriculotomy: a study of select cases. In: Proceedings of the Association of Avian Veterinarians. pp. 195–200.

Case 2.13 *P. Sandmeier*

Clinical history

A female Papua hornbill (*Aceros plicatus*) of unknown age (Fig. 2.27), weighing 1220 g was presented with the following clinical signs of a few weeks' duration:

- Slight general listlessness
- Reduced feather quality.

The hornbill had been kept in the same breeding facility for over 10 years and was fed a diet of mixed fruit and vegetables, a commercial hornbill diet (Nutribird®) and a vitamin mineral supplement.

Clinical examination

On presentation, the bird had a good body condition. The feather condition was poor with dull contour feathers and many broken flight and tail feathers. Abdominal palpation was unremarkable. Under general anaesthesia using isoflurane, survey radiographs were taken and blood samples were collected for haematology and blood chemistry. A faecal sample was collected to examine for endoparasites.

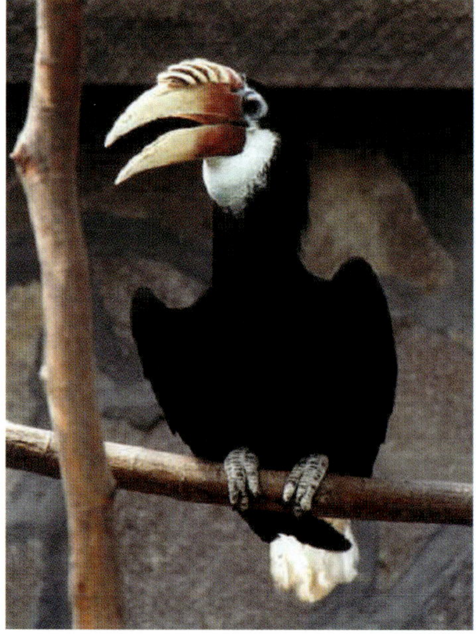

Fig. 2.27 Female Papua hornbill.

Clinical diagnosis examination

Radiology (Fig. 2.28)

Q 1. *What is your interpretation of the radiographs in Fig. 2.28a, b?*

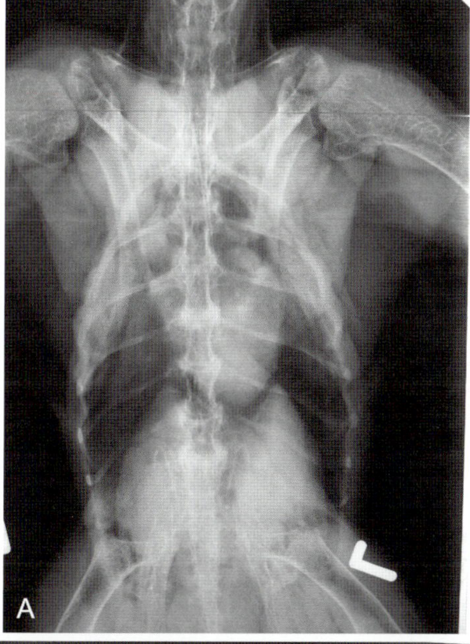

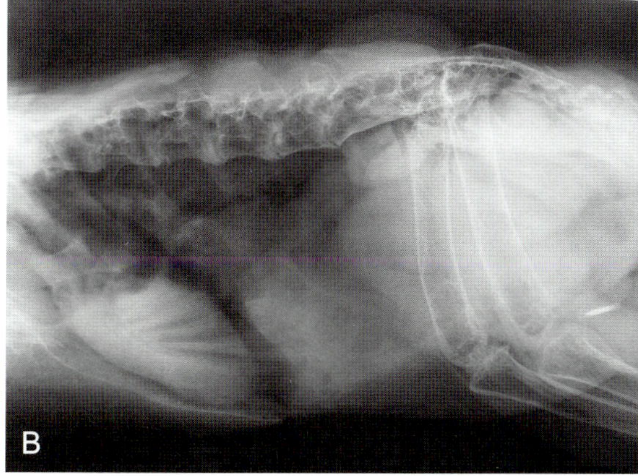

Fig. 2.28 (a) Ventrodorsal and (b) lateral survey radiographs of the Papua hornbill.

Clinical diagnosis laboratory

The results of the laboratory assays are shown in Tables 2.22 and 2.23.

2. What is your interpretation of the haematology and blood chemistry values shown in Tables 2.22 and 2.23?

Results

- Faecal examination negative for the presence of endoparasites
- Radiographic findings included a slightly enlarged liver shadow

Table 2.22 Haematology values of the Papua hornbill

Parameters	Results (absolute)	Results (%)	Morphology
Hct		43	
WBC ($\times 10^9$/l)	28.8		
Heterophils ($\times 10^9$/l)	21.25	72.4	Physiological
Lymphocytes ($\times 10^9$/l)	3.52	12	Physiological
Monocytes ($\times 10^9$/l)	2.9	9.9	Physiological
Eosinophils ($\times 10^9$/l)	0.81	3.6	
Basophils ($\times 10^9$/l)	0.61	2.1	
Thrombocytes ($\times 10^9$/l)	54.7		Activated

No reference values available.

Table 2.23 Blood chemistry values of the Papua hornbill

Parameter	Results
Albumin (g/l)	16
AST (U/l)	94
Bile acids (μmol/l)	95
Calcium (mmol/l)	2.27
Globulin (g/l)	39
Glucose (mmol/l)	13.86
LDH (U/l)	478
Total protein (g/l)	55
Total iron (μmol/l)	128
Uric acid (μmol/l)	352

No reference values available.

- Haematology analysis showed a moderate leucocytosis with a relative and absolute heterophilia/monocytosis/eosinophilia, a relative lymphopenia and a physiological morphology
- Blood chemistry analysis showed suspected elevated bile acids

Please evaluate the clinical history, the radiographic findings, Fig. 2.28a, b, the results of the physical examination and clinical diagnosis laboratory tests.

Q *3. List your differential diagnoses.*

Q *4. List your plan for further diagnostics.*

Differential diagnoses

- Hepatopathy:
  - Viral hepatitis
  - Bacterial hepatitis
  - Iron storage disease
  - Fatty liver degeneration
  - Toxic liver degeneration
  - Liver neoplasia
  - Liver amyloidosis
- Systemic chronic infectious disease:
  - Viral, chlamydial, bacterial, mycobacterial, fungal

Further diagnostics

- Liver biopsy (Fig. 2.29)
- MRI

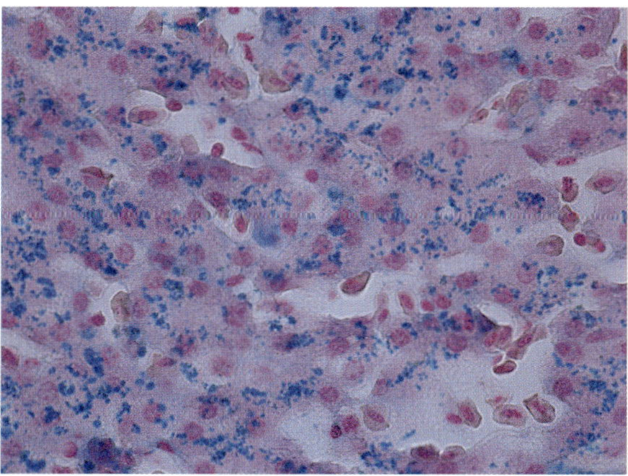

Fig. 2.29 Prussian blue-stained liver histology sample.

Final diagnosis

- Iron storage disease

4. List your therapeutic strategy and your strategy to monitor the therapeutic success.

Therapy (Table 2.24)

Therapy monitoring

- Serial liver biopsies to monitor liver iron content (Table 2.25)
- Magnetic resonance imaging (MRI) (Table 2.26).

Table 2.24 Therapy

Enrofloxacin	10 mg/kg PO BID until results of liver biopsy obtained
Deferiprone (Ferriprox®), oral iron chelator	75 mg/kg PO SID 3 months
Milk thistle extract	350 mg PO SID 3 months
Replace mineral supplement with iron-free supplement	

Table 2.25 Serial liver biopsies

Method	Time	Result (%)
Quantitative image analysis	Pre-treatment	35.5
	30 days into treatment	4.1
	60 days into treatment	3.7
	90 days into treatment	0.3

Table 2.26 MRI

Method	Time	Result
MRI	Pre-treatment	7260±1675 mg/kg tissue
	70 days into treatment	1675±1117 mg/kg tissue

Discussion

Successful treatment of iron storage disease is only possible if diagnosed before the patient develops liver failure and ascites. In susceptible species such as hornbills, toucans, mynahs, starlings or birds of paradise showing non-specific signs of disease and with a non-diagnostic basic database, iron storage disease should always be considered. Due to the fact that serum iron levels do not correlate with liver iron content, a diagnosis can only be made based on liver biopsies or MRI. Being non-invasive, MRI has become the method of choice for calculating liver iron content in human patients. If available, this diagnostic option can also be considered in avian patients.

Treatments described include weekly phlebotomies as well as daily injections of the iron chelator deferoxamine. Both of these methods involve regular and severe stress for the patient. The oral iron chelator deferiprone (Ferriprox®), used in this case, has proven to be very effective in reducing the liver iron content and can be administered with food. In all cases, the iron content of the diet must be assessed and, if necessary, corrected. Factors influencing iron uptake (high levels of ascorbic acid, stress, chronic inflammation) should be addressed if possible.

Treatment success can be monitored by quantifying the liver iron content in serial liver biopsies using quantitative image analysis. The mean percentage of blue-staining (iron) area in a Prussian blue-stained histological sample is determined using a PC-based image analysis system. For each liver sample, ten randomly chosen areas are examined and the mean percentage calculated.

Further reading

Cork, S.C., Alley, M.R., Stockdale, P.H.G., 1995. A quantitative assessment of hemosiderosis in wild and captive birds using image analysis. Avian Pathol. 24, 239–254.

Gandon, Y., Olivié, D., Guyader, D., et al., 2004. Non-invasive assessment of hepatic iron stores by MRI. The Lancet 363, 357–362.

Lowenstine, L.J., Munson, L., 1999. Iron overload in the animal kingdom. In: Fowler, M.E., Miller, R.E. (Eds.), Zoo and Wild Animal Medicine, Current Therapy 4. WB Saunders, Philadelphia, pp. 260–268.

Sandmeier, P., Clauss, M., Donati, O.F., et al., The use of deferiprone in the treatment of iron storage disease in three hornbills. Sequential monitoring of the liver iron content by quantitative image analysis, quantitative chemical analysis and magnetic resonance imaging. J. Am. Vet. Med. Assoc. accepted for publication.

Case 2.14 *T. A. Bailey*

Clinical history

An adult female trumpeter hornbill (*Bycanistes bucinator*) weighing 410 g (weight 12 months earlier at a health check when healthy was 430 g), was presented with the following non-specific clinical signs of unknown duration:

- Lethargy
- Decreased appetite.

The bird had been part of a shipment of wild caught birds that were confiscated by Custom authorities. It had been in the zoological collection for more than 5 years. It had been housed alone in a large outdoor aviary since its partner died of iron storage disease the previous year.

Clinical examination

On physical examination, she weighed 410 g, was in fair body condition and had a quiet demeanour. No neurological or behavioural abnormalities were recorded.

Survey radiographs were taken while the bird was under anaesthesia (Fig. 2.30a, b). Blood samples were collected for haematology and blood chemistry. Subsequently, endoscopy was performed through the left caudal thoracic air sac. Two liver biopsies were collected. Aerobic bacteriology and cytology were conducted on the first sample. The second biopsy was fixed in neutral 10 % buffered formalin and submitted for histology.

Parasitology crop swabs for wet preparation and faecal samples for direct smear and flotation were performed.

A rapid antigen capture test (Speed CHLAM, BVT, France) was performed on a swab of the faecal sample for chlamydophilosis.

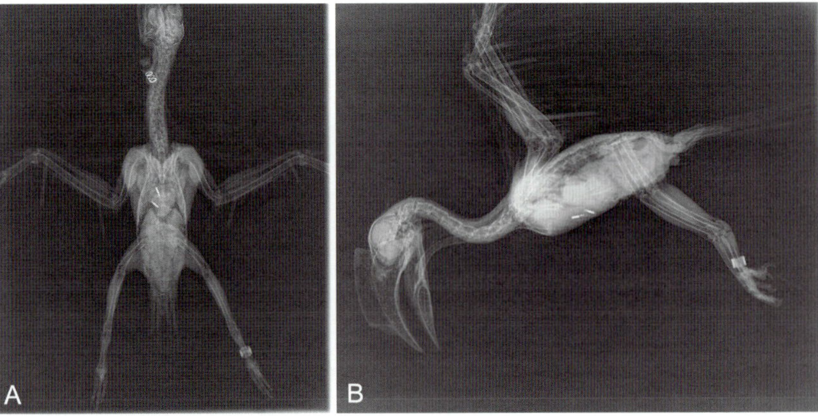

Fig. 2.30 (a) Ventrodorsal survey radiograph of trumpeter hornbill; (b) lateral survey radiograph of the trumpeter hornbill.

Radiology (see Fig. 2.30a, b)

Q *1. What is your interpretation of the radiographs in Fig. 2.30a, b?*

- Radiographic findings included a grossly enlarged liver shadow causing loss of the cardiohepatic "waist", cranial and dorsal displacement of the liver, distinct hepatic margins and outline and increased radio-opacity of the liver. The dorsal displacement of the liver has also displaced the proventriculus dorsally and there is compression of the area of the caudal thoracic air sacs

Endoscopy findings

- Endoscopy examination was challenging because of difficulty accessing the caudal thoracic air-sac space resulting from a liver that was displaced dorsally and cranially. The air sacs, lungs and intestines appeared normal in colour, shape and texture. The liver was enlarged with rounded margins and the surface was moderately congested. The liver texture was friable when biopsied (Fig. 2.31).

Clinical diagnosis laboratory results

- Faecal examination was negative for the presence of endoparasites
- Examination of saline crop swabs was negative for the presence of parasites
- The antigen capture test for chlamydophilosis was negative
- Aerobic bacteriology and fungal culture on hepatic biopsy material yielded no growth

The results of the clinical diagnosis laboratory assays are shown in Tables 2.27 and 2.28.

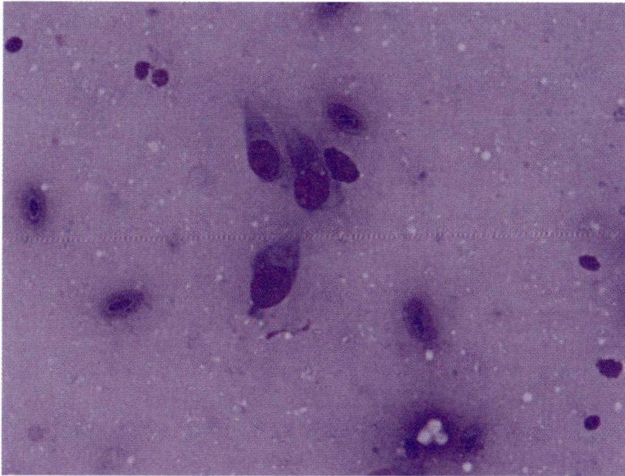

Fig. 2.31 Liver imprint cytology of trumpeter hornbill.

Table 2.27 Haematology values of the trumpeter hornbill (mean±standard deviation)

Parameters	Results	Reference values*	Reference values** (ISIS)
Hb (g/dl)	15.9	16.1±2.1	17.0±5.2
Hct (l/l)	38	46.7±5.2	53.6±4.3
MCHC (g/dl)	41.84	33.9±3.3	31.2±2.4
WBC (×10⁹/l)	7.5	11.65±5.4	8.8±5.2
Heterophils (×10⁹/l)	4.95	6.2±3.8	3.4±2.3
Lymphocytes (×10⁹/l)	1.13	4.4±3.4	4.1±4.1
Monocytes (×10⁹/l)	1.35	0.8±0.9	0.6±0.5
Eosinophils (×10⁹/l)	0.08	0.4±0.4	0.3±0.2
Basophils (×10⁹/l)	0	0.3±0.2	0.3±0.3

**Values for the great Indian hornbill as no data available for trumpeter hornbill (Dutton, 2003).*
***ISIS values are for trumpeter hornbills (n 3–29).*

Table 2.28 Blood chemistry values of the trumpeter hornbill

Analysis	Results	Reference values* (ISIS)
Albumin (g/l)	9	13±2
Bile acid (μmol/l)	9	nd
Calcium (mmol/l)	2.4	2.1±0.2
Chloride (μmol/l)	119	117±5
CK (U/l)	3183	729±409
GGT (U/l)	2	6±2
AST (U/l)	305	147±53
ALT (U/l)	104	68±44
Glucose (mmol/l)	22.6	17.21±6.7
Iron (μmol/l)	7	nd
Phosphorus (mmol/l)	0.62	1.0±0.9
Potassium (mmol/l)	2.37	4.1±2.9
Sodium (mmol/l)	166	156±5
Total protein (g/l)	26	36±6
Total urea (mmol/l)	0.9	1.5±0
Uric acid (mmol/l)	0.188	0.46±0.28

**ISIS values are for trumpeter hornbills (n 3–29).*

RBC, WBC and thrombocyte morphology

- Nothing abnormal detected

Cytology (Fig. 2.31)

2. What is your interpretation of the haematology and blood chemistry values shown in Tables 2.27 and 2.28 and the cytology in Fig. 2.31?

Results

- Impression smears of liver showed hepatocytes with signs of metaplasia, nuclear pleomorphism, dispersed chromatin and multiple nucleoli. Many mononuclear cells resembling reactive lymphocytes were apparent in other fields
- Haematology analysis showed a mild monocytosis, a lymphopenia and a low PCV and a raised MCHC
- Blood chemistry analysis showed elevated levels of ALT, CK and AST. While high AST levels may result from liver pathology, the elevated CK and AST levels can also occur following muscle damage (perhaps in this case associated with the stress of catching the bird). Therefore, in this case, while elevated AST levels may be associated with liver pathology, the elevated CK confuses the situation. ALT is a non-specific enzyme and is present in most avian tissues so the raised levels indicate non-specific cell damage. Although there are no normal values for trumpeter hornbills for bile acids, the level in this bird appears normal when compared to levels in other avian species.

3. How reliable is the negative rapid Chlamydia spp. antigen capture test on the faecal sample?

Pooled choanal and oropharyngeal swabs are considered to be more consistent for the isolation of the agent than faecal swabs, especially in the early stages of infection. Consequently, swabs from the choana and cloaca should be collected for *Chlamydophila* spp. antigen testing. Conducting a rapid antigen test on a faecal sample may not be sensitive enough if a bird is in the early stages of infection.

An ocular–choanal–cloacal swab submitted from this bird for *Chlamydophila* spp. ELISA antigen testing was negative.

Please evaluate the clinical history, Figs 2.30a, b and 2.31, the results of the physical examination and clinical diagnosis laboratory tests.

4. List your differential diagnoses.

Findings of hepatomegaly with an inflammatory process in the liver of a hornbill would be consistent with:

- Chlamydophilosis
- Viral hepatitis (herpes, adenovirus, polyomavirus)
- Bacterial hepatitis including mycobacteria
- Fungal hepatitis

- Parasitic disease (toxoplasmosis, sarcocystosis)
- Neoplasia
- Metabolic disease – haemochromatosis.

Histopathology findings (Fig. 2.32)

Please evaluate the histopathology photomicrograph (Fig. 2.32) and re-evaluate your differential diagnosis list.

Liver histology revealed some heterophils, mild interstitial hepatitis, a mild haemosiderosis of Kupffer cells, and some hepatocytes containing large, pale intranuclear (arrow) (polyomavirus-like) inclusions were seen (Fig. 2.32). A provisional diagnosis of viral hepatitis was made.

5. What further diagnostic testing should be undertaken to investigate a suspected viral hepatitis?

In this case, the bird was re-admitted for endoscopy and another liver biopsy was collected. An unfixed fresh liver biopsy was submitted for virology and another was fixed in ethanol 70% and sent for viral PCR testing.

Laboratory findings

The liver biopsy submitted for virus isolation was negative.

The sample submitted for PCR analysis tested as avian polyomavirus negative and adenovirus negative. Herpesvirus PCR was positive and sequencing showed homology with several herpesviruses (equine, human, vulture). There was high identity with vulture herpesvirus DNA polymerase (73%).

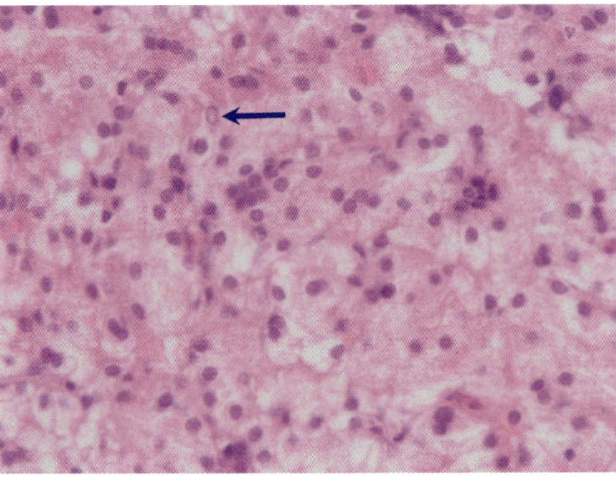

Fig. 2.32 Photomicrograph of the liver biopsy from the trumpeter hornbill.

Q *6. What is your diagnosis?*

➤ Herpes virus hepatitis

Q *4. List your therapeutic strategy.*

Initially, the finding of hepatomegaly in a known susceptible species is highly suggestive of iron storage disease, especially given the fact that the cage-mate of this bird had died of this condition the previous year. Initial stabilization of the bird with fluid therapy, chelation therapy with defroxamine and a low iron diet would be prudent.

Once the diagnosis of (herpes) virus hepatitis is confirmed, treatment with the antiviral agents may be attempted. No licensed drugs are available for the treatment of herpesvirus-induced diseases in birds. Acyclovir and gancyclovir are recommended for treatment of cutaneous herpetic lesions in humans. Treatment options in parrots with herpesvirus include acyclovir administration in the water (1 mg/ml) or orally (80 mg/kg q8h or 330 mg/kg q12h). Avian interferon may be helpful, but surprisingly few antiviral treatment protocols are available to the avian practitioner.

Supportive therapy for birds with hepatic damage includes reducing stress, fluid therapy, and nutritional support. Lactulose and echinacea are used as hepatoprotectants by some clinicians. Isolation of the bird from other conspecifics is appropriate once a viral aetiology has been confirmed.

Colchicine may be useful as this drug prevents fibrosis by a variety of inhibitory actions and may protect the liver by stabilization of the hepatocyte plasma membrane.

Free herpesviruses are very sensitive to all disinfectants with virucidal properties and appropriate steps should be taken to ensure that cages and facilities linked with this bird are disinfected.

Discussion

This case shows the lengthy diagnostic steps needed to investigate an inclusion body hepatitis caused by a herpesvirus in a hornbill. The difficulty in diagnosing herpesviruses is emphasized. Interestingly, this bird responded positively to non-specific supportive therapy, was not given any antiviral medication and remains healthy and is alive 3 years later. Follow-up PCR analysis of a liver biopsy 12 months later was PCR negative for herpesvirus.

Avian herpesviruses are double-stranded DNA viruses that cause a variety of disease conditions in birds and those individuals that recover tend to establish latent infections for prolonged times.

In many cases of herpesvirus infection, concomitant infections by other agents, environmental factors and social or reproductive stress contribute to the development of forms of overt disease. During periods of stress the virus may be reactivated in asymptomatic hosts and shedding of infectious virions occurs. Shedding can occur without overt clinical signs of disease in hosts. What is interesting about this case is the long period of latency in a bird that had been kept in an isolated aviary with no other birds for many years.

Herpesviruses generally produce Cowdry type A intranuclear inclusion bodies in target cells. Herpesvirus inclusion bodies associated with hepatitis have been reported in psittaciformes (Pacheco's disease virus), raptors (as variations of the inclusion body hepatitis of the falcon), in cranes and storks, and in quail and pheasants. Vulture herpesvirus (VUHV) is an alphaherpesvirus along with Marek's disease virus and turkey herpesvirus (HVT).

Although transmission routes for avian herpesviruses in companion birds have not been well investigated, it is likely that the gastrointestinal and respiratory tract are the primary points of entrance and release of the virus. While herpesviruses are usually associated with liver pathology, herpesviruses have been associated with pathology of other organ systems (e.g. pancreas).

This case report illustrates the problem in achieving a rapid diagnosis so that appropriate treatment can be started as quickly as possible. It has been found that psittacid herpesviruses (PsHV) persist in the oral and cloacal mucosa of carrier birds and PCR testing of swabs of these surfaces has been recommended as a way of detecting PsHV in psittacines.

Acknowledgements

Thanks to Kassy Sainsbury, Christudas Silvanose, Joerg Kinne and Gerry Dorrestein for their contribution to this case.

Further reading

Dutton, C., 2003. Coraciformes, (Kingfishers, Motmots, Bee-eaters, Hoopoes, Hornbills). In: Fowler, M., Miller, R.E. (Eds.), Zoo and Wildlife Medicine, fifth ed. Elsevier Science, Philadelphia, pp. 254–260.

Gerlach, H., 1994. Viruses. In: Ritchie, B., Harrison, G., Harrison, L. (Eds.), Avian Medicine: Principles and Application. Wingers Publishing, Lake Worth, pp. 862–948.

International Species Information System, 12101 Johnny Cake Ridge Road, USA. www.worldzoo.org.

Kaleta, E.F., Docherty, D.E., 2007. Avian herpesviruses. In: Thomas, N.J., Hunter, D.B., Atkinson, C.T. (Eds.), Infectious Diseases of Wild Birds. Blackwell Publishing, Ames, pp. 63–86.

Lazic, T., Ackermann, M.R., Drahos, J.M., et al., 2008. Respiratory herpesvirus infection in two Indian ringneck parakeets. J. Vet. Diagn. Invest. 2, 235–238.

Phalen, D., Tomaszewski, E., Styles, D., 2003. Psittacid herpesviruses correlation of genotype and phenotype implications for control. In: Proceedings of the 7th European AAV conference. Loro Parque, pp. 58–63.

Phalen, D., 2006. Implications of viruses in clinical disorders. In: Harrison, G., Lightfoot, T. (Eds.), Clinical Avian Medicine. Spix Publishing, Palm Beach, pp. 721–746.

Phalen, D.N., Falcon, M., Tomaszewski, E.K., 2007. Endocrine pancreatic insufficiency secondary to chronic herpesvirus pancreatitis in a cockatiel (*Nymphicus hollandicus*). J. Avian Med. Surg. 21 (2), 140–145.

Sandmeier, P., 2009. The use of deferiprone in the treatment of iron storage disease in three hornbills. Sequential monitoring of the liver iron content by quantitative analysis. In: Proceedings of the European College of Avian Medicine and Surgery, pp. 27–28.

Wernery, U., 2008. Viral diseases. In: Samour, J. (Ed.), Avian Medicine, second ed. Mosby Elsevier, London, pp. 358–373.

Case 2.15 *L. Crosta*

Clinical history

An adult female toco toucan (*Ramphastos toco*) was presented because of lameness and the presence of bilateral swelling on the volar aspect of both tarsi-metatarsi, just under both tarsal joints.

Apparently, the problem started after a male had been introduced into the aviary (4×4 m, ×2 m height). The owner believed the female was stressed by the male's continuous chasing and he thought the male was pecking at the legs, leading to small wounds that eventually became infected.

Clinical examination

The bird was alert and in good body condition (3/5) and weighed 630 g. It was able to fly properly and was actively trying to escape from capture and jumping from perch to perch. There were massive swellings on both legs of about 1 cm diameter (Figs 2.33–2.35); the tail was not well feathered and it was dirty with faeces.

Clinical diagnosis examination

Radiographs of the body and detailed radiographs of legs and joints were taken while the bird was anaesthetized. Blood samples were collected for haematology, blood chemistry and plasma protein electrophoresis analyses.

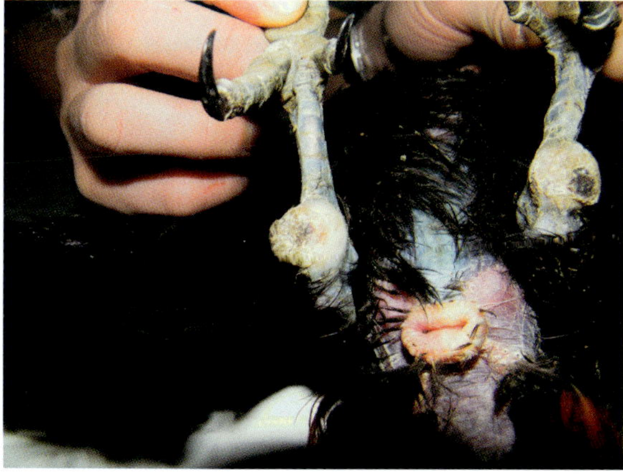

Fig. 2.33 Lesions on the legs of the female toco toucan.

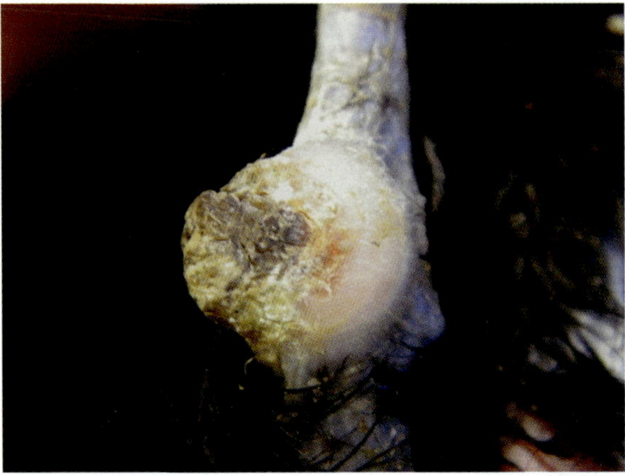

Fig. 2.34 Detail of the lesion on the right leg.

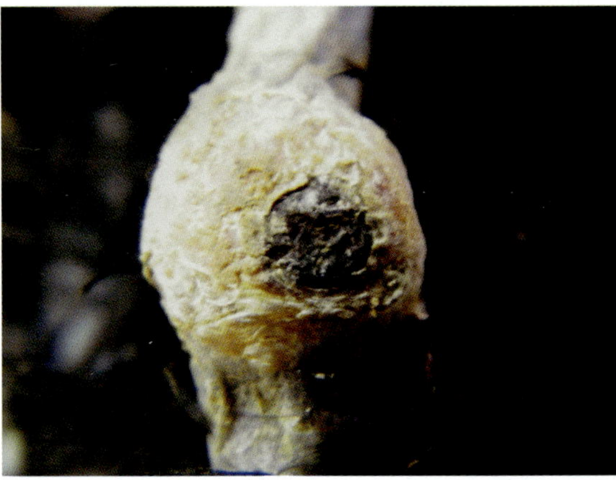

Fig. 2.35 Detail of the left leg lesion.

Radiology (Figs 2.36–2.39)

1. What is your interpretation of the radiographs in Figs 2.36–2.39?

Clinical diagnosis laboratory

The results of the clinical diagnosis laboratory assays are shown in Tables 2.29–2.31 and Fig. 2.40.

RBC, WBC and thrombocyte morphology

- Reactive monocytes

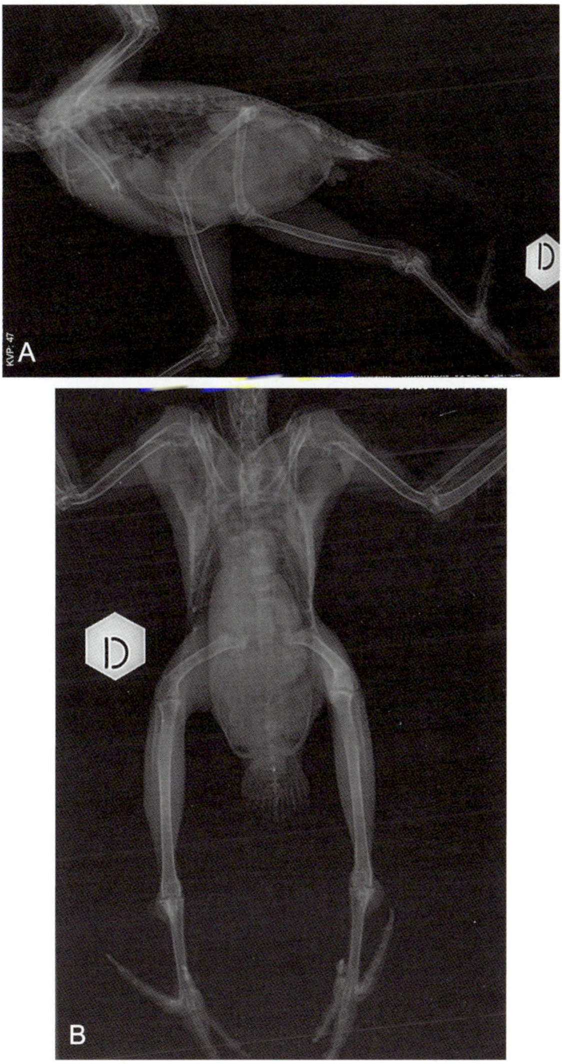

Fig. 2.36 (a) Lateral view of the toco toucan female; (b) ventrodorsal view of the toco toucan female.

Cytology

- Right tarsal lesion: scanty cells and scanty heterophils, slightly degenerated. Scanty macrophages and scanty bacterial forms (cocci)
- Left tarsal lesion: no cells, inconclusive

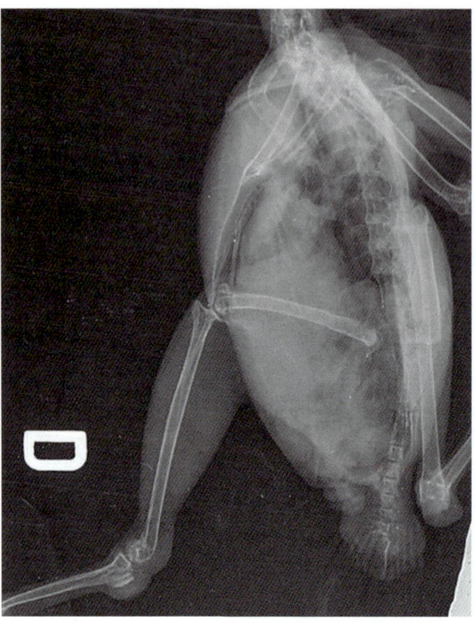

Fig. 2.37 Detail of the right hip of the toucan.

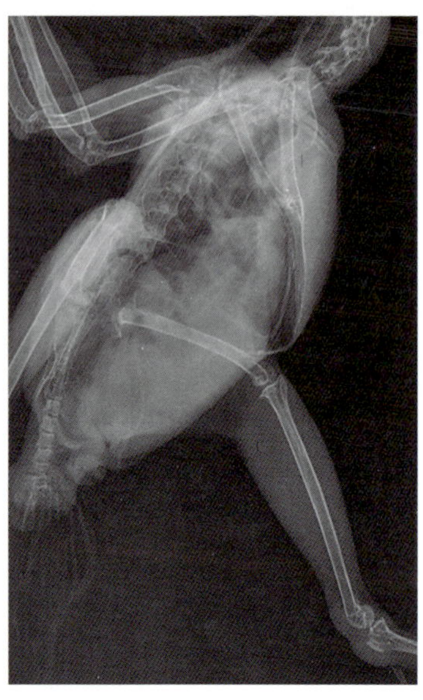

Fig. 2.38 Detail of the left hip of the toucan.

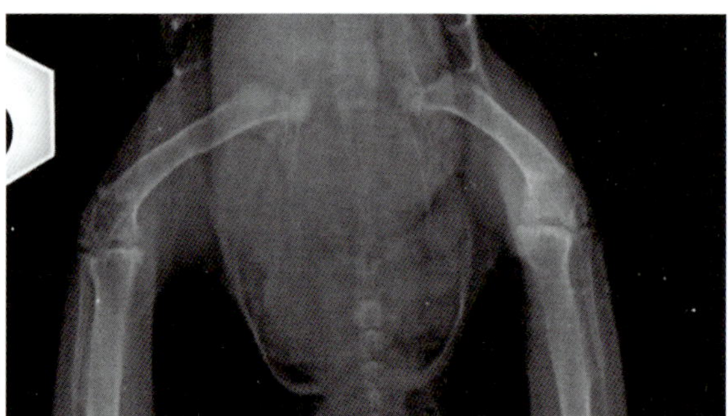

Fig. 2.39 Detail of the knees of the toucan.

Comment: picture compatible with a chronic, non-specific, granulomatous inflammatory process.

Q *2. What is your interpretation of the haematology, blood chemistry, protein electrophoresis values shown in Tables 2.29–2.31 and Fig. 2.40 and the cytology examination?*

Table 2.29 Haematology values of the toco toucan

Parameters	Results	Reference values
RBC ($\times10^{12}$/l)	2.470	(2.500–4.500)
Hb (g/dl)	18.3	(14.0–19.5)
Hct (%)	49	(45–60)
MCV (fl)	198	(148–210)
MCH (pg)	74	(55.0–70)
MCHC (g/dl)	37.1	(30–39.8)
WBC ($\times10^{9}$/l)	13.00	(8.0–18.0)
Heterophils (%)	40	(41–62)
Lymphocytes (%)	30	(36–70)
Monocytes (%)	30	(0–2)
Eosinophils (%)	0	(0–3)
Basophils (%)	0	(0–1)
Thrombocytes (k/µl)	8.960	

Table 2.30 Blood chemistry values of the toco toucan

Analysis	Results	Reference values
Bile acids (µmol/l)	10	(n.d.)
Cholesterol (mg/dl)	166	(n.d.)
CK (U/l)	3.593	(3.440–3.948)
GOT (U/l)	193	(130–330)
Glucose (g/dl)	286	(220–350)
LDH (U/l)	544	(200–400)
Total protein (g/l)	50	(30–50)
Uric acid (mg/dl)	7.14	(4.0–14.0)

Results

- Lesions are bilateral and symmetrical. Apparently infected
- Cytology revealed a chronic inflammatory process, with few bacteria (cocci)
- Radiographic findings included decreased bone density of the right hip and proximal portion of the right femur, which also looks distorted; furthermore, the right knee is clearly altered and looks very different from the left one

Table 2.31 Plasma protein electrophoresis of the toco toucan

Parameters	Fractions (%)	Concentrations (g/l)
Total protein		50.0
Pre-albumin	7.7	3.9
Albumin	22.7	11.4
Alpha 1 globulins	7.3	3.7
Alpha 2 globulins	16.9	8.5
Beta globulins	43.4	21.7
Gamma globulins	2.0	0.9
A:G ratio		0.44

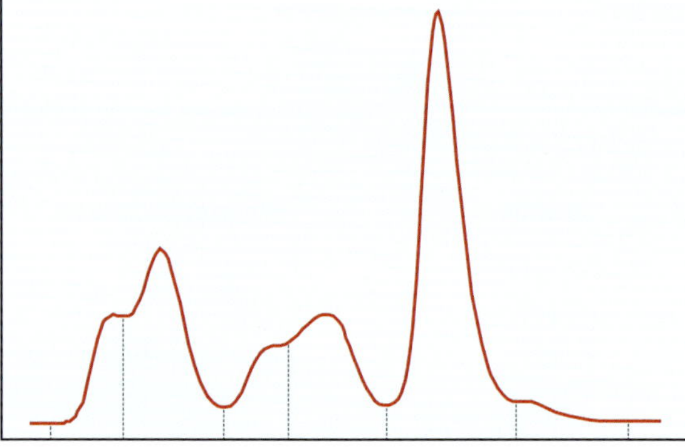

Fig. 2.40 Expression of plasma protein electrophoresis of the toucan.

- Haematology analysis showed slightly decreased RBC, slight heteropenia and marked monocytosis
- Blood chemistry analysis showed elevated LDH levels
- Plasma protein electrophoresis showed a marked beta globulin peak and low albumin:globulin ratio

Please evaluate the clinical history, Figs 2.33–2.35, the results of the physical examination and clinical diagnosis laboratory tests.

Q *3. List your differential diagnoses.*

Q *4. List your therapeutic strategy.*

Differential diagnoses

- Bilateral bumblefoot/septic arthritis/tenosinovitis
- Poxvirus infection

Therapy (Table 2.32)

Final diagnosis

- Skeletal abnormalities
- Chronic localized abscesses

Discussion

This case, while appearing as a simple chronic undiagnosed bumblefoot, provides interesting factors for a discussion and is a good example of the difficulties encountered with captive management:

1. A first important fact is that the lesions had not been observed by the owner until a few weeks before presentation
2. Lesions occurred after a male had been introduced into the aviary
3. There are obvious skeletal lesions in the patient
4. Blood testing and especially protein electrophoresis indicates a chronic or subacute inflammatory process.

The most important question here is: were the bone lesions indirectly caused by the inflammatory process, or were they the main problem and, in a certain way, the cause of the bumblefoot? First, the skeletal lesions could have been caused by the misuse of the right leg, which apparently was the most seriously affected. Secondly, pre-existing skeletal lesions, which were not symptomatic because the bird was alone and quiet, under the stress caused by the chasing male became acute and painful again, the female toucan started bearing her weight on the tarsal bones, instead of using only the feet, the soft skin cracked, in addition to the cold winter temperature, and the bumblefoot started. In either of the two cases, surgery was an option and would correct the problem, at least temporarily, but adequate diagnosis was considered very important to select the most appropriate treatment. If the bumblefoot was the primary lesion, surgical resolution would possibly be definitive

Table 2.32 Therapy

Consider surgery	
Enrofloxacin	15 mg/kg BID, PO, × 1 week
Meloxicam	0.2 mg/kg SID, PO
Gentamycin cream	Locally, BID, TID

and maybe the bone lesions would improve, bringing the bird back to normality. However, if the bone lesions were the main cause of the bumblefoot, treating the bumblefoot would not correct the problem permanently and seasonal recurrences could be expected.

Further reading

Cornelissen, H., Ritchie, B.W., 1994. Ramphastidae. In: Ritchie, B.W.; Harrison, G.J., Harrison, L.R. (Eds.), Avian Medicine: Principle and Application. Wingers Publishing Inc., Lake Worth, pp. 1276–1283.

Crosta, L., Timossi, L., Bürkle, M., 2006. Management of zoo and park birds. In: Harrison, G.J., Lightfoot, T. (Eds.), Clinical Avian Medicine. Spix Publishing Inc., Palm Beach, pp. 991–1003.

Crosta, L., Timossi, L., 2009. The management of a multi-species bird collection in a zoological park. In: Tully, T.N., Dorrestein, G.M., Lawton, M. (Eds.), Handbook of Avian Medicine, second ed. Saunders Elsevier, Edinburgh, pp. 404–435.

Cubas, Z.S., 2007. Piciformes (Tucano, Araçari, Pica-Pau). In: Cubas, Z.S., Ramos da Silva, J.C., Catão-Dias, J.L. (Eds.), Tratado de Medicina Veterinária de Animais Selvagens. Editora Roca Ltda, São Paulo, pp. 210–221.

Worrell, A.B., 2009. Ramphastids. In: Tully, T.N., Dorrestein, G.M., Lawton, M. (Eds.), Handbook of Avian Medicine, second ed. Saunders Elsevier, Edinburgh, pp. 335–349.

Case 2.16 *P. Sandmeier*

Clinical history

A 9-year-old female Bali or Rothschild's mynah (*Leucopsar rothschildi*), weighing 90g, was presented with the following clinical signs of a few weeks' duration:

- Open-mouthed breathing
- Occasional coughing and shaking of the head.

The female Bali mynah (Fig. 2.41) was part of a breeding facility and had bred successfully for the last 2 years. Roughly 6 months earlier two new birds had been introduced to the breeding collection.

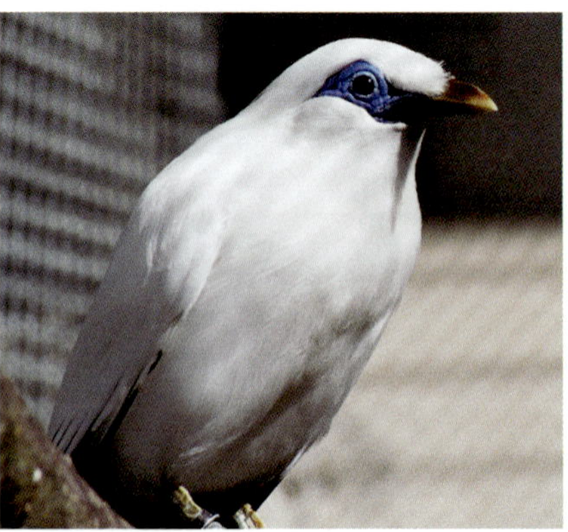

Fig. 2.41 Female Bali mynah (courtesy of Andy Fuchs).

Clinical examination

On presentation, the bird had a good body condition. The feather condition was excellent. The eyes were clear and without discharge. No nasal discharge could be observed. The bird had a slightly extended recovery time after handling and during this time it breathed with an open beak.

Please evaluate the clinical history and the results of the physical examination.

 *1. List your differential diagnoses.*

 *2. List your plan for further diagnostics.*

Differential diagnoses

Upper respiratory tract disease

- Viral infections (PMV, poxvirus, other viruses)
- Bacterial infections (*Pseudomonas* spp., *Mycoplasma* spp., *Chlamydophila psittaci*, other bacteria)
- Fungal infections (*Aspergillus* spp.), possible fungal granuloma in trachea
- Parasitic infections
  - *Syngamus trachea*
  - *Sternostoma tracheocolum*
  - *Trichomonas gallinae*
- Foreign body inhalation
- Inhalant toxins
- Lower respiratory tract disease
- Abdominal distension
  - Iron storage disease
  - Ascites
  - Organomegaly
  - Neoplasia
  - Egg binding

Further diagnostics

- Radiology (Fig. 2.42)
- Rhinoscopy, pharyngoscopy, tracheoscopy (Fig. 2.43)

Final diagnosis

- *Syngamus trachea* infestation

Q *3. List your therapeutic strategy and your strategy to monitor the therapeutic success for this individual bird and for the complete breeding collection.*

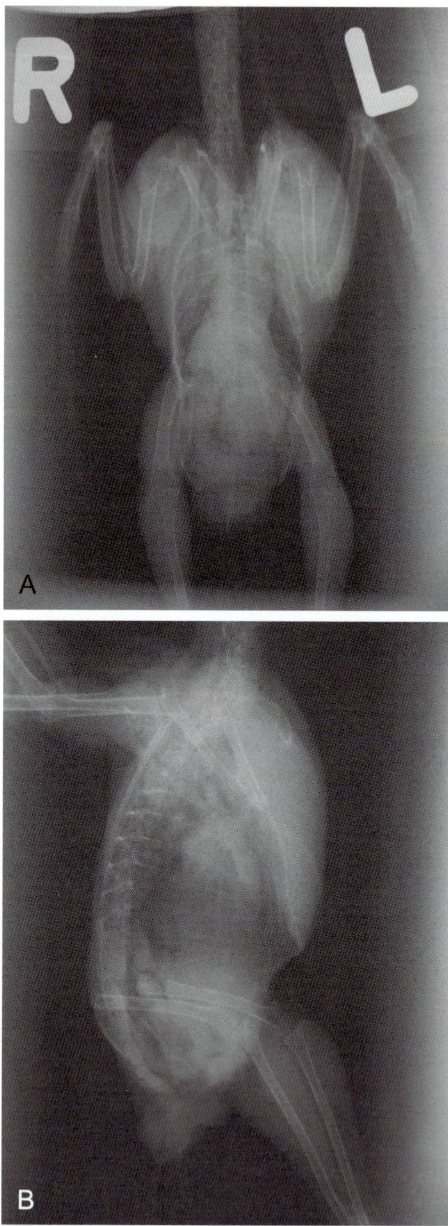

Fig. 2.42 (a) Ventrodorsal radiograph of the Bali mynah revealing no signs of abdominal distension or lower respiratory tract disease; (b) latero-lateral radiograph of Bali mynah revealing no signs of abdominal distension or lower respiratory tract disease.

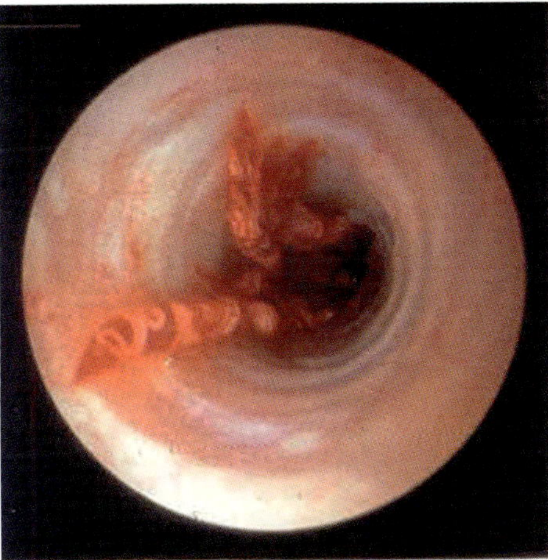

Fig. 2.43 *Syngamus trachea* recognized on tracheoscopy.

Therapy (Table 2.33)

Therapy monitoring

- Tracheoscopy in individuals showing clinical signs of gape worm disease
- Serial faecal flotation until three negative samples
- Regular annual or biannual testing or deworming programme should be instituted

Table 2.33 Therapy

Endoscopic removal of the most cranial gape worms from the trachea	
Fenbendazole	20–40 mg/kg SID, 3 days' duration
Doramectin	Dilute 1:10 in sesame oil. Spot on treatment 1 drop/50 g. Repeat after 10 days
	Repeat cycle until serial faecal flotations remain negative
Decontamination of aviary	p-Chlor-m-kresol (Interkokask®) 2% solution, leave for 2 hours
Prevent contact with natural soil and earthworms	

Discussion

Syngamus trachea is a common parasite in starlings and crows and must be considered in all passerines, especially those housed in outdoor aviaries. The clinical signs with respiratory distress, gasping, coughing and head shaking are typical. The life cycle of *S. trachea* is direct, but earthworms can act as transport and accumulation hosts. Adult worms live in permanent copulation within the trachea causing the clinical signs. Diagnosis is based on visualization of the adult worms within the trachea using tracheoscopy or tracheal transillumination. Asymptomatically infected birds are recognized by identifying the ovoid eggs on faecal flotation. Treatment is performed using fenbendazol, flubendazole, doramectin, ivermectin or similar products. Monitoring the therapeutic success using regular faecal flotation is mandatory. Important differential diagnoses include poxvirus, *Chlamydophila psittaci*, tracheal mites (*Sternostoma tracheocolum*), bacterial tracheitis and abdominal distension (especially due to iron storage disease in this species).

Further reading

Beck, W., Pantchev, N., 2006. Praktische Parasitologie bei Heimtieren. Schlütersche Verlag, Germany.

Sandmeier, P., Coutteel, P., 2006. Management of canaries, finches and mynahs. In: Harrison, G.J., Lightfoot, T.L. (Eds.), Clinical Avian Medicine. Spix Publishing, Inc., Palm Beach, pp. 879–913.

Case 2.17 *N. A. Forbes*

Clinical history

A 5-year old hyacinth macaw (*Anodorhynchus hyacinthinus*) was presented for examination. The captive-bred bird was one of four pet macaws owned by a client who had all recently been cared for by the breeder while the owner was on holiday. The breeder had phoned the owner reporting that while the other birds were fine, that this bird had become unwell, showing the following signs:

- Inappetence
- Sudden weight loss
- Increased dark-green coloration in the faeces
- Weakness
- Mild incoordination, difficulty remaining on the perch.

Physical examination

On examination, the macaw was subdued although still vocal. The bodyweight was 1220 g with a body condition of 2/5 (thin) and was mildly dehydrated. The bird was weak and moderately incoordinated and had difficulty perching unassisted.

Clinical diagnosis examination

Survey radiographs were taken (Fig. 2.44) while the bird was under anaesthesia.

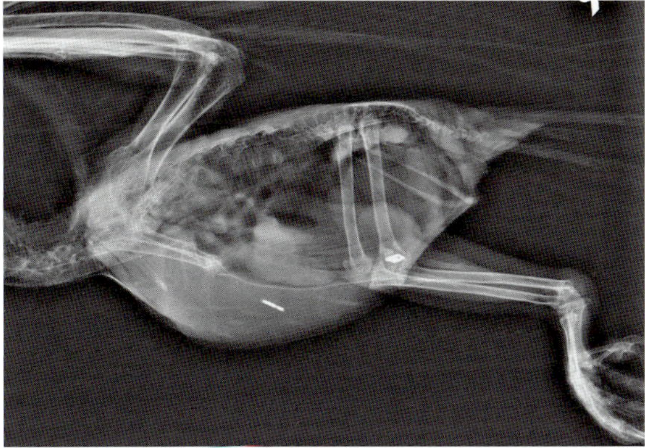

Fig. 2.44 Lateral survey radiograph of this macaw.

Radiology (Fig. 2.44)

 *1. What is your interpretation of the radiograph in Fig. 2.44?*

Clinical diagnosis laboratory examination

Blood samples were collected for haematology and blood chemistry analyses.

The results of the clinical diagnosis laboratory assays are shown in Tables 2.34 and 2.35.

RBC, WBC and thrombocyte morphology

- Nothing abnormal detected

 *2. What is your interpretation of the haematology and blood chemistry analyses results?*

 *3. In view of the clinical signs and radiographic findings, what are your differential diagnoses?*

Summary of diagnosis results

- Radiographic findings indicate a metallic item in the ventriculus. On questioning, the breeder who had been caring for the bird explained that the bird had chewed up a toy, remnants were not available. The lead level is normal, while the zinc level shows moderate elevation, but not to a level where one would anticipate clinical signs
- Haematology analyses showed marginally low RBC, low Hb and low Hct. The WBC was elevated, although within normal range, as a physiological stress leucogram is common in macaws, in particular after lengthy journeys (this macaw had travelled for 2.5 hours prior to examination)

Table 2.34 Haematology values of the hyacinth macaw

Parameters	Results (absolute)	Results (%)	Reference values
RBC (×10[12]/l)	2.6		(2.7–4.5)
Hb (g/dl)	12.8		(15.0–17.0)
Hct (l/l)	0.43		(0.47–0.55)
MCV (fl)	130		(125–170)
MCHC (g/dl)	29.5		(29–35)
WBC (×10[9]/l)	17.3		(7–22)
Heterophils (×10[9]/l)	3.98	23	55.3±10.0 (37–75)
Lymphocytes (×10[9]/l)	12.8	74	39±10 (20–60)
Monocytes (×10[9]/l)	0.17	1	4.4±2.9 (1–10)
Eosinophils (×10[9]/l)	0	0	0±0.2 (0.0–1.0)
Basophils (×10[9]/l)	0.34	2	0.5±1.0 (0.0–3.0)
Chlamydophila serology	0		<3

Table 2.35 Blood chemistry values of the hyacinth macaw

Analysis	Results	Reference values
Total protein (g/l)	38	34–42
Globulin (g/l)	22	25–38
Albumin (g/l)	16	12–31
A/G ratio	0.73	0.7–1
Bile acids (μmol/l)	11	25–71
Calcium (mmol/l)	2.1	2.37–2.62
Cholesterol (mmol/l)	4.7	2.59–7.76
CK (U/l)	1033	180–500
AST (U/l)	208	90–180
Glucose (mmol/l)	12.6	12–18
LDH (U/l)	285	40–250
Phosphorus (mmol/l)	1.24	1.49–2.07
Total urea (mmol/l)	1.5	0.04–1.68
Uric acid (μmol/l)	66	109–231
Zinc (μmol/l)	57.8	<32
Lead (μmol/l)	0.75	<1.12

- Chlamydophila serology negative
- Blood chemistry analysis showed elevated levels of CK, AST and LDH, which are most likely due to muscle (condition) loss

Please evaluate the clinical history, radiograph, clinical findings and laboratory diagnostic testing results.

Q *4. List your differential diagnoses.*

 *5. List your therapeutic strategy.*

Differential diagnoses

- Heavy metal poisoning, not involving lead or zinc
- Psittacine proventricular dilation syndrome – showing central or peripheral signs rather than GIT signs

Therapy

The macaw was placed on therapeutic management (Table 2.36).

Response to therapy

The bird became stronger, perching better, vocalizing and brighter in herself.

The radiograph was repeated and the metal links had not moved from the ventriculus.

Q *6. What are your next diagnostic and therapeutic steps?*

Diagnostic and therapeutic options

- Test for copper and iron
- Magnetic or endoscopic recovery of metal particles from the ventriculus
- Serological and PCR test for bornavirus or ganglioside antibody ELISA

Table 2.36 Therapy

Marbofloxacin 10%	15 mg/kg IM SID
Sodium calcium EDTA	35 mg/kg IM BID
D-Penicillamine	40 mg/kg BID PO
MgSO4 (pinch) and peanut butter	10 ml BID by gavage
Fluids	Ringer's lactate 15 ml/kg IV TID
Forced feeding	Harrison's recovery diet mixed to porridge consistency and fed by gavage tube 25 ml QID PO

Action taken

- General anaesthetic, ingluviotomy, attempted magnetic recovery (using micromagnets fixed with glue within a tube which could be passed into the ventriculus) was not effective. Endoscopic recovery of metal particles from the ventriculus was achieved without complication
- Metal particles comprised links of a copper chain
- Chelation with NaCa EDTA was maintained BID IM for 5 further days, plus D-penicillamine for a further 10 days PO BID
- The bird made an uneventful recovery

Q ***7. If endoscopic recovery or referral had not been an option, what surgical approach would have been appropriate?***

Surgery

- Left lateral coeliotomy, with left leg abducted dorsally and an incision from the ischium to the sixth rib
- The fascia of lateral wall of the ventriculus is identified, and stay sutures are placed in this to effect the exteriorization (out of or tight against) of the laparotomy incision
- The coelom, anterior and adjacent to the proventriculo-ventricular isthmus is packed off with surgical swabs and suction equipment is made ready. The caudal triangular lobe of the liver, covering the isthmus is elevated with a cotton bud, and a 1 cm incision is made into the isthmus. As the incision is made, it is likely that fluid will rise up from the GIT, the surgeon or surgical assistant should be ready for this with suction equipment to collect any such fluid
- Suction is then used to aspirate the gut lumen craniad and caudad to the incision. The ventricular contents are visualized, if necessary with an endoscope, and the foreign body removed
- The GIT incision is closed in two layers using PDS 4/0. The first layer is opposed and the second layer inverted. After this, the elevated liver lobe is tacked down in place over the incision. Surgical swabs are removed. The laparatomy wound is closed in a routine manner

Discussion

The clinician should never forget the possibility of copper or iron toxicosis as well as the more common zinc or lead. All toys and equipment in any psittacines environment should be safe for purpose.

Further reading

Forbes, N.A., 2008. Soft tissue surgery. In: Samour, J. (Ed.), Avian Medicine, second ed. Mosby Elsevier Ltd., Oxford, p. 161.

Lloyd, C., 2009. Staged endoscopic ventricular foreign body removal in a gyr falcon (*Falco rusticolus*). J. Avian Med. Surg. 23 (4), 314–319.

Samour, J., 2008. Toxicology. In: Samour, J. (Ed.), Avian Medicine, second ed. Mosby Elsevier Ltd., Oxford, p. 275.

Case 2.18 *N. A. Forbes*

Clinical history

A regular breeder client presents two breeding pairs of macaws for examination, which he had purchased at a very good price from a breeder who was giving up keeping birds, some 4 months previously.

Physical examination

The birds appeared fit and well, but one scarlet macaw (*Ara macao*) demonstrated a choanal papilloma (Fig. 2.45a) and one blue and gold macaw (*Ara ararauna*) had a cloacal papilloma (Fig. 2.45b). One of the blue and gold macaws appeared to be in poor condition, with weight loss and poor plumage.

Clinical diagnosis examination

Survey radiographs were taken while the blue and gold macaw was under anaesthesia.

Radiology

➤ The blue and gold macaw appears to have an enlarged liver

Endoscopy

➤ Visualization and biopsy collection from the liver

Clinical diagnosis laboratory examination

Blood samples were collected for haematology and blood chemistry analyses.

The results of the clinical diagnosis laboratory assays are shown in Tables 2.37 and 2.38.

RBC, WBC and thrombocyte morphology

➤ Nothing abnormal detected

Q *1. What is your interpretation of the haematology and blood chemistry results?*

Q *2. In view of the clinical signs and radiographic findings, what are your differential diagnoses?*

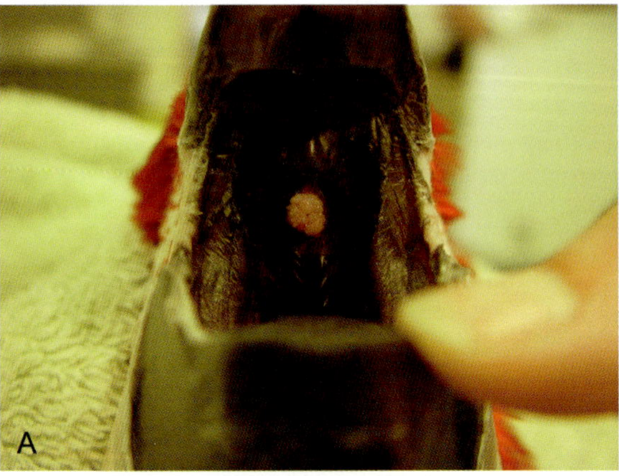

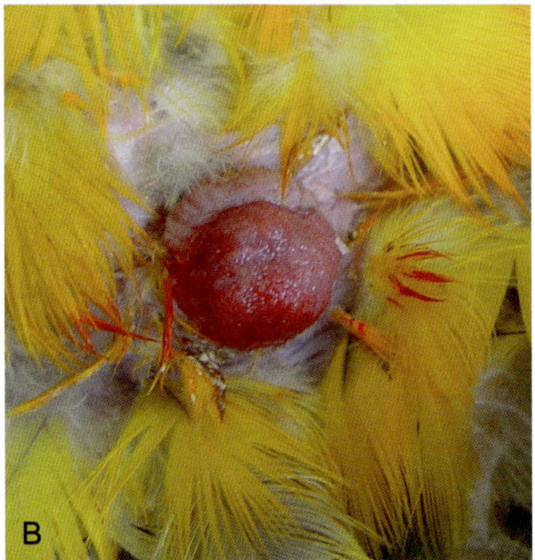

Fig. 2.45 (a) Choanal papilloma in the scarlet macaw; (b) cloacal papilloma in the blue and gold macaw.

Summary of diagnostic results

- Radiographic findings indicate an enlarged liver
- Haematology analysis shows a regenerative anaemia, with a marginally low RBC, low Hb and low Hct, but raised MCV. The WBC was elevated, although within normal range, as a physiological stress leucogram is common in macaws, in particular after lengthy journeys
- Chlamydia serology negative
- Blood chemistry analysis showed reduced albumin, albumin/globulin ratio, elevated bile acid, reduced calcium, elevated CK, AST and LDH
- Liver biopsy indicates hepatobiliary adenocarcinoma

Please evaluate the clinical history, radiographic findings, clinical findings and laboratory diagnostic tests.

Table 2.37 Haematology values of the blue and gold macaw

Parameters	Results (absolute)	Results (%)	Reference values
RBC ($\times10^{12}$/l)	2.45		(2.7–4.5)
Hb (g/dl)	12.2		(15.0–17.0)
Hct (l/l)	0.37		(0.47–0.55)
MCV (fl)	172		(125–170)
MCHC (g/dl)	29.5		(29–35)
WBC ($\times10^{9}$/l)	16.8		(7–22)
Heterophils ($\times10^{9}$/l)	3.53	21	55.3±10.0 (37–75)
Lymphocytes ($\times10^{9}$/l)	12.77	76	39±10 (20–60)
Monocytes ($\times10^{9}$/l)	0.168	1	4.4±2.9 (1–10)
Eosinophils ($\times10^{9}$/l)	0	0	0±0.2 (0.0–1.0)
Basophils ($\times10^{9}$/l)	0.336	2	0.5±1.0 (0.0–3.0)
Chlamydia serology	0		<3

Table 2.38 Blood chemistry values of the blue and gold macaw

Analysis	Results	Reference values
Total protein (g/l)	38	34–42
Globulin (g/l)	28	25–38
Albumin (g/l)	10	12–31
A:G ratio	0.35	0.7–1
Bile acids (μmol/l)	145	25–71
Calcium (mmol/l)	1.9	2.37–2.62
Cholesterol (mmol/l)	4.5	2.59–7.76
CK (U/l)	1275	180–500
AST (U/l)	255	90–180
Glucose (mmol/l)	13	12–18
LDH (U/l)	351	40–250
Phosphorus (mmol/l)	1.24	1.49–2.07
Total urea (mmol/l)	1.5	0.04–1.68
Uric acid (μmol/l)	225	109–231
Zinc (μmol/l)	15	<32

Q *3. What is your diagnosis and are the liver and cloacal findings linked?*

Q *4. List your therapeutic strategy.*

Diagnoses

➤ Cloacal papilloma with a secondary viral oncogenic hepatobiliary adenocarcinoma

Therapy

There is no recommended treatment for this bird. Psittacine cloacal and choanal papilloma are herpesvirus induced. Once infected, the birds maintain a lifelong infection, moreover, the virus is oncogenic and all infected birds eventually go on to develop hepatobiliary, renal or pancreatic adenocarcinoma.

Discussion

The following issues need to considered:

- Was the client's collection already infected with psittacine herpesvirus prior to these macaws arriving?
- Could infection have been spread from these birds to the rest of the collection in the last 4 months?
- Could these new birds be kept (isolated) and eggs from them artificially incubated and reared without risk of the chicks being infected with herpesvirus?
- How can prevention of spread of disease between birds best be achieved?
- Are the effected bird's mates inevitably infected?
- Are previous offspring of effected birds inevitably infected?

New world psittacines (macaws and parrots) are typically susceptible. All new susceptible birds should always be checked for papilloma. If cloacal lesions are suspected but not obvious, the cloacal lining can be painted with acetic acid (vinegar) and, if positive, the surface will become white.

Birds may be asymptomatic carriers in the absence of clinical signs. Most parrots are infected by direct contact with infected mates, or by ingestion of infected faeces (as contamination of food), as such, all in contact birds should be considered infected.

In poor hygiene establishments, especially where air flow is restricted, birds may become infected from faecal dust. Direct vertical spread via the egg has been reported, so collection of eggs from infected breeding adults, for artificial incubation, should be discouraged.

Herpesviridae are enveloped viruses and hence relatively unstable outside the host, being susceptible to heat and most disinfectants. If infected birds are kept well away from other stock, with no possibility of air spread, and good hygiene, e.g. good aviary cleaning and effective foot baths, infection between groups should be possible to prevent. However, as infected birds cannot be bred from, and still pose a risk to other birds, the general advice is to remove all clinically affected birds and their contacts. PCR testing of cloacal smears and faeces may be valuable.

Acyclovir may be effective at preventing infection, but is not effective at clearing the virus from the body.

Further reading

Johne, R., Konrath, A., Krautwald-Junghanns, M.E., et al., 2002. Herpesviral, but no papovaviral sequences, are detected in cloacal papillomas of parrots. Arch. Virol. 147 (10), 1869–1880.

Ritchie, B.R., 1995. Herpesviridae. Avian Viruses: function and control. Wingers Publishing, Inc., Lake Worth.

Case 2.19 *L. Crosta*

Clinical history

A blue-fronted Amazon parrot (*Amazona aestiva*) was presented for examination. This bird was the female of a pair acquired recently as a breeding pair from an important bird dealer. The birds were kept in a 2 × 1 × 2 m outdoor aviary and fed on a blend of cooked beans and cereals, sprouted-soaked seeds and a few dry seeds in the evening.

Soon after arrival, the female bird started showing respiratory sounds, but maintained normal behaviour and good appetite. It was climbing and flying normally. The bird was examined by a first veterinarian but, during clinical examination, she had a seizure and the veterinarian stopped the procedure. No samples were collected, with the exception of a faecal sample for parasitology examination. The examination did not reveal the presence of endoparasites. A suspect diagnosis of aspergillosis was done and the bird was sent home on itraconazole and fluconazole orally, plus nebulization therapy with F10, aminophylline and acetylcysteine.

Clinical diagnosis examination

The bird was thin (2/5), but the upper part of the thorax was rounded and very firm, as if there was an abscess underneath. Considering the seizures observed by the first veterinarian, it was agreed with the owner to take the risk of anaesthesia with isoflurane for further investigations. The induction of anaesthesia was not smooth, even in the induction chamber, and maintaining an appropriate anaesthetic plan was challenging. However, the main gross abnormality was the presence of whitish exudates from the oropharynx close to the entrance of the trachea. Samples were taken for basic haematology and blood chemistry analyses and a deep tracheal swab for microbiology.

Radiology (Fig. 2.46a, b)

Q *1. What is your interpretation of the radiographs in Fig. 2.46a, b?*

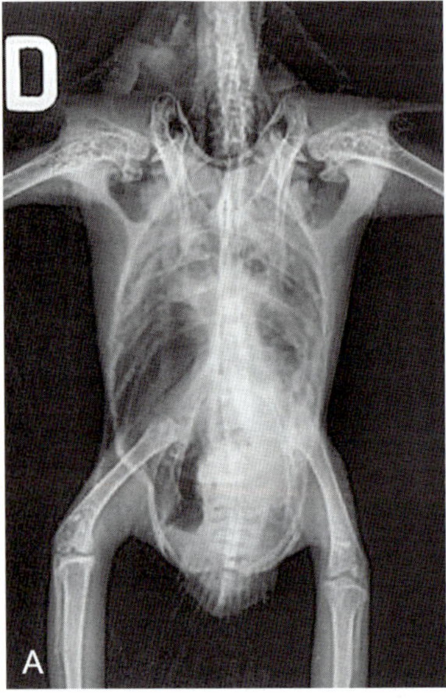

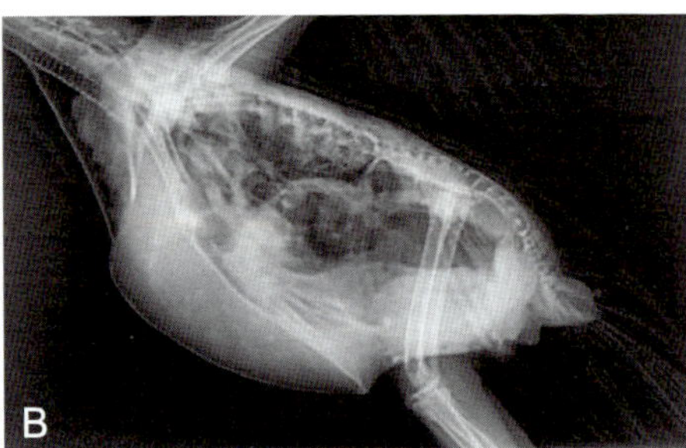

Fig. 2.46 (a) Ventrodorsal survey radiograph of the adult female blue-fronted Amazon parrot; (b) lateral survey radiograph of the adult female blue-fronted Amazon parrot.

Clinical diagnosis laboratory examination

The results of the clinical diagnosis laboratory assays are shown in Tables 2.39 and 2.40.

RBC, WBC and thrombocyte morphology

- Large, reactive lymphocytes

2. What is your interpretation of the haematology, blood chemistry and protein electrophoresis values shown in Tables 2.39 and 2.40?

Clinical diagnosis results

- Radiology revealed a large mass between the pectoral muscles and the thorax. A cardiac involvement was considered possible
- Air sacs were opaque, especially on the right side
- Haematology analysis showed slightly low RBC, with mildly elevated WBC and slight heteropenia. Also a thrombocytopenia was evident
- Blood chemistry analysis showed reduced levels of GOT, glucose and uric acid

Table 2.39 Haematology values of the blue-fronted Amazon parrot

Parameters	Results (absolute)	Results (%)	Reference values
RBC (×10[12]/l)	2.48		(2.6–3.5)
Hb (g/dl)	16.8		(13.8–17.9)
Hct (l/l)	0.42		(0.42–0.53)
MCV (fl)	169.3		(156–194)
MCH (pg)	67.7		(44.7–58.6)
MCHC (g/dl)	40		(28.9–35.8)
WBC (×10[9]/l)	18.300		(6.0–13.0)
Heterophils (×10[9]/l)	5.856	32	(33–72)
Lymphocytes (×10[9]/l)	10.980	60	(22–65)
Monocytes (×10[9]/l)	0	0	(0–1)
Eosinophils (×10[9]/l)	1.464	8	(0–1)
Basophils (×10[9]/l)	0	0	(0–1)
Thrombocytes (×10[9]/l)		3.79	(10–67)

Table 2.40 Blood chemistry values of the blue-fronted Amazon parrot

Analysis	Results	Reference values
Calcium (mg/dl)	8.33	(8.2–13.2)
Cholesterol (mg/dl)	192	(100–270)
AST/GOT (U/l)	133	(146–408)
Glucose (mg/dl)	216	(246–389)
Zinc (μg/dl)	105	<200
Uric acid (mg/dl)	1.2	(2.3–10.0)

- Microbiology: from the tracheal swab *E. coli* was cultured, sensitive to most antibiotics, but resistant to cephalotin, cefazolin and cefadroxil. No fungi were cultured from the tracheal swab
- Endoscopy examination was not performed, since it was considered too risky

Please evaluate the clinical history, Fig. 2.46a, b, the results of the clinical examination and clinical diagnosis laboratory tests.

Q *3. List your differential diagnoses.*

Q *4. List your therapeutic strategy.*

Differential diagnoses

Several diagnostic hypotheses were taken into consideration:

- Local infection, possibly after IM injection
- Very large fungal granulomas
- Tumour
- Generalized tracheitis and airsacculitis, possibly mycotic in origin.

Therapy (Table 2.41)

Table 2.41 Therapy

Itraconazole	10 mg/kg PO BID
Enrofloxacin	15 mg/kg PO BID
Meloxicam	2 mg/kg PO BID
Aerosol therapy (mixture):	20 minutes BID
F10 (diluted 1:250)	
Enilconazole	
Gentamycin	
Diet	Boiled cereals and legumes, fresh fruits and greens

Post-mortem findings

Unfortunately the bird died on the second day of admission. A thorough post-mortem examination was performed (Fig. 2.47a–d). Samples from different organs were collected for microbiology and histopathology analyses.

 *5. What lesions can you observe in the post-mortem photographs?*

 *6. What is your provisional post-mortem diagnosis?*

Summary of post-mortem examination findings

- Large thoracic mass, involving the pectoral muscles, sternum and protruding into the coelomic cavity and connecting to the base of the heart
- The mass is filled with a whitish-yellow exudate
- Apparently no other gross lesions of clinical significance were seen

Provisional post-mortem diagnosis

- Bacterial/mycotic mass
- Neoplasm

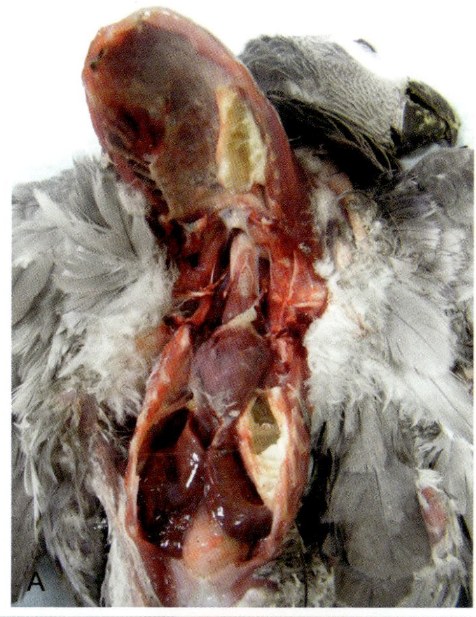

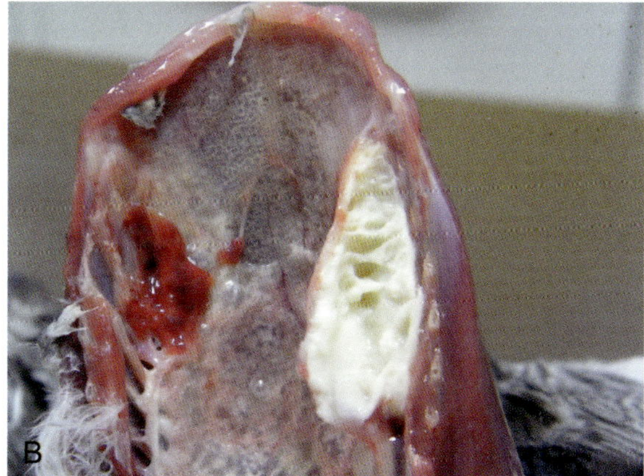

Fig. 2.47 (a–d) Post-mortem examination photographs of the blue-fronted Amazon parrot.

Laboratory findings

Histology

No changes in the myocardium. Severe atherosclerosis in the larger vessel with cartilage formation and possible beginning of mineralization. Further, there were two different pieces of abnormal tissue: (1) a large bean-shaped piece, which looked more like a myofibroma-type tissue and (2) a smaller part, more fibroma-like, with necrosis and areas with mucine-like material between the cells.

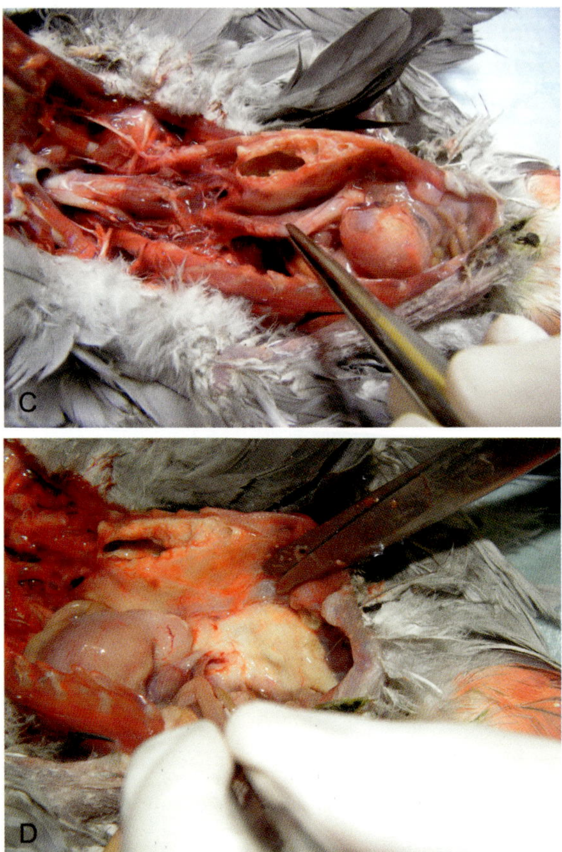

Fig. 2.47—cont'd

Special staining

In the van Gieson staining (for connective tissue) there were fibres of connective tissues in all parts. The PAS was negative, therefore no mucine.

Microbiology

Cultures from the exudate did not show any fungal growth, but *Pseudomonas aeruginosa* was isolated, sensitive to amikacin, clindamycin, gentamycin, tobramycin and piperacillin.

Final diagnosis

➤ Fibroma with different amounts of connective tissue

Discussion

Respiratory symptoms in parrots are often perceived as having only two causes: psittacosis and aspergillosis. It is obviously not that simple and clinical and laboratory testing is imperative to reach the precise diagnosis.

In this case, the first attending veterinarian suspected the parrot to have aspergillosis due only to the symptoms observed. Because of the severe seizure, no other tests were run. When the bird was referred, a more comprehensive approach to the diagnosis was deemed necessary. Results of the blood diagnosis analyses were not typical of any severe infection, with only an elevated WBC. In this case, radiology was carried out and the presence of the mass became clear.

General anaesthesia in patients is commonly required by veterinarians to carry out diagnostic testing. This very often carries a degree of risk, but it is often necessary in order to reach a correct diagnosis. There was very little that could have been done for this bird. However, without a radiograph, detection of the tumour would have been impossible. This case shows that with a little extra cost, even if the life of the patient was not saved, the owner felt he was provided with the right assistance and a complete diagnostic scenario was offered.

Further reading

Amann, O., Meij, B.P., Westerhof, I., et al., 2007. Giant cell tumor of the bone in a scarlet macaw (*Ara macao*). Avian Dis. 51 (1), 146–149.

Kogekar, N., Spurgeon, T.L., Simon, M.C., et al., 1987. Proliferative fibromatosis in avian skeletal muscle caused by cloned recombinant avian leukosis viruses. Cancer Res. 47 (8), 2083–2091.

Kubo, M., Kobayashi, K., Masegi, T., et al., 2007. A case of chondrosarcoma in a free-flying great egret. J. Wildl. Dis. 43 (3), 542–544.

Razmyar, J., Dezfoulian, O., Peighambari, S.M., 2008. Ossifying fibroma in a canary (*Serinus canaria*). J. Avian Med. Surg. 22 (4), 320–322.

Rothschild, B.M., Panza, R.K., 2005. Epidemiologic assessment of trauma-independent skeletal pathology in non-passerine birds from museum collections. Avian Pathol. 34 (3), 212–219.

Schmidt, R.E., Reavill, D.R., Phalen, D.N., 2008. Pathology of Pet and Aviary Birds. Blackwell Publishing, Ames.

Case 2.20 *J-M. Hatt*

Clinical history

An 11-year-old, female red-lored Amazon parrot (*Amazona autumnalis*) weighing 416 g was presented with the clinical signs of lameness of the left leg. The bird had been presented regularly during the previous 3 years for nail trimming because of deformations on the distal phalanges of all toes on both feet.

The animal lived alone, could move around the owner's flat freely with supervision. The diet consisted of seed mixture for parrots, fruits, vegetable and nuts.

Clinical examination

On presentation, the animal was alert and had a body condition of 3/5. Chronic feather loss was noted around the sternum and the animal showed severe lameness of the left leg. Both intertarsal joints showed mild swelling, appeared painful and felt warm. Auscultation of the heart and the lungs did not reveal any abnormalities.

Radiography (Fig. 2.48)

Q *1. What is your interpretation of the radiographic image in Fig. 2.48a, b?*

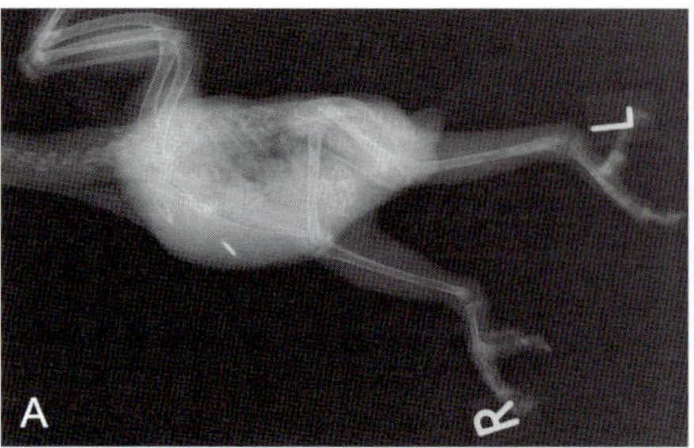

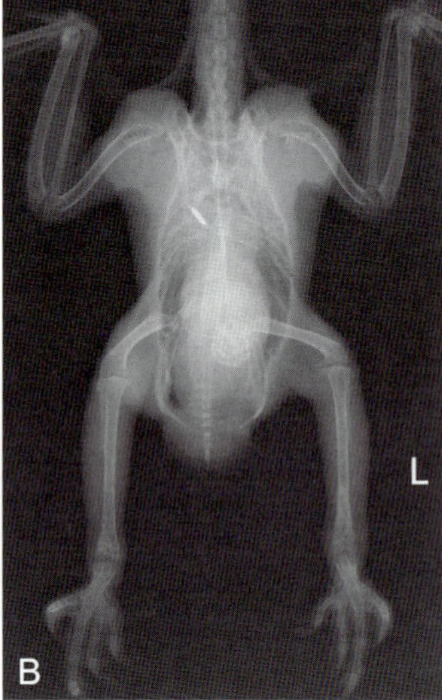

Fig. 2.48 (a) Latero-lateral radiographic overview of the red-lored Amazon; (b) ventrodorsal radiographic overview of the red-lored Amazon.

Clinical diagnosis laboratory

The results of the clinical diagnosis laboratory assays are shown in Tables 2.42 and 2.43.

RBC morphology

➤ Polychromasia index 2

2. What is your interpretation of the haematology and the blood chemistry values shown in Tables 2.42 and 2.43?

Table 2.42 Haematology values of the red-lored Amazon

Parameters	Results (absolute)	Results (%)	Reference values
Hb (g/dl)	13.9		11.3±3.1
Hct (l/l)	0.45		0.51±0.05
Erythrocytes (×10^6/μl)	Not evaluated due to agglutination		3.2±0.4
MCHC (g/dl)	31		24.2±3.1
WBC (×10^9/l)	24.8		12.2±5.0
Heterophils (×10^9/l)	17.9	72	50% (33–73)
Lymphocytes (×10^9/l)	4.1	16.5	46% (22–66)
Monocytes (×10^9/l)	2.7	11	0.03% (0–1)
Eosinophils (×10^9/l)	0.12	0.5	0% (0)

Table 2.43 Plasma blood chemistry values of the red-lored Amazon

Analysis	Results	Reference values
Albumin (g/l)	14	19 (10–24)
Albumin:globulin ratio	0.3	1.1 (0.7–1.4)
Bile acids (μmol/l)	13.4	69 (24–120)
Calcium (mmol/l)	2.3	2.3±0.15
Creatine kinase (U/l)	341	403±57
Globulin (g/l)	47	21 (19–23)
Glucose (mmol/l)	13.9	13.6±3.80
GOT (U/l)	147	320±111
Total protein (g/l)	61	39±8
Urea (mmol/l)	0.6	1.1±0.3
Uric acid (μmol/l)	220	327±107

Reference values: ISIS Physiological Reference Values, 2002; Fudge, AM (2000), Laboratory Medicine Avian and Exotic Pets. W.B. Saunders Company, Philadelphia.

Results

- Radiography revealed mild soft tissue swelling around intertarsal joints (left > right), severe bony destruction of left distal tibiotarsus and mild bony destruction of right distal tibiotarsus, suggestive for osteomyelitis or neoplasia. In the coelomic cavity, the signs of organomegaly, possibly hepatomegaly. Large amount of grit in the ventriculus
- Haematology revealed a moderate leucocytosis with heterophilia, monocytosis and lymphopenia, suggestive for a granulomatous inflammation
- Chemistry revealed a mild elevation of total protein, hyperglobulinemia, mild decrease of urea and bile acids

Please evaluate the clinical history, Fig. 2.48a, b, the results of the physical examination and clinical diagnosis laboratory tests.

3. List your differential diagnoses.

Differential diagnoses

- Bacterial infection (*Chlamydophila psittaci*, *Mycobacteria* spp., other)
- Neoplasia
- Metabolic bone disease

4. What would be your next diagnostic steps to ascertain the diagnosis?

Further diagnostic steps

- Antigen testing for *Chlamydophila psittaci*
- Cytology and microbiology of bone marrow aspirate of tibiotarsus (including acid-fast staining)
- Cytology and microbiology of intertarsal joint aspirate of tibiotarsus (including acid-fast staining)
- Cytology and microbiology of liver biopsy (including acid-fast staining)
- Endoscopic evaluation of the coelomic cavity
- Faecal analysis for *Mycobacteria* spp.

Endoscopy and faecal analysis were not performed.

Chlamydophila psittaci detection (oral/conjunctiva/cloacal swab)

- Negative for antigen (IDEIA-Antigen-ELISA)

Cytology and microbiology of intertarsal joint and bone marrow aspirate of tibiotarsus (including acid-fast staining)

- Negative for signs of infection or neoplasia

Cytology and microbiology of liver biopsy (including acid-fast staining)

➤ Mild to moderate multifocal, histiocytic hepatitis and detection of acid-fast rods

 *5. What therapy would you propose?*

Therapy (Table 2.44)

Table 2.44 Therapy

Clarithromycin	55 mg/kg PO SID × 12 months
Ethambutol	30 mg/kg PO SID × 12 months
Rifabutin	6 mg/kg PO SID × 12 months
Enrofloxacin	30 mg/kg PO SID × 12 months
Meloxicam	1 mg/kg PO SID × 4 weeks
Vitamin A	5000 IU/kg IM once
Vitamin K	3 mg/kg IM once
Repeat liver biopsy	After 12 months
Information for owner	Zoonotic risk and potential complications due to fungal respiratory tract disease

Final diagnosis

➤ Mycobacteriosis

Discussion

Avian mycobacteriosis is a frequent disease and is caused by several different species of the genus *Mycobacterium*, typically *Mycobacterium avium* or *Mycobacterium genavense*. Infection occurs by ingestion or inhalation of Mycobacteria which can contaminate soil, water or other matter. The disease is typically slowly progressing and may lead to a variety of clinical signs, depending on the affected organs. Typically, there is a granulomatous inflammation. Organs that are frequently affected are the intestine, liver and spleen, the skin and long bones. Reliable intra vitam diagnosis is hampered because of lack of sensitive diagnostic tests. Detection of acid-fast rods followed by culture is the diagnostic method of choice. In the present case, diagnosis could only be made by a liver biopsy which revealed acid-fast bacteria. Ideally, the mycobacteria should be cultured and differentiated. Treatment is controversial due to the lack of scientific data regarding the outcome and the potential zoonotic risk that an infected bird may represent. In the present case, treatment was elected since the owner was living on her own and had only one bird.

Further reading

Lennox, A.M., 2007. Mycobacteriosis in companion psittacine birds: a review. J. Avian Med. Surg. 21, 181–187.

Witte, C.L., Hungerford, L.L., Papendick, R., et al., 2010. Investigation of factors predicting disease among zoo birds exposed to avian mycobacteriosis. J. Am. Vet. Med. Assoc. 236, 211–218.

Case 2.21 *A. Montesinos*

Clinical history

A 12-year-old female orange-winged Amazon parrot (*Amazona amazonica*) weighing 380 g was presented with the following clinical signs observed in the past 5 days:

- Dyspnoea
- Inappetence
- Lack of vocalization
- Overgrowth of the beak.

The wild-caught parrot was the only pet in the house and was offered commercially available avian food supplemented with fruits and vegetables daily.

Physical examination

On presentation, the bird had a body condition of 4/5 and all the symptoms were exacerbated during the handling. The parrot was put into an oxygen chamber and nebulizated with salbutamol. After 2 hours, whole body radiographs were taken and blood samples were collected for haematology, blood chemistry, blood gas analyses, plasma protein electrophoresis and serology and antigen detection test against *Chlamydophila psittaci*.

Clinical diagnosis examination

Radiology (Fig. 2.49)

1. What is your interpretation of the radiographs of Fig. 2.49a, b?

Clinical diagnosis laboratory examination

The results of the clinical diagnosis laboratory assays are shown in Tables 2.45–2.48.

RBC, WBC and thrombocyte morphology

➤ Activated lymphocytes +++

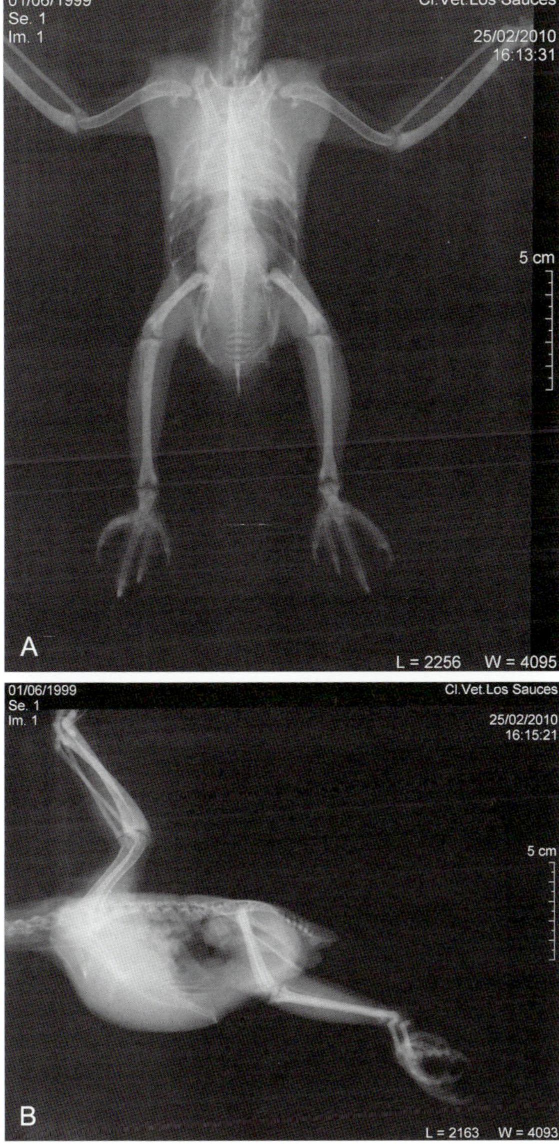

Fig. 2.49 (a) Ventrodorsal survey radiograph of a 12-year-old orange-winged parrot; (b) lateral survey radiograph of a 12-year-old orange-winged parrot.

Table 2.45 Haematology results of the orange-winged Amazon parrot

Parameters	Results (absolute)	Results (%)	Reference values
RBC ($\times10^{12}$/l)	2.24		2.4–4.1
Hb (g/dl)	13.9		12.6–17
Hct (l/l)	0.48		0.48–0.56
MCV (fl)	214.29		
MCH (pg)	79.91		
MCHC (g/dl)	37.29		
WBC ($\times10^{9}$/l)	6.125		4–11
Heterophils ($\times10^{9}$/l)	37.97	62	30–65%
Lymphocytes ($\times10^{9}$/l)	18.98	31	20–75 %
Monocytes ($\times10^{9}$/l)	3.06	5	0–3 %
Eosinophils ($\times10^{9}$/l)	0	0	0–1 %
Basophils ($\times10^{9}$/l)	1.22	2	0–5 %
Thrombocytes ($\times10^{9}$/l)	15.75		

Table 2.46 Blood chemistry results of the orange-winged Amazon parrot

Assays	Results	Reference values
Albumin (g/l)	15.9	19–35
ALKP (U/l)	230.6	15–150
Bile acids (µmol/l)	290	19–144
Calcium (mg/dl)	9.5	8–12
Cholesterol (mg/dl)	233.7	130–250
CK (U/l)	581	45–265
GGT (U/l)	12.5	0–15
GOT (U/l)	106	130–350
Glucose (mg/dl)	272	220–350
Lactate (mg/dl)	72.21	8–30
Phosphorus (mg/dl)	2.3	2–5
Potassium (mmol/l)	5.2	2.5–4.5
Sodium (mmol/l)	150	136–152
Total protein (g/l)	27	25–40
Tryglycerides (mg/dl)	91.4	85–170
Uric acid (mg/dl)	2	2–10

Table 2.47 Plasma protein electrophoresis results of the orange-winged Amazon parrot

Parameters	Fractions (%)	Concentration (g/l)
Total protein	100	27
Pre-albumin	18.1	5.1
Albumin	58.8	15.9
Alpha 1 globulins	2.59	0.7
Alpha 2 globulins	6.6	1.8
Beta globulins	7.03	1.9
Gamma globulins	5.92	1.6
A:G ratio		2.64

Table 2.48 Blood gases results of the orange-winged Amazon parrot

Parameters	Results FIO_2 100%, 38°C	Reference values
Ionized calcium (mmol/l)	1.21	
pH	7.201	7.3–7.48
PCO_2 (mmHg)	72.9	24–30
PO_2 (mmHg)	88	>200
TCO_2 (mmol/l)	33	
HCO_3 (mmol/l)	31	25–30
BEecf	3	0–20
SO_2 (%)	94	99–100
Plasma osmolality (mOsm/kg)	303.06	336±6.38

Serology against *Chlamydophila* spp. using Inmunocomb® (Biogal laboratories)

➤ Strong positive result

Detection of LPS antigen of *Chlamydophila* spp. using Speed Chlam test®

➤ Strong positive result

2. What is your interpretation of the haematology, blood chemistry and protein electrophoresis values shown in Tables 2.45–2.48?

Summary of diagnostic results

- Faecal examination showed negative result for the presence of endoparasites
- Radiographic findings included increased radiodensity on the cranial part of the heart, enlarged kidney shadow, especially in the cranial lobe, presence of opacities in the bronchial tree and enlarged spleen shadow
- Haematology analysis showed low RBC and low Hct. There were also slight heterophilia and monocytosis
- Blood chemistry analysis showed elevated levels of bile acids, CK, ALKP, L-lactate and potassium
- Plasma protein electrophoresis showed low total protein and low levels of albumin
- Blood gases analysis showed marked respiratory acidosis with good level of oxygenation

Please evaluate the clinical history, Fig. 2.49a, b, the results of the physical examination and clinical diagnostic tests.

Q *3. List your differential diagnoses.*

Q *4. List your diagnostic strategy.*

Q *5. List your therapeutic strategy.*

Differential diagnoses

- Hepatopathy and splenomegaly due to *Chlamydophila* infection
- Renal disease
- Respiratory disease due to *Chlamydophila* or complicated with concurrent *Aspergillus* spp. infection
- Precardiac neoplasia

Further clinical diagnosis examination

If the owner agrees and the health status of the bird improves, an endoscopic examination could reveal more details about the disease of the parrot. An exploratory coelomic endoscopy was programmed 3 days after admission.

Therapy

Since the bird was positive in two tests against *Chlamydophila*, a treatment with doxycycline was started awaiting the results of histopathology (Table 2.49).

Further clinical diagnosis examination

Endoscopy

Consent was obtained from the owner and the endoscopy examination carried out. Figures 2.50–2.52 are images obtained during the procedure.

Table 2.49 Therapy

Doxycycline 20 mg/ml	100 mg/kg IM one dose every week, 6 weeks
Meloxicam	1 mg/kg IM BID one week
Nebulization	Salbutamol 250 µg (0.5 ml) + saline 5 ml for 30 min
Fluids	Saline 50 ml/kg/day IV IRC

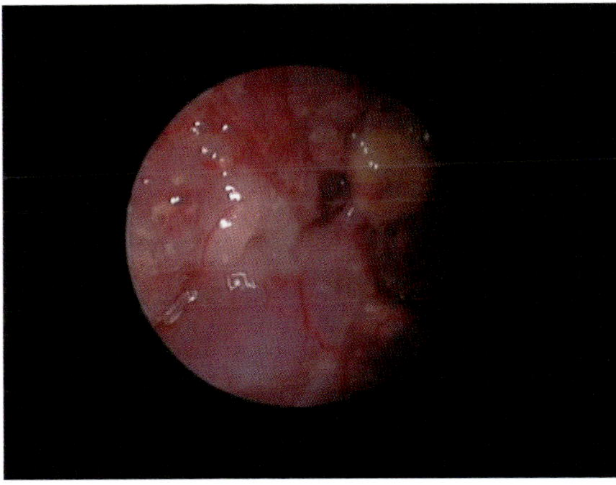

Fig. 2.50 View of the cranial thoracic air sac showing an amorphous mass surrounding the base of the heart in the orange-winged Amazon parrot.

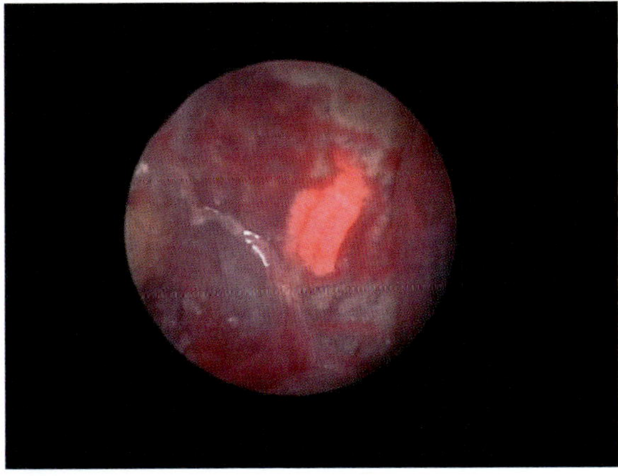

Fig. 2.51 View of the caudal thoracic air sac showing a marked congestion of the lung parenchyma.

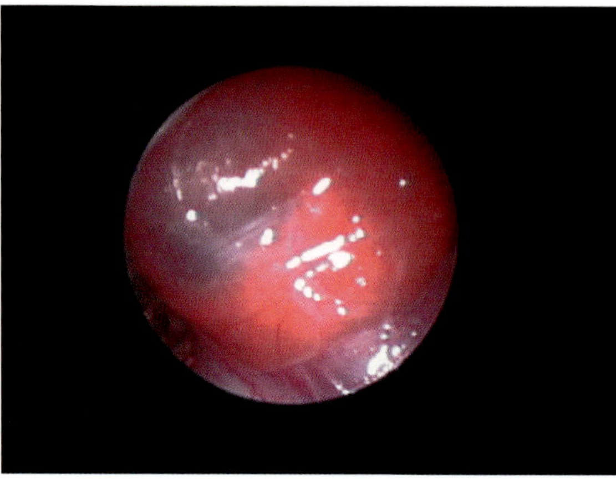

Fig. 2.52 View of the cranial lobe of the left kidney through the left abdominal air sac showing a cystic dilatation of the cranial lobe.

Biopsy

Lung, precardiac mass and kidney biopsies were taken during the endoscopy procedure.

Biopsy findings

The precardiac mass was an air sac carcinoma. Renal dilatation showed normal renal tissue and polycystic kidney.

Post-mortem findings

Because of the reserved prognosis and the gradual deterioration in the condition of the bird, the owner elected for euthanasia and allowed a full post-mortem examination. Samples from different organs were collected for histopathology analysis (Figs 2.53–2.55).

 *6. What is your provisional post-mortem diagnosis?*

Summary of post-mortem examination findings

- Coelomic cavity wall: medium to big size granulomatous masses on the thoracic air sacs
- Pancreas: enlarged with few focal haemorrhagic foci
- Great vessels: enlarged and firm when touched
- Lung: bilateral mild congestion
- Kidney: fluid-filled cavities in left kidney

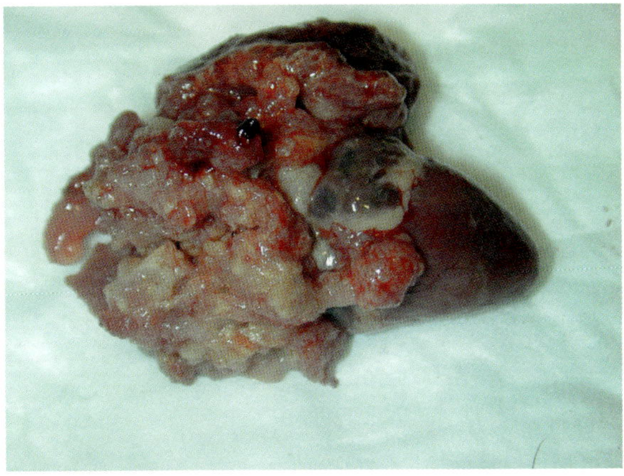

Fig. 2.53 View of the neoplastic mass surrounding the heart of the orange-winged Amazon parrot.

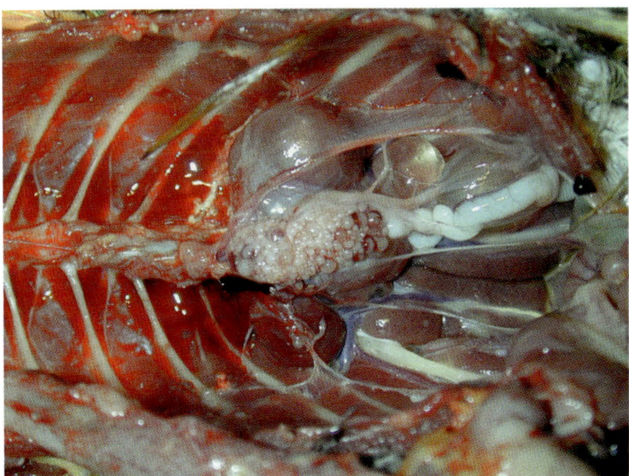

Fig. 2.54 View of the left kidney showing the cystic dilatation of the whole organ.

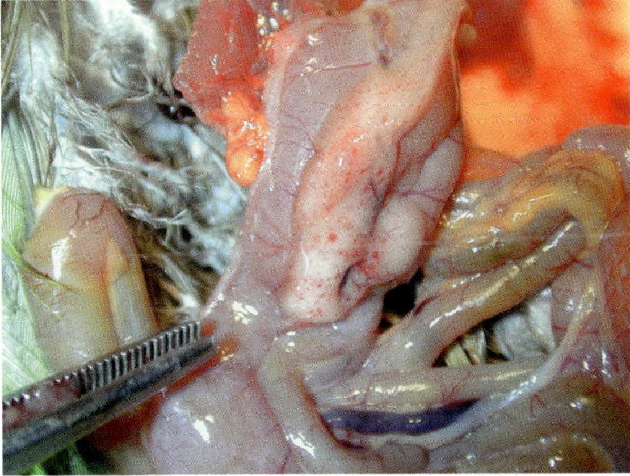

Fig. 2.55 Image of the pancreas of the orange-winged Amazon parrot.

Provisional post-mortem diagnosis

- Respiratory neoplasia
- Respiratory granulomatous disease
- Renal failure

Post-mortem laboratory findings

Post-mortem laboratory analyses confirmed the same results obtained from the endoscopic-guided biopsies.

- Histology
  - Air sac carcinoma
  - Air sac carcinoma metastasis to pancreas
  - Neoplastic cells embolism in lung
  - Great vessels arteriosclerosis
  - Polycystic kidney

Final diagnosis

- Air sac carcinoma with metastasis in pancreas
- Polycystic kidney

Discussion

Air sac carcinomas have been described in the avian literature affecting humeral bone and interclavicular air sac but not producing precardiac masses. However, this kind of neoplasia has to be included in the differential diagnoses of precardiac masses seen in the radiographs. The latest imaging diagnostic techniques will help in the differentiation of neoplasia and granulomas although endoscopic biopsy remains the gold standard for ante-mortem diagnosis. Assessment of blood gases status in the bird patient could help to differentiate between oxygenation problems (primary respiratory disease) or ventilation problems (anaesthesia, compressive masses).

Further reading

Bateman, S.H., 2008. Making sense of blood gas results. Vet. Clin. North Am. Small Anim. 28, 543–557.

Baumgartner, W.A., Sanchez-Migallon, D., et al., 2008. Bronchogenic adenocarcinoma in a Hyacinth macaw. J. Avian Med. Surg. 3, 218–225.

Garner, M., 2003. Air sac carcinomas in bird: 7 clinical cases. In: Proceedings of the Association of Avian Veterinarians. pp. 55–57.

Hunter, D.B., Taylor, M., 1992. Lung biopsy as a diagnostic technique in avian medicine. In: Proceedings of the Association of Avian Veterinarians. pp. 233–245.

Jones, M.P., Orosz, S.E., Richman, L.K., et al., 2001. Pulmonary carcinoma with metastases in a Moluccan cockatoo. J. Avian Med. Surg. 15, 107–113.

Marshall, K., Daniel, G., Patton, C., 2004. Humeral air sac mucinous adenocarcinoma in a Moluccan cockatoo. J. Avian Med. Surg. 18, 167–174.
Powers, L.V., Merrill, C.L., Degernes, L.A., 1998. Axillary cystoadenocarcinoma in a Moluccan cockatoo. Avian Dis. 42, 408–412.

Case 2.22 *N. A. Forbes*

Clinical history

A 25-year-old blue-fronted Amazon parrot (*Amazona aestiva*) was presented for examination. The wild-caught and previously imported bird was a single pet bird owned by the family. The bird was reported to have developed a significant swelling under its lower beak (Fig. 2.56). The bird was apparently otherwise bright, lively and behaving normally. The bird was reported to eat very well, having been on a seed-based diet, with minimal fruit supplementation for the past 25 years. History:

- Swelling under the lower beak
- Otherwise apparently normal
- Mild URT infection.

Physical examination

On examination, the parrot was bright, lively, but with a gross swelling under the beak measuring 2 cm × 1 cm. The bird was slightly overweight, bodyweight was 557 g with a body condition of 3/5 (slightly overweight).

Clinical diagnosis examination

Survey radiographs were taken while the bird was under anaesthesia, which were found to be normal. Routine CBC was carried out, which demonstrated a mild leucocytosis 10.5×10^9/l (n=5–8.5), but was otherwise normal.

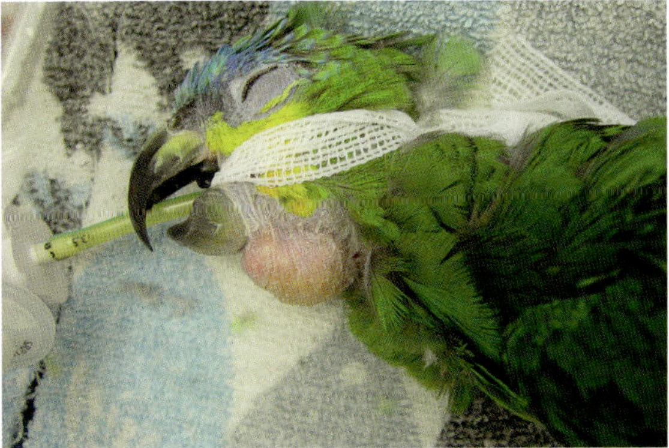

Fig. 2.56 Visible swelling under the beak of the blue-fronted Amazon parrot.

Q *1. What condition do you believe this bird is suffering from?*

Q *2. What tissue is affected?*

Q *3. How could you confirm the diagnosis?*

Q *4. What secondary problems can occur in this condition?*

Q *5. What treatments are indicated?*

Q *6. What foods are low in the dependent nutrient?*

Q *7. What foods are high in the dependent nutrient?*

Answers

- Chronic hypovitaminosis A
- Squamous metaplasia of the submandibular or sublingual salivary glands
- Blood vitamin A levels are not diagnostically useful. Confirmation of the diagnosis is achieved on clinical signs, history, or liver biopsy and analysis or salivary gland biopsy and histopathology
- Vitamin A plays the role of protecting the bird against mouth, respiratory or renal disease, so in deficiency cases the patient is prone to these diseases. Many affected birds will demonstrate a wide open choana. Loss of vision, reduced reproduction, increased periosteal bone deposition, impaired immune function have all also been noted
- Vitamin A supplementation (<50 KIU/kg once parenterally), conversion onto a better diet. Some granuloma will fail to resolve subsequent to correct nutrition and may need to be surgically removed. Granuloma are also prone to secondary bacterial infection which, if present, will require medical treatment
- Nut- and seed-based diets are low in vitamin A, any psittacine bird on an unsupplemented seed- or nut-based diet will eventually suffer from vitamin A deficiency, although it may take years (often 10 or more years) to occur, so long as they live long enough
- Fresh fruit and highly coloured vegetables tend to be high in vitamin A, e.g. sweetcorn, apricots, cantaloupe, kiwi, mango, watermelon.

Differential diagnoses

- Foreign body, trauma, bacterial or yeast infection of the salivary gland

Therapy

The parrot was placed on therapeutic management shown in Table 2.50.

Table 2.50 Therapy

Vitamin A injection	40 KIU/kg IM once, plus change onto a quality proprietary commercial pelleted diet, plus fresh coloured fruit
Baytril	5 mg/kg BID PO for 5 days
Surgery	Removal of the granuloma 10 days later

Response to therapy

The bird was noted by the owner to be much stronger, boisterous and noisy following treatment.

The skin and plumage appeared much brighter and healthier after the subsequent moult.

Discussion

There is a fundamental need for avian clinicians to council all parrot-owning clients in relation to the feeding of an appropriate diet.

Further reading

Hensel, P., 2010. Nutrition and skin diseases in veterinary medicine. Clin. Dermatol. 28 (6), 686–693.

McDonald, D., Nutritional considerations. In: Harrison, G.J., Lightfoot, T.L. (Eds.), Clinical Avian Medicine. Spix Publishing, Inc., Palm Beach, pp. 92–95.

Phalen, D.N., 2000. Respiratory medicine of cage and aviary birds. Vet. Clin. North Am. Exot. Anim. Pract. 3 (2), 423–452.

Case 2.23 *L. Crosta*

Clinical history

An 8-year-old African grey parrot (*Psittacus erithacus*), of unknown gender, was brought to our veterinary clinic for a second opinion. The first attending veterinarian examined the bird and ran haematology and blood chemistry diagnostic analyses. After evaluating the history, clinical symptoms and blood diagnostic results, the veterinarian suggested aspergillosis and psittacosis as possible aetiologies.

After a short course with doxycycline and ketoconazole the owner decided to seek a second opinion as the treatment did not lead to any visible improvement.

Physical examination

The bird had a history of living in a small cage and had been fed almost exclusively on sunflower seeds for the past 6–7 years.

At presentation, the bird appeared very depressed. The main reported symptoms were:

- Anorexia
- Severe weakness
- Progressive weight loss.

Clinical diagnosis examination

Since the owner had a limited budget, and due to the fact that the blood samples were going to be submitted to the same laboratory as the first samples, it was decided to accept the blood analyses results and opt for a radiographic study only.

Radiology (Fig. 2.57)

1. What is your interpretation of the radiographs in Fig. 2.57a, b?

Clinical diagnosis laboratory examination

The results of the clinical diagnosis laboratory assays are shown in Tables 2.51 and 2.52.

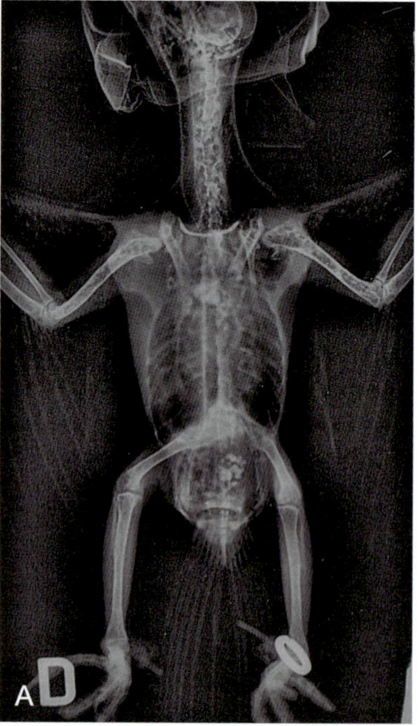

Fig. 2.57 (a) Ventrodorsal survey radiograph of the African grey parrot ("D" stands for "right");

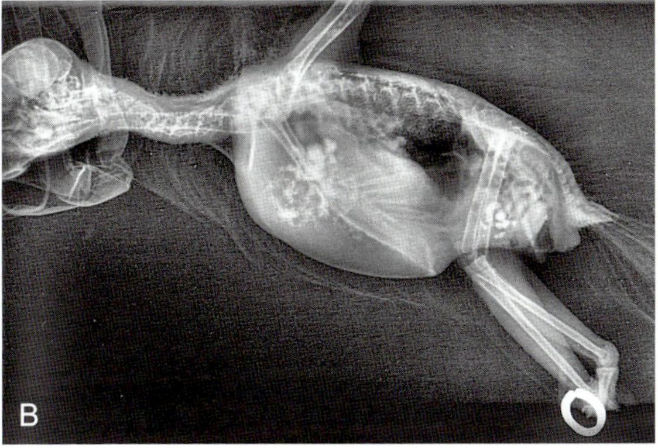

Fig. 2.57—cont'd (b) left lateral survey radiograph of the 8-year-old African grey parrot.

Blood film comments

➤ No haemoparasites were observed. Moderate anisocytosis and moderate poikilocytosis

2. What is your interpretation of the haematology and blood chemistry values shown in Tables 2.51 and 2.52?

Table 2.51 Haematology values of the African grey parrot

Parameters	Results (absolute)	Results (%)	Reference values
RBC (×10^{12}/l)	2.72		3.0–3.6
Hb (g/dl)	17.4		14.2–17.0
Hct (l/l)	0.44		0.43–0.51
MCV (fl)	161		137–155
MCH (pg)	64.1		41.9–52.8
MCHC (g/dl)	39.5		28.9–34.0
RDW (%)	12.8		
WBC (×10^{9}/l)	61.7		6.0–12.0
Heterophils (%)	55.53	90	45–73
Lymphocytes (%)	61.7	10	19–50
Monocytes (%)		0	0.03–0.9
Eosinophils (%)		0	0.0–0.68
Basophils (%)		0	0.0–0.29
Thrombocytes k/μl	14.6		11–42

Table 2.52 Blood chemistry values of the African grey parrot

Analysis	Results	Reference values
Uric acid (mg/dl)	3.7	2.2–11.0
AST (U/l)	96	110–340
CK (U/l)	544	140–411
LDH (U/l)	875	154–378
Total Protein (g/dl)	3.1	2.7–4.4
Calcium (mg/dl)	7.39	8.0–14.0
Glucose (mg/dl)	199	256–360

Summary of diagnostic results

- Radiographic findings included increased diffused radio-density of the left cranial thoracic air sacs and increased definition of the margins of the right air sacs
- Haematology analysis showed low RBC, slightly elevated Hb and normal Hct. There was a severe leucocytosis with absolute heterophilia
- Blood chemistry analysis showed elevated levels of CK and LDH and reduced levels of glucose and calcium

Please evaluate the clinical history, Fig. 2.57a, b, the results of the physical examination and clinical diagnosis laboratory tests.

Q *3. List your differential diagnoses.*

Q *4. List your therapeutic strategy.*

Differential diagnoses

- Aspergillosis
- *Ab ingestis* pneumonia/airsacculitis
- Psittacosis

Therapy

The parrot was immediately placed on treatment (Table 2.53).

Post-mortem findings

Unfortunately, the bird died on the second day of admission. A thorough post-mortem examination was performed (Fig. 2.58a–e). Due to budget limitations, samples were collected only for microbiology, while histopathology samples were stored.

Table 2.53 Therapy

Voriconazole	10 mg/kg IM BID × 1 week, then orally for at least one month
Doxycycline	100 mg/kg IM q7d
Vitamin ADE	Vitamin A 20 000 IU/kg IM once
Fluids/Vitamin B complex	Ringer's lactate 20 ml/kg with 30 mg/kg thiamine SC BID
Forced feeding	Harrison's Recovery formula + Avix booster BID

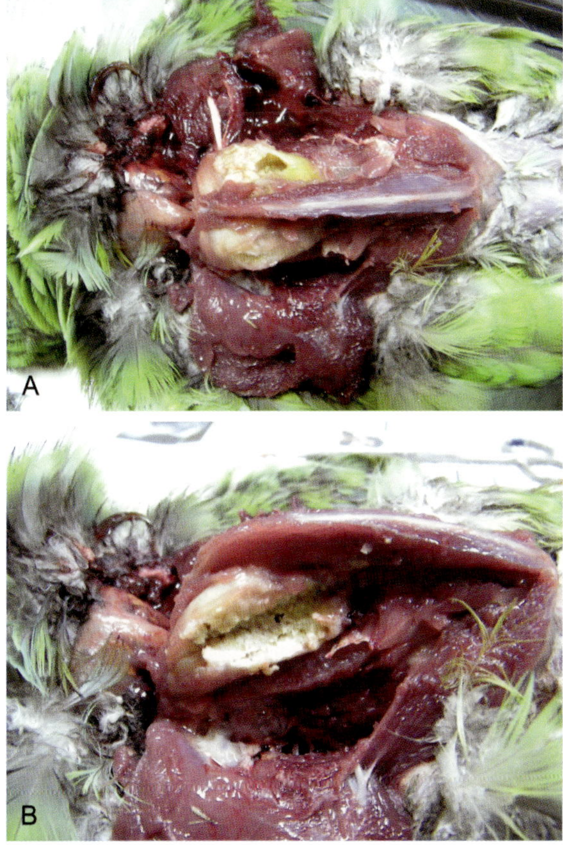

Fig. 2.58 (a–e) Post-mortem photographs of the African grey parrot.

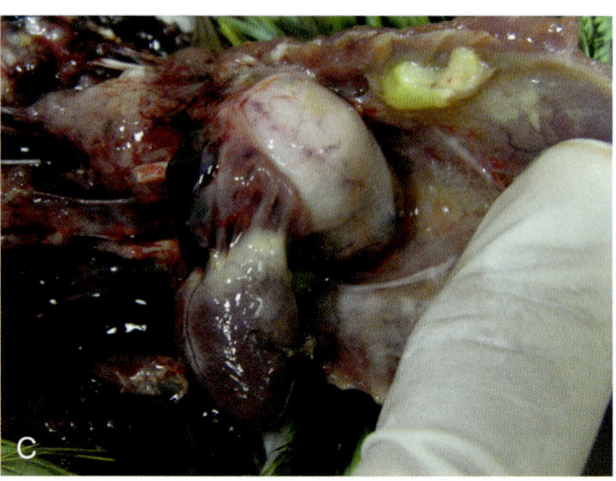

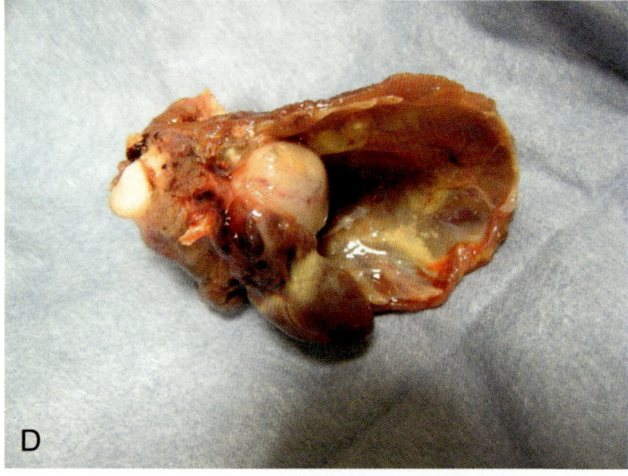

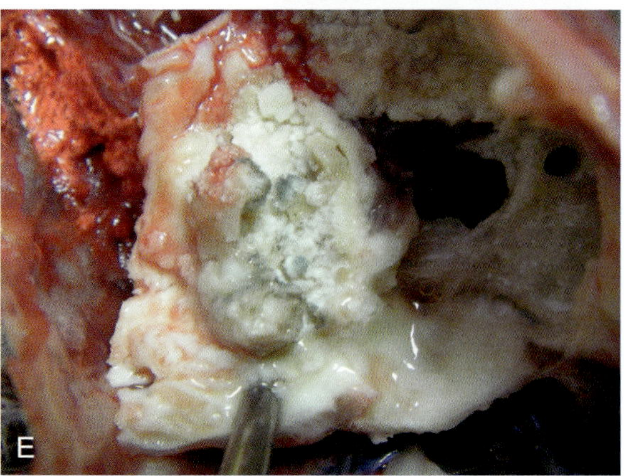

Fig. 2.58—cont'd

Q *5. What lesions can you observe in the post-mortem photographs?*

Q *6. What is your provisional post-mortem diagnosis?*

Summary of post-mortem examination findings

- Liver: nothing remarkable
- Coelomic cavity: presence of a large granuloma involving all the air sacs of the left side. At opening, a carpet of grey-bluish tissue was evident
- Intestines: no direct involvement of the GI tract by the granulomatous lesions
- Left kidney: whitish and enlarged, almost not recognizable

Provisional post-mortem diagnosis

- Aspergillosis

Laboratory findings

- Microbiology: *Aspergillus fumigatus* was isolated from the coelomic cavity wall lesion

Final diagnosis

- Aspergillosis

Discussion

The bird was presented for a second opinion with an already advanced disease. Taking into consideration the radiology, haematology and blood chemistry results, there were not many differential diagnoses on the list. However, there are several interesting facts in this case:

- Although for the inexperienced eye, the right air sac system may look more severely affected, the left side was worse at necropsy. This is due to the mild fibrin deposits over the right side coelomic walls, which defined the air sacs very well radiologically. The right side, instead, appears more as a diffused problem which tends to happen when the air sacs are filled with exudates, as in this case
- Even if the left kidney was literally destroyed by the pathological process, blood uric acid level was not elevated. This happens when the disease is unilateral and the contralateral organ is still able to support the function of both sides
- Such a high WBC with absolute heterophilia is typical of two diseases in psittacines, psittacosis and aspergillosis, but a low glucose level may indicate a chronic disease highly suggestive of a fungal infection.

This is the typical second opinion case, when the first veterinarian made a correct diagnosis, but possibly the therapy was not aggressive enough or, more than likely, the condition of the bird was already too advanced to have a positive resolution.

A common problem facing the private practitioner is the limited budget of some customers. This normally leads to having the first consultation from a local veterinarian and eventually asking for a second opinion from a more experienced/certified/well-known professional. In most cases, this does not work as pathological conditions in birds tend to develop very fast.

Further reading

Beernaert, L.A., Pasmans, F., Van Waeyenberghe, et al., 2009. Avian *Aspergillus fumigatus* strains resistant to both itraconazole and voriconazole. Antimicrob. Agents Chemother. 53 (5), 2199–2201.

Beernaert, L.A., Pasmans, F., Baert, K., et al., 2009. Designing a treatment protocol with voriconazole to eliminate *Aspergillus fumigatus* from experimentally inoculated pigeons. Vet. Microbiol. 139 (3–4), 393–397.

Beernaert, L.A., Pasmans, F., Van Waeyenberghe, et al., 2010. Aspergillus infections in birds: a review. Avian Pathol. 39 (5), 325–331.

Cray, C., Watson, T., Arheart, K.L., 2009. Serosurvey and diagnostic application of antibody titers to Aspergillus in avian species. Avian Dis. 53 (4), 491–494.

Di Somma, A., Bailey, T., Silvanose, C., et al., 2007. The use of voriconazole for the treatment of aspergillosis in falcons (Falco species). J. Avian Med. Surg. 21, 307–316.

Redig, P., 2008. Fungal Disease – Aspergillosis. In: Samour, J. (Ed.), Avian Medicine, second ed. Mosby Elsevier, Oxford, pp. 373–387.

Schmidt, R.E., Reavill, D.R., Phalen, D.N., 2008. Pathology of Pet and Aviary Birds. Blackwell Publishing, Ames.

Case 2.24 *M. Hochleithner*

Clinical history

A 17-month-old African grey parrot (*Psittacus erithacus*), of unknown gender, was presented with the history of seizures within the last 4 days.

Q *1. What further information do you need from the owner?*

- What is the diet?
- How many birds are in the collection?
- How many juvenile birds?
- Are there any other birds sick?

The owner had two African grey parrots of the same age, the second bird had no clinical signs. The diet contained a seed mixture together with some pellets he bought in a pet shop, but the birds did not eat them. On further questioning, the owner said that the bird had not eaten well for about 10 days.

Physical examination

On presention, the bird's bodyweight was 359 g with a body condition of 3/5. During examination the bird suddenly started seizuring (Fig. 2.59).

2. What do you think this condition can be and what can we do as first aid?

African grey parrots are known for the so-called "hypocalcaemic syndrome" where plasma calcium concentration drops below normal. First aid would consist of administering calcium injection IM. The use of steroids in this case is not recommended as they will further decrease the plasma calcium.

Clinical diagnosis examination

3a. What diagnostic tests can and/or should be considered?

- Radiology
- Ultrasound
- Faecal examination for parasites including flotation

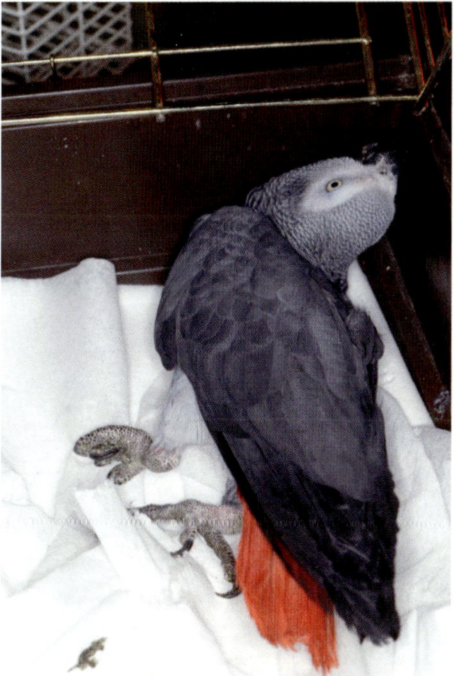

Fig. 2.59 African grey parrot seizuring.

- PCR for
  - Polyomavirus
  - Psittacine beak and feather disease (PBFD)
  - *Chlamydophila*
  - Bornavirus
- Bacteriological examination, including *Salmonella*
- Haematology and blood chemistry
- Endoscopy
- Computed tomography

Q ***3b. What are the advantages and disadvantages of each in this special case?***

- *Radiology*: heavy metal intoxication can be the cause of seizures in parrots. The mineralization of bones as well as old fractures due to secondary hyperparathyroidism should be evaluated especially in African grey parrots
- *Ultrasound*: in birds, the air sacs limit the use of ultrasound in many cases. In this special case, ultrasound would not be first choice, although congenital cardiac diseases have been described and could be the reason for seizures
- *Faecal examination for parasites including flotation*: endoparasites are seen very rarely in parrots within the EU as no more wild-caught birds are imported
- *PCR for polyomavirus, PBFD,* Chlamydophila, *bornavirus*: many laboratories have combinations of these tests. With such a history, it is important to test for these diseases
- *Bacteriological examination of faeces and maybe a swab from throat including* Salmonella: although the information about the microbiological status would be interesting, it is not very likely that a certain bacterial infection will cause the seizures without any other symptoms
- *Haematology*: a haemogram is very useful, however, one has to be careful with interpreting avian leucograms, because there is a wide variation in the normal leucogram among birds of the same species. Blood parasites are very seldom seen in captive-bred psittacines
- *Blood chemistry*: a minimum panel including calcium, AST, CK, total protein and uric acid should be done
- *Endoscopy*: with the history of seizures, the sex should be known. Intoxications can be the cause of seizures, however, in many cases, it is hardly detected by other diagnostic procedures
- *Computed tomography*: the history of this case does not require CT

Results

Radiology

- No signs of heavy metal. No abnormal signs

PCR

- Polyomavirus, PBFD, *Chlamydophila*, bornavirus: negative

Bacteriological swabs

- Choana: + *E. coli*
- Cloaca: negative

Blood chemistry (Tables 2.54 and 2.55)

Table 2.54 Haematology

Parameter	Results	Reference range
RBC ($\times 10^{12}$/l)	2.71	2.7–3.6
HB (g/dl)	153	142–171
Hct (l/l)	0.46	0.43–0.51
WBC ($\times 10^{9}$/l)	9.7	3.3–10.3

Table 2.55 Blood chemistry

Parameter	Results	Reference range
AST (U/l)	1413	28–200
CK (U/l)	8332	71–800
Total protein (g/l)	41	26–49
Uric acid (mmol/l)	243	100–500
Calcium (mmol/l)	1.7	1.9–2.4

Endoscopy (Fig. 2.60)

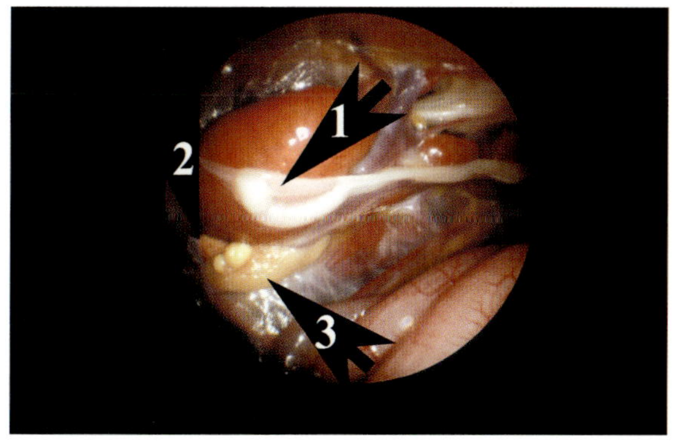

Fig. 2.60 Endoscopic *in situ*.

Q *4. Name the structures 1, 2, 3.*

- 1: Dorsal ligament of the oviduct across the kidney, this only can be seen in female birds and can be the only structure to differentiate between male and female birds in very young individuals
- 2: Adrenal gland
- 3: Juvenile ovary

Juvenile ovary, airsacs and internal organs appear normal.

Q *5. How would you interpret these results?*

The finding of some *E.coli* in a choanal swab is not normal, however, it does not mean that the bird has an *E.coli* infection. There are many possible reasons for this finding, including contamination of the swab when taking the sample. In many psittacine birds, we find Gram-negative bacteria, which are not normal, without any clinical signs. In these cases we do not recommend any antibiotic treatment.

Blood chemistry

Although the bird did get a calcium injection, the calcium concentration is still low; it is very likely that the symptoms are due to hypocalcaemia. Usually, the plasma calcium concentration would be low for 24–48 hours even when injecting calcium twice a day, however, seizuring usually stops.

AST and CK are both very much elevated. AST is not liver specific and also will be increased when muscle cells are damaged. CK is specific for muscle cell damage so the increase of both enzymes is suspicious for muscle cell damage.

6. How could the bird have got the muscle cell damage and is this the reason for the seizures?

Usually it is the other way around. Birds with seizures will have elevated enzymes because they often fall down from the perch. Although the measurement of enzymes is not quantitative method, the high concentration of CK could indicate that there is severe muscle damage.

Therapy

The treatment of the bird was proceeded with calcium injections (calcium gluconolactobionate 10%, 2 ml/kg), tube feeding using a formulated diet and SC infusions with lactated Ringer's Vitamin ADEC.

The bird did not stop seizuring and continued with 3–4 seizures a day.

7. What is your next step?

Re-check calcium and CK.

- CK (U/l): 10 235 (day 1: 8332) 71–800
- Calcium (mmol/l): 2.0 (day 1: 1.7) 1.9–2.4

 *8. What next?*

It is very unlikely that this is a case of hypocalcaemia only. Although PCR for viral infections was negative, any of the above mentioned diseases could be involved. However, the high CK is a sign for severe muscle damage, which can be seen in juvenile birds due to vitamin E deficiency, often in combination with selenium deficiency. In such a case, the intramuscular injection of calcium twice daily would worsen the situation.

 *9. How can we diagnose the problem?*

Further laboratory diagnosis examination

A muscle biopsy could confirm the diagnosis of vitamin E deficiency. However, in this case, it is most important to avoid any further muscle damage by giving any intramuscular injection. As the blood calcium concentration was within the reference values, no more calcium injections were needed. A dietary change was deemed necessary.

Final diagnosis

➤ The case was confirmed by muscle biopsy as vitamin E deficiency

Discussion

Although this case looks very easy and with all the characteristic symptoms of the "hypocalcaemic syndrome" in African grey parrots, there are cases which are always different. Hypocalcaemia is usually a dietary problem and birds who are on a calcium deficient diet can also easily have other deficiencies, like in this case, vitamin E and selenium. There is always the possibility of having two different problems at the same time in the same patient. In cases when there is muscle damage due to any disease (e.g. vitamin E–selenium deficiency), intramuscular injections will worsen the case.

Further reading

Harrison, G.J., Lightfoot, T.L., 2006. Clinical Avian Medicine. Spix Publishing, Inc., Palm Beach.
Samour, J., 2008. Avian Medicine, second ed. Mosby Elsevier, London.

Case 2.25 *P. Sandmeier*

Clinical history

A 7-year-old female African grey parrot (*Psittacus erithacus*) weighing 485 g was presented for unilateral feather plucking of a few weeks' duration (Fig. 2.61).

The captive-bred parrot was kept together with a male African grey parrot of the same age as a pet. Both birds were hand raised and very tame. Their aviary was in the living room, they had regular free flight within the house and their diet was a varied mixture of cooked beans and vegetables, fresh fruit, pellets and a small number of seeds.

Clinical examination

On presentation, the African grey parrot had a good body condition. The left side of the body and the left leg were plucked. All other feathers were normal and there was no sign of skin disease. The bird showed no obvious signs of malnutrition with a good feather quality, clear eyes and nostrils, no hyperkeratosis of the feet or cloaca and no dandruff or overly dry skin.

To collect a basic database, the African grey parrot was anaesthetized using isoflurane. Blood samples were taken for haematology, blood chemistry, zinc levels, galactomannan levels and PCR testing for circovirus and polyomavirus. Survey radiographs were taken. A faecal sample was collected to examine for the presence of endoparasites (wet mount and faecal flotation).

Radiology (Fig. 2.62a, b)

1. What is your interpretation of the radiographs in Fig. 2.62a, b?

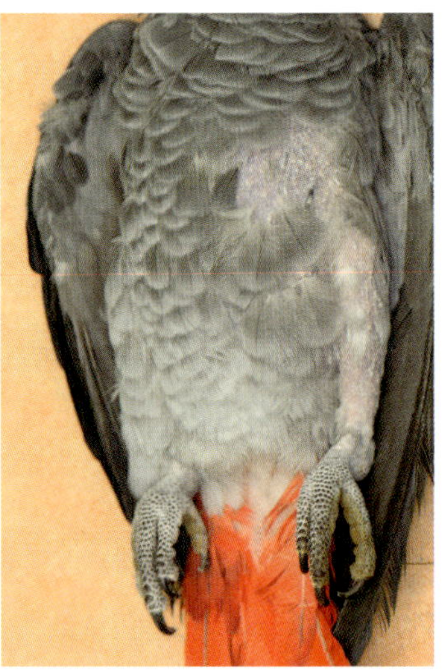

Fig. 2.61 Unilateral feather plucking in the female African grey parrot.

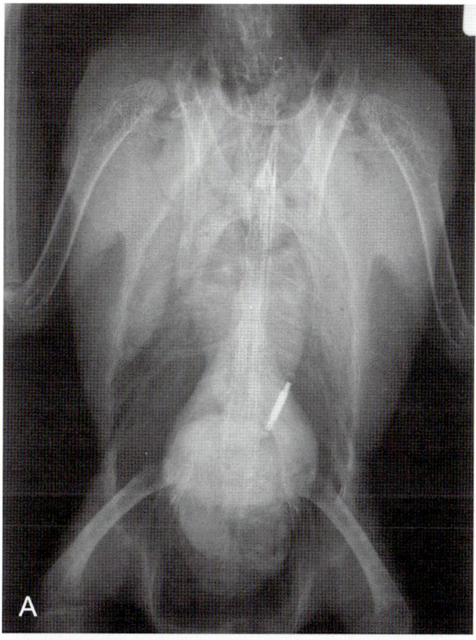

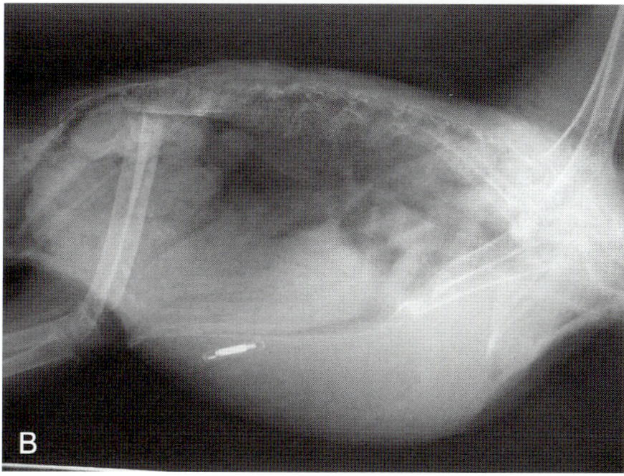

Fig. 2.62 (a) Ventrodorsal survey radiograph of a 7-year-old African grey parrot; (b) lateral survey radiograph of the African grey parrot.

Clinical diagnosis laboratory

The results of the clinical diagnosis laboratory assays are shown in Tables 2.56 and 2.57.

RBC, WBC and thrombocyte morphology

- Slight leucocytosis with an even increase in heterophils, monocytes and lymphocytes, relative and absolute eosinophilia

Table 2.56 Haematology values of the African grey parrot

Parameters	Results (absolute)	Results (%)
Hct (l/l)	0.45	
WBC (×10⁹/l)	22.75	
Heterophils (×10⁹/l)	15.58	68.5
Lymphocytes (×10⁹/l)	5.35	23.5
Monocytes (×10⁹/l)	0.774	3.4
Eosinophils (×10⁹/l)	0.774	3.4
Basophils (×10⁹/l)	0.296	1.3
Thrombocytes (×10⁹/l)	93.625	
Fibrinogen (g/l)	4.0	

Table 2.57 Blood chemistry values of the African grey parrot

Analysis	Results	Reference values
Albumin (g/l)	8	8–49
Amylase (U/l)	237	211–519
Bile acids (μmol/l)	10.6	
Calcium (mmol/l)	2.46	1.85–2.38
Cholesterol (mmol/l)	6.01	5.61–8.53
Triglycerides (mmol/l)	1.55	0.58–1.58
CK (U/l)	340	71–408
AST (U/l)	185	28–200
Glucose (mmol/l)	12.45	12.44–17.11
LDH (U/l)	490	105–420
Globulin (g/l)	29	21–32
Total protein (g/l)	33	26–49
Uric acid (μmol/l)	442	184–416
Zinc (μmol/l)	16.4	
Galactomannan	0.1	< 0.3

2. What is your interpretation of the haematology, blood chemistry, zinc and galactomannan levels shown in Tables 2.56 and 2.57?

Results

- Faecal examination showed negative result for the presence of endoparasites
- Circovirus-PCR and polyomavirus-PCR were both negative
- On radiographs no changes could be observed

- Haematology analysis revealed a slight eosinophilia
- Blood chemistry analysis showed minimally increased uric acid
- Zinc plasma level was within normal limits
- Galactomannan plasma level was normal

Please evaluate the clinical history, the results of the physical examination, Fig. 2.62a, b and clinical diagnosis laboratory tests.

Q *3. List your differential diagnoses.*

Q *4. List your next diagnostic steps.*

Differential diagnoses

- Feather plucking, not induced by a medical problem (psychological plucker)
- Disease process within left side of the coelomic cavity, not detectable by the above diagnostics
- Allergy-induced feather plucking (eosinophilia)

Next diagnostic steps

- Endoscopic evaluation of the coelomic cavity (Fig. 2.63).

Final diagnosis

- Subclinical *Aspergillus* granuloma causing unilateral feather plucking in the region of the granuloma

Q *5. List your therapeutic plan.*

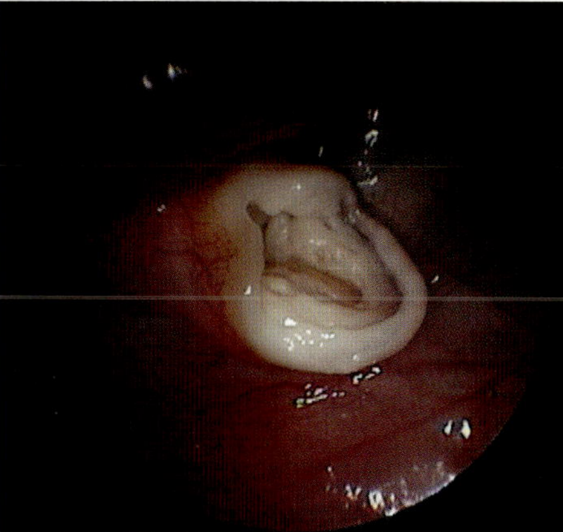

Fig. 2.63 *Aspergillus* granuloma in the left caudal thoracic air sac.

Therapy (Table 2.58)

Table 2.58 Therapy

Vitamin A	Vitamin A 20 000 IU/kg IM once
Vitamin B complex	Thiamine 30 mg/kg IM once
Amphotericin B	One time application directly onto the granuloma during endoscopy
Terbinafine hydrochloride	10 mg/kg PO BID, 8 weeks
Nebulization	F10 SC™ 0.1 ml + normal saline 25 ml for 30 min BID

Discussion

This case proves that it is very difficult to rule out aspergillosis in patients without signs of respiratory disease. Many parrots living in indoor aviaries, especially in heated apartments during the cold season show sporadic signs of respiratory disease, but will recover, and appear clinically normal. Diagnostic testing in these birds is normally unrewarding.

The classical changes on haematology and electrophoresis with high white blood cell counts including monocytosis and increases in the beta globulin fraction and the specific but not sensitive high galactomannan level, are normally only observed in birds with invasive aspergillosis and clinically severely ill. *Aspergillus* antibody titres also only have a low predictive value.

Radiography is also of limited diagnostic value until late in the disease. Signs such as asymmetry, hyperinflation, focal air sac densities indicating granulomas, or diffuse visualization of the air sac walls must be considered.

Computed tomography is useful for demonstrating small lesions not visible on radiography but is often not available in a private practice situation.

Endoscopy remains the diagnostic tool of choice for diagnosing subclinical aspergillosis in birds. Minimal airsacculitis and small granulomas not visible on radiography can be observed, biopsy samples for histopathology or culture can be taken and initial therapy with amphotericin B, applied directly into the coelomic cavity, can be performed.

All cases of plucking parrots, especially those with atypical distribution of plucking patterns, and those past puberty need a very thorough work up before they can be diagnosed as "psychological".

Further reading

Dahlhausen, R.D., 2006. Implications of mycoses in clinical disorders. In: Harrison, G.J., Lightfoot, T.L. (Eds.), Clinical Avian Medicine. Spix Publishing Inc., Palm Beach, pp. 691–709.

Gray, C., Reavill, D., et al., 2009. Galactomannan assay and plasma protein electrophoresis findings in psittacine birds with aspergillosis. J. Avian Med. Surg. 23 (2), 125–135.

Wilson, L., Lightfoot, T.L., 2006. Concepts in behavior: pubescent and adult psittacine behavior. In: Harrison, G.J., Lightfoot, T.L. (Eds.), Clinical Avian Medicine. Spix Publishing Inc., Palm Beach, pp. 74–84.

Case 2.26 *R. J. Doneley*

Clinical history

A 2-year-old male African grey parrot (*Psittacus erithacus erithacus*) was presented for lethargy, poor body condition and a prominent swelling on the neck. As the bird was housed outdoors in a large aviary complex, the owner was unsure of the bird's appetite as well as the duration of the illness. The bird was lethargic for approximately 12 hours prior to presentation. According to the client, the bird had no known prior health concerns and had been fed a seed-based diet with fresh fruit and vegetables and a vitamin and mineral powder supplement (Soluvet®, Vetafarm).

Clinical examination

On examination, the bird was alert and active. The faecal component of its droppings appeared dark green and had increased fluid content. The bird weighed 557 g (normal weight 400–500 g). The physical exam revealed significant pectoral muscle wasting, and multiple firm smooth nodules along the ventral neck (measuring approx. 5–20 mm in diameter). The masses were easily visible through the skin and could be palpated as separate from the crop and underlying muscle. No other abnormalities were noted on examination. Seed was palpable in the crop.

Clinical diagnosis laboratory

Blood was collected for in-house blood smear evaluation and biochemistry (Vetscan®, Abaxis).

Haematology

The PCV (37%) was mildly reduced (reference interval 43–55%). Examination of a blood smear revealed normal erythrocyte morphology with minimal anisocytosis and polychromasia. A profound lymphocytic leucocytosis was present, with greater than 20 lymphocytes visible per high power field, and few other leucocytes seen (Table 2.59).

Table 2.59 Blood chemistry values of the African grey parrot

Analysis	Results	Reference values
Bile acids (μmol/l)	>200	12–96
Calcium (mmol/l)	2.19	2–3.49
CK (U/l)	>2000	123–875
AST (U/l)	1766	100–350
Glucose (mmol/l)	6	14.21–19.98
Total protein (g/l)	29	27–44
Uric acid (μmol/l)	548	117.8–648.3

 *1. What is your interpretation of the haematology and blood chemistry values shown in Table 2.59?*

Results

- The haematology suggested either a marked inflammatory response or a leukaemic condition. The lack of polychromasia and anisocytosis suggested the anaemia was due to chronic disease
- The elevated bile acids, coupled with low protein and glucose, indicated hepatic disease. Elevated CK levels were attributable to muscle damage or wasting, and elevated AST indicated either muscle or hepatic tissue damage. In light of this bird's poor body condition, the interpretation of this pattern of biochemical abnormalities pointed to severe hepatic disease coupled with significant muscle catabolism

Please evaluate the clinical history, the results of the physical examination and clinical diagnosis laboratory tests.

 *2. List your differential diagnoses.*

 *3. List your therapeutic strategy.*

Differential diagnoses

- Neoplasia
- Chlamydiosis
- Aspergillosis
- Mycobacteriosis
- Other hepatopathies (i.e. hepatic lipidosis, bacterial or viral hepatitis, amyloidosis)

Therapy

A therapeutic plan was instituted (Table 2.60).

The bird appeared reasonably bright, alert and responsive, and was placed in a heated cage overnight. Unfortunately, it died overnight.

Table 2.60 Therapy

Antibiotic therapy	Piperacillin and tazobactam (Tazocin®, Wyeth) at 100 mg/kg IM Doxycycline (Doxycycline Injection, Vetafarm) at 100 mg/kg IM
Supportive care	Subcutaneous fluids Gavage feeding with a hand-feeding formula (Roudybush Formula 3®, Roudybush, Inc., USA) Warmth

Post-mortem findings (Figs 2.64–2.66)

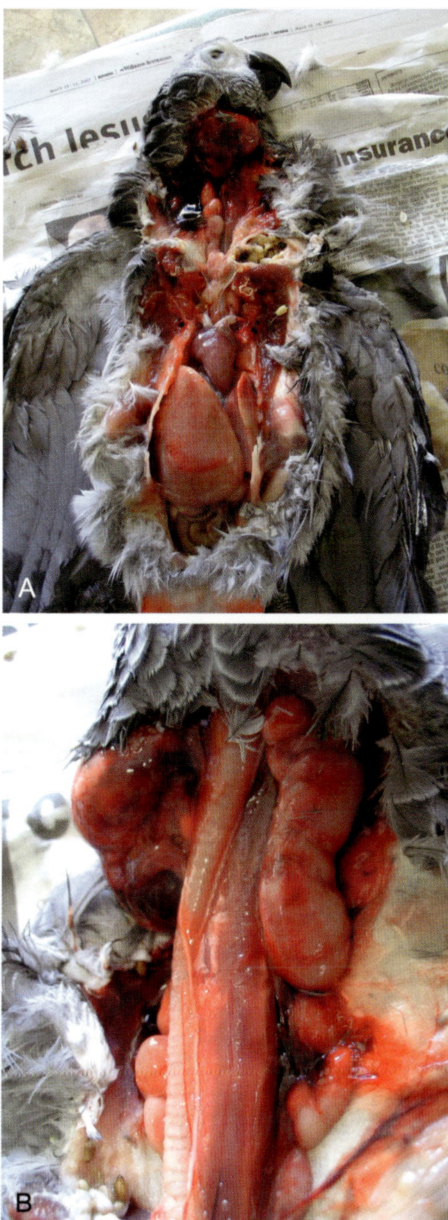

Fig. 2.64 (a) Post-mortem photograph of the African grey parrot. General view; (b) post-mortem photograph of the African grey parrot. Close-up view of the neck.

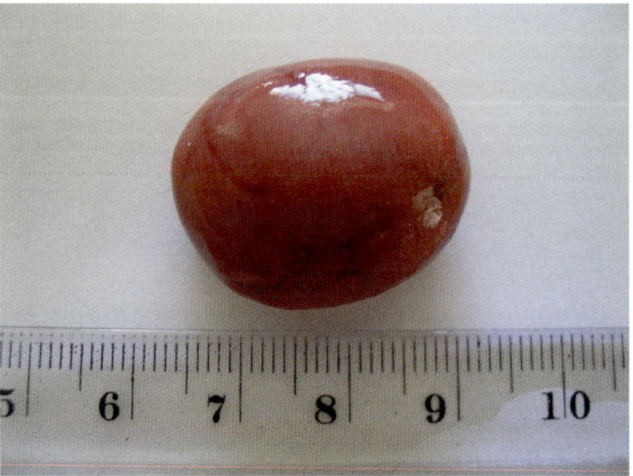

Fig. 2.65 Post-mortem photograph of the exceedingly enlarged spleen of the African grey parrot.

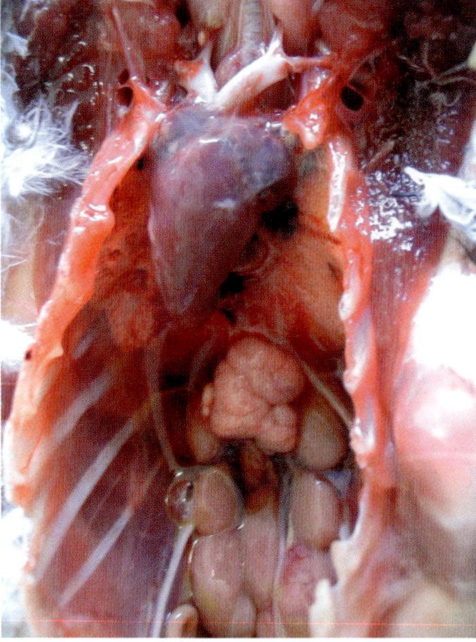

Fig. 2.66 Irregular round mass, suspected to be either a testicle or adrenal gland, found at the cranial-most aspect of the left kidney.

Q *4. What lesions can you observe in the post-mortem photographs?*

Q *5. What is your provisional post-mortem diagnosis?*

Summary of post-mortem examination findings

- The liver and kidneys were markedly enlarged and pale
- The spleen measured 2.7 cm in length (normal <1 cm)

- Numerous smooth tan nodules (measuring 5–20 mm in diameter), believed to be the thymus, were found running in bilateral chains from the thoracic inlet to the submandibular areas
- A 1 cm round mass with an irregular surface, suspected to be either a testicle or adrenal gland, was found at the cranial-most aspect of the left kidney

Provisional post-mortem diagnosis

- Thymic neoplasia

Laboratory findings

Histopathology of multiple organs (liver, kidney, thyroid, lung, heart, skeletal muscle, bursa and gastrointestinal tract) using haematoxylin and eosin showed infiltration by neoplastic round cells. These cells were characterized as having a moderate amount of homogeneous eosinophilic cytoplasm with distinct borders. Their nuclei were round and paracentral with a dense chromatin pattern and a single small deeply eosinophilic nucleolus. There was moderate anisokaryosis and up to three mitotic figures per high power field (400×).

Immunohistochemical staining using T-cell marker (CD3) showed a marked predominance of neoplastic T-cell lymphocytes which were infiltrating and effacing tissue parenchyma of multiple organs.

The particular severity of splenic, liver and kidney effacement explained the multiple organ dysfunctions and was the probable cause of death of this bird.

Final diagnosis

- Disseminated lymphosarcoma with leukaemia

Discussion

In birds, lymphocytes originate either in the thymus or the bursa of Fabricius, producing T- and B-cell lymphocytes, respectively. The thymus is found in the neck and may have multiple sites extending from the angle of the jaw to the thoracic inlet. It is at its largest size in the sexually immature bird. It processes and serves as the source of T-cell lymphocytes, the circulating cells responsible for cell-mediated immune responses. Approximately 65% of mononuclear cells in the spleen and 80% in the blood of chickens are T cells, although a small number of B lymphocytes are also present.

Lymphoid neoplasia in some birds is suspected to be linked to viral infections. A classic example of this is Marek's disease in chickens. The herpesvirus responsible causes T-cell lymphoma with lymphoid infiltration of internal organs and nervous tissue. Another example is lymphoid leukosis, caused by oncogenic poultry retroviruses. Lesions similar to those found in chickens infected with retroviruses have been described in passerine and psittacine birds, however, there is currently no evidence of viral involvement in the development of lymphoid tumours in non-poultry species.

Lymphosarcoma is one of the most common neoplastic conditions found in pet birds, and is the most common lymphoid neoplasia among the psittacine species. It can present in either disseminated (i.e. multicentric) or nodular forms, and has been well documented in canaries, doves, mynahs and a broad range of psittacine species. The average age of onset across all species is 8 years, however, it has been found in birds as young as 5 months of age.

Common clinical signs of lymphosarcoma consist of lethargy, depression, anorexia, weight loss, periorbital, cutaneous or abdominal swellings, dyspnoea, feather loss, folliculitis, blindness, paresis, lameness, diarrhoea, and regurgitation. Haematology often reveals anaemia (PCV <35%). While a lymphocytic leucocytosis is commonly found in canaries, parrots appear rarely to display a leukaemic component to lymphoid disease. However, a few documented cases of leukaemic blood profiles in psittacine lymphoma patients exist in the literature.

Lymphosarcoma infiltrates a broad range of organ systems. The tumours develop in primary and secondary lymphoid organs (thymus, bursa of Fabricius, spleen) and spread to other tissues. Tissues most commonly affected include the liver, kidneys, spleen, gastrointestinal tract, pancreas, thyroid, lung, brain, sinuses, adipose tissue, testes and oviduct. Post-mortem examination often reveals internal organs to be grossly enlarged and pale in colour, and the lesions may appear similar to various hepatopathies, amyloidosis, mycobacteriosis, and other types of neoplastic disease.

Few reports of lymphoid neoplasia in grey parrots exist in the literature. The most commonly cited case involves periocular lymphoma with disseminated disease in a 1.5-year-old male. Radiation therapy in that case resulted in a short-lived remission followed by euthanasia.

In addition to radiation therapy, various chemotherapeutic agents have been utilized in the treatment of lymphoid neoplasia in birds. Protocols used in birds have been extrapolated from those used in human and small animal oncology. Prednisolone, chlorambucil, cyclophosphamide, doxorubicin, vincristine, and L-asparaginase have all been employed in avian cancer treatment with highly variable and often unfavourable results.

There are few case reports in the literature where the cell line responsible for an avian lymphoma case has been identified. The identification of cell lines in canine lymphoma cases enables the clinician to predict remission and survivability rates, with T-cell lymphoma having a significantly more guarded prognosis than B-cell neoplasia. Similar correlations do not exist for the cat. Clearly, more data are needed to make correlations between cell lines and prognosis in avian species. However, immunohistochemical staining may allow a more targeted approach to avian lymphoma treatment.

Further reading

Bauck, L., 1986. Lymphosarcoma/leukosis in pet birds – case reports. In: Proceedings of the Association of Avian Veterinarians Conference. pp. 241–245.

Campbell, T.W., 1984. Lymphoid leukosis in an Amazon parrot – a case report. In: Proceedings of the International Conference on Avian Medicine, Association of Avian Veterinarians. pp. 229–234.

Coleman, C.W., 1995. Lymphoid neoplasia in pet birds: a review. J. Avian Med. Surg. 9 (1), 3–7.

Greenacre, C.B., 2005. Viral diseases of companion birds. Vet. Clin. North Am. Exot. Anim. Pract. 8, 85–105.

Hill, J.E., Burke, D.L., Rowland, G.N., 1986. Hepatopathy and lymphosarcoma in a mynah bird with excessive iron storage disease. Avian Dis. 30 (3), 634–636.

Latimer, K.S., Ritchie, B.W., Campagnoli, R.P., et al., 1998. Cutaneous T-cell rich B-cell lymphoma and leukemic blood profile in an umbrella cockatoo. In: Proceedings of the International Virtual Conference Veterinary Medicine, Diseases of Psittacine Birds. http://www.vet.uga.edu/vpp/ivcvm/1998/latimer01/index.php.

Paul-Murphy, J., Lowenstine, L., Turrel, J.M., et al., 1985. Malignant lymphoreticular neoplasm in an African gray parrot. J. Am. Vet. Med. Assoc. 187, 1216–1217.

Ramos-Vara, J.A., Smith, E.J., Watson, G.L., 1997. Lymphosarcoma with plasmacytoid differentiation in a scarlet macaw (*Ara macao*). Avian Dis. 41 (2), 499–504.

Reavill, D.R., 2001. Pet bird oncology. In: Proceedings Association of Avian Veterinarians Conference. pp. 29–43.

Reavill, D.R., 2004. Tumors of pet birds. Vet. Clin. North Am. Exot. Anim. Pract. 537–560.

Ritchie, B.W., 1995. Avian Viruses, Function and Control. Wingers Publishing, Lake Worth.

Rivera, S., McClearen, J.R., Reavill, D.R., 2009. Treatment of nonepitheliotropic cutaneous B-cell lymphoma in an umbrella cockatoo (*Cacatua alba*). J. Avian Med. Surg. 23 (4), 294–302.

Teske, E., van Heerde, P., Rutteman, G.R., et al., 1994. Prognostic factors for treatment of malignant lymphoma in dogs. J. Am. Vet. Med. Assoc. 205, 1722–1728.

Case 2.27 *R. J. Doneley*

Clinical history

A 4-year-old male African grey parrot (*Psittacus erithacus erithacus*) was presented for generalized weakness. The bird had been obtained some 18 months previously from another breeder and was housed in a large single flight suspended aviary with a hen (obtained at the same time from a different breeder). It was fed a diet of sunflower seed, fruit and vegetables with no vitamin or mineral supplementation. The pair had not yet bred.

The bird had appeared unwell for the last week, although the owner (who had been away for 5 weeks) conceded it could have been unwell for much longer. The owner reported the bird had been fluffed and lethargic, with its wings drooping. It was unable to fly and appeared very weak, dragging itself along on the floor of the cage. Its appetite and thirst appeared unchanged, but the owner could not be certain about this.

Clinical examination

On presentation, the bird was in good body condition, weighing 365 g. It had great difficulty perching, preferring to lie on the floor of the cage. It displayed increased respiratory effort at rest, evidenced by open mouth breathing and exaggerated inspiratory effort (Fig. 2.67).

The bird was anaesthetized with isoflurane and oxygen via a face mask, and survey radiographs were taken.

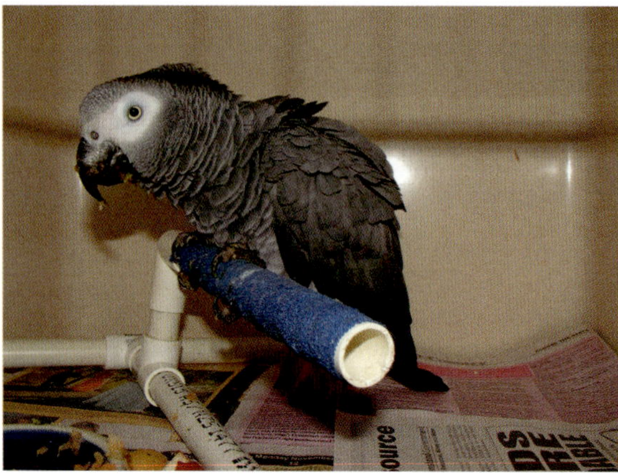

Fig. 2.67 Grey parrot on initial presentation.

Radiology (Fig. 2.68a, b)

1. What is your interpretation of the radiographs in Fig. 2.68a, b?

Clinical diagnosis laboratory

The results of the clinical diagnosis laboratory assays are shown in Tables 2.61 and 2.62.

RBC, WBC and thrombocyte morphology

- Cellular morphology was normal

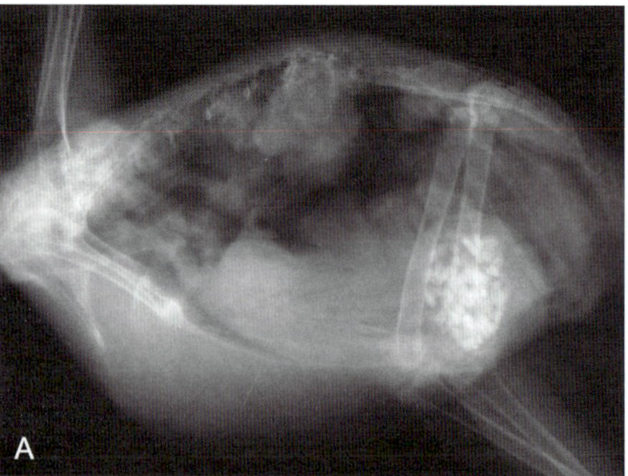

Fig. 2.68 (a) Lateral survey radiograph of the African grey parrot;

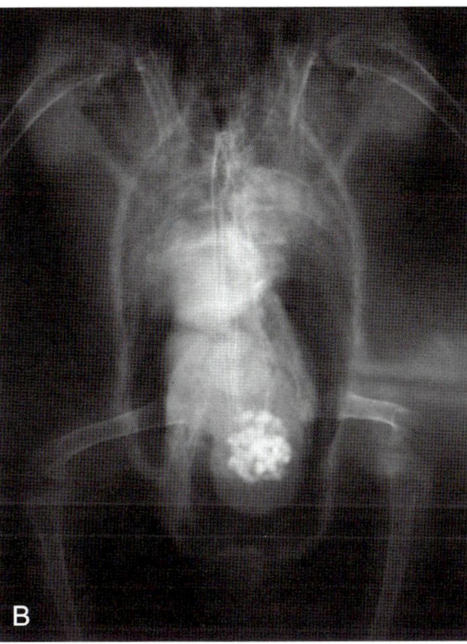

Fig. 2.68—cont'd (b) ventrodorsal survey radiograph of the African grey parrot.

2. What is your interpretation of the haematology and blood chemistry values shown in Tables 2.61 and 2.62?

Results

- Radiographic findings included a large mass in the region of the lung that appeared to be invading the vertebral column
- Haematology analysis showed a high normal PCV. The WBC was elevated with predominantly a heterophilia

Table 2.61 Haematology values of the African grey parrot

Parameters	Results	Reference values
PCV (%)	55	41.1–53.5
Estimated WBC (%)	23.2	6–13
Heterophils (%)	82	45–73
Lymphocytes (%)	16	20–54
Monocytes (%)	2	1–3
Eosinophils (%)	0	1–2
Basophils (%)	0	0–1

Table 2.62 Blood chemistry values of the African grey parrot

Analysis	Results	Reference values
Bile acids (μmol/l)	<35	12–96
Calcium (mmol/l)	2.17	2–3.49
CK (U/l)	5431	123–875
AST (U/l)	178	100–350
Glucose (mmol/l)	12.4	14.21–19.98
Total protein (g/l)	50	27–44
Uric acid (μmol/l)	378	117.8–648.3

- Blood chemistry analysis showed elevated levels of total protein and CK. This suggested a catabolic process and possible dehydration

Please evaluate the clinical history, Fig. 2.68a, b, the results of the physical examination and clinical diagnosis laboratory tests.

 *3. List your differential diagnoses.*

 *4. What would be your next diagnostic step?*

Differential diagnoses

- Neoplasia
- Aspergillosis
- Mycobacteriosis
- Bacterial granuloma
- Aspiration pneumonitis

Endoscopy

The bird was anaesthetized with isoflurane and oxygen via a face mask. A 2.7 mm rigid endoscope was introduced into the left caudal thoracic air sac. There was no evidence of airsacculitis, and the liver appeared normal. A large mass was visible in the pulmonary parenchyma, but was not accessible for biopsy.

Post-mortem findings

Based on the severity of the lesions seen radiographically and endoscopically, the owner elected for euthanasia. A thorough post-mortem examination was performed (Fig. 2.69). Samples from different organs were collected for histopathology.

Q *5. What lesions can you observe in the post-mortem photograph?*

Q *6. What is your provisional post-mortem diagnosis?*

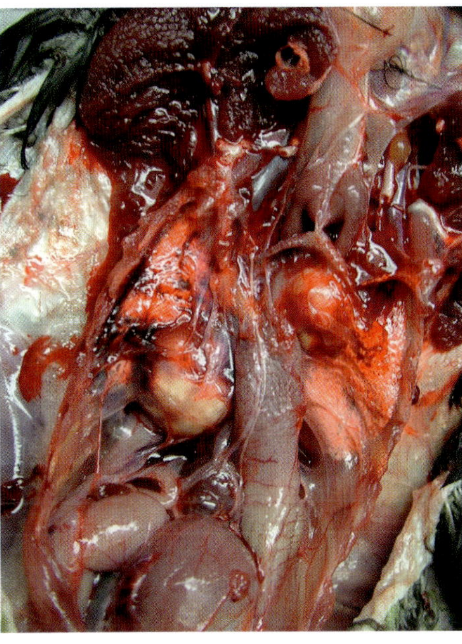

Fig. 2.69 Post-mortem photograph of the African grey parrot.

Summary of post-mortem examination findings

- Two large caseated masses were found, one in each lung. These masses were invading the ribs on both sides and the spine

Provisional post-mortem diagnosis

- Pulmonary abscess
- Osteomyelitis of the spine and ribs

Histopathology findings

- Lung: within the lung, there is a focally extensive lesion of eosinophilic and granulocytic debris (necrosis) which is surrounded by marked infiltrates of macrophages, granulocytes, lymphocytes, plasma cells and multinucleated histiocytic giant cells within fibrillar eosinophilic material (fibrin) and more peripherally, concentrically arranged fibrous tissue. Some small nodular aggregates of macrophages and giant cells are noted within the latter tissue (microgranulomas). Moderate numbers of branching fungal hyphae are noted within the necrotic debris in several fields
- Thoracic spine: there is local destruction and fragmentation of the lateral processes and vertebral bodies by the underlying inflammatory lung mass, which

is causing compression of the spinal cord. Inflammatory cells are expanding the meninges and extending into parenchymal perivascular spaces in small numbers. Small to moderate amounts of woven bone are deposited on some surfaces of vertebral process fragments

- Spleen: the capsule and surrounding adipose tissue contains multifocal, mild infiltrates of lymphocytes, plasma cells and macrophages surrounding but not involving nerve bundles
- Liver: one portal tract and surrounding tissue are expanded and replaced by fibrous tissue containing moderate numbers of granulocytes, lymphocytes and macrophages with hyperplastic bile ducts
- Pancreas, ventriculus, proventriculus, small intestine, colon, cloaca, testes, heart, and brain: significant lesions are not noted in these tissue sections

Final diagnosis

- Aspergillosis:
  - Severe chronic-active, pulmonary granulomas with intralesional fungal elements
  - Granulomatous, chronic-active, extensive osteomyelitis of the vertebral column, with spinal cord compression, meningomyelitis, and vertebral bone destruction

Discussion

Aspergillus spp. are ubiquitous environmental fungi found worldwide, growing readily in bird faeces and warm, moist environments and in substrates such as wood shavings, corn cob bedding and seed hulls. *A. fumigatus* is the species most commonly associated with birds, although *A. flavus, A. glaucus, A. niger, A. terreus* and *A. nidulans* have also been reported. They are non-contagious opportunistic pathogens often associated with disease in immunocompromised individuals; however, apparently healthy birds exposed to high concentrations of fungal spores can also develop disease. Some species of birds, e.g. the African grey parrot, the pionus parrot (*Pionus* spp.), ostriches (*Struthio camelus*), penguins (*Sphenisciformes* spp.), waterfowl and many raptors, appear to be particularly prone to infection and disease.

Infection can occur in the skin, the respiratory tract and the digestive tract, although haematogenous dissemination and localized invasion can blur these distinctions and lead to disease in other organ systems including muscles, bone and the nervous system. Respiratory infection, the most common presentation in birds, can localize in the sinuses, the trachea, the lungs or the air sacs.

Ante-mortem diagnosis can be difficult. As with many clinical conditions, the combination of a detailed history and thorough physical examination, augmented by radiology, haematology and endoscopy can lead the clinician to a tentative diagnosis of aspergillosis.

Treatment of aspergillosis is often frustrating, especially when an individual is acutely compromised. Both acute and chronic forms of disease are recognized; acute infection, with miliary abscess formation in the parenchyma of the lung, is almost invariably fatal. More chronic infections (in the sinuses, trachea and air sacs) are sometimes treatable if diagnosed early and treated aggressively.

Although treatment of this bird with an appropriate antifungal therapy may have inhibited or even killed the fungi within the granulomas, it is unlikely that, given the extent of skeletal invasion and collapse, the bird would have been able to regain normal neurological function. Chronic invasive aspergillosis carries a guarded prognosis at best.

Further reading

Dahlhausen, R.D., 2006. Implications of mycoses in clinical disorders. In: Harrison, G.J., Lightfoot, T.L. (Eds.), Clinical Avian Medicine. Spix Publishing Inc., Palm Beach, pp. 691–704.

Case 2.28 *M. Hochleithner*

Clinical history

A 9-year-old female Major Mitchell`s cockatoo (*Cacatua leadbeateri*) (Fig. 2.70) from a breeding facility was presented with the history of enteritis for 4 days.

Q ***1. Give some information about the natural environment of the Major Mitchell`s cockatoo (Cacatua leadbeateri).***

The Major Mitchell's cockatoo, (*Cacatua leadbeateri*), also known as Leadbeater's cockatoo or pink cockatoo, is a medium-sized cockatoo restricted to arid and semi-arid inland areas of Australia. Unlike the galah, Major Mitchell's cockatoo has declined rather than increased as a result of man-made changes to the arid interior of Australia. Where galahs readily occupy cleared and part-cleared land, Major Mitchell's cockatoo requires extensive woodlands, particularly favouring *Callitris*, *Allocasuarina* and *Eucalyptus*. In contrast to other cockatoos, Major Mitchell's pairs will not nest close to one another; in consequence, they cannot tolerate fragmented, partly-cleared habitats, and their range is contracting.

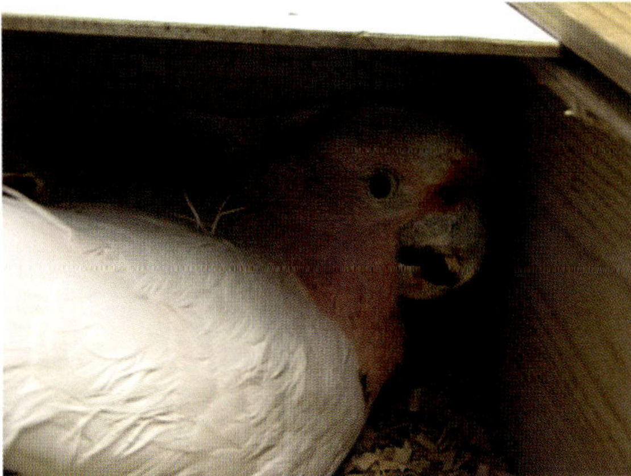

Fig. 2.70 Major Mitchell's cockatoo (*Cacatua leadbeateri*).

Q *2. Can you give some information about aviculture?*

Breeding success is not easy, finding compatible pairs is often difficult, and male aggression can be a significant problem. During the breeding season, male Major Mitchell's cockatoos can become very aggressive to any humans who enter their aviary, and they often do not tolerate nest inspections. Two or three, rarely four eggs are laid, with incubation by both parents taking around 25 days. The young fledge after 7 to 8 weeks, and are fed for a further 8 weeks by the parents. They should be removed from their parents by 6 months of age, and birds are mature enough to breed at 3 to 4 years, although breeding success may often take another year or two.

Clinical examination

The bird's weight was 367 g, body condition 5/5. Faeces were as seen in Fig. 2.71.

Q *3. Interpret the finding of the faeces.*

Yellow discoloration of faeces and urates is suggestive of hepatitis. The consumption of some yellow-pigmented vegetables and administration of parenteral B vitamins can cause a similar discoloration of the urates. In this case biliverdinuria was presented.

 *4. What further diagnostic tests would you recommend?*

Clinical diagnosis examination

- Radiology
- Faecal examination for parasites including flotation
- PCR for polyomavirus, PBFD, *Chlamydophila*, bornavirus
- Bacteriological examination including *Salmonella*
- Haematology and blood chemistry

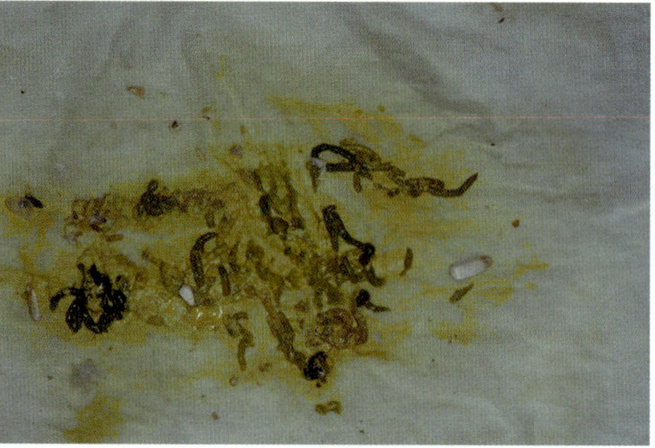

Fig. 2.71 Yellow discoloration of faeces and urates.

Results

Parasitology

- Negative

Radiology

- No abnormal signs

PCR

- Polyomavirus, PBFD, bornavirus: negative
- *Chlamydophila*: positive

Bacterial swabs

- Choana: + *Streptococcus* spp.
- Cloaca: negative

Haematology and blood chemistry (Tables 2.63 and 2.64)

Table 2.63 Haematology results

Parameter	Results	Reference range
RBC ($\times 10^{12}$/l)	2.70	2.7–3.6
HB (g/dl)	142	142–171
Hct (l/l)	0.42	0.43–0.51
WBC ($\times 10^{9}$/l)	15.9	3.3–10.3

Table 2.64 Blood chemistry results

Parameters	Results	Reference range
AST (U/l)	987	28–200
CK (U/l)	498	71–800
Total protein (g/l)	35	26–49
Uric acid (mmol/l)	321	100–500
Calcium (mmol/l)	2.2	1.9–2.4

Q 5. *Interpretation of the result?*

An infection with *Chlamydophila* is very likely. Also the WBC and the AST point to this direction.

 6. *What therapy would you recommend?*

We used doxycycline, 100 mg/kg intramuscular once a week for a minimum of 5 weeks. After 3 days, the bird behaved normally and the discoloration of faeces disappeared. The bird was sent home on day 7, shortly after the second injection. The partner bird was tested for *Chlamydophila* but was negative so the male bird was not treated.

After 2 weeks (third injection of doxycycline), the owner reported that the bird was in perfect health and started to go into the nest box with the male. Mating was observed.

After 5 weeks, the bird suddenly got worse, stopped feeding, feathers were fluffed. No changes on faeces.

Q 7. *What happened? Is this change on the health status of the bird still related to the infection with Chlamydophila?*

Multiple injections of doxycycline can have severe side effects, like muscle bleeding at the injection site or immune suppression with following fungal infections. The infection with *Chlamydophila* is usually not a problem after the first injection.

Q 8. *What is next?*

Further diagnostic testing

PCR

- *Chlamydophila:* negative

Bacterial swabs

- Choana: negative
- Cloaca: negative

Haematology and blood chemistry (Tables 2.65 and 2.66)

Table 2.65 Haematology results

Parameters	Results	Reference range
RBC ($\times10^{12}$/l)	2.97	2.7–3.6
HB (g/dl)	146	142–171
Hct (l/l)	0.48	0.43–0.51
WBC ($\times10^{9}$/l)	10.7	3.3–10.3

Table 2.66 Blood chemistry results

Parameters	Results	Reference range
AST (U/l)	387	28–200
CK (U/l)	1264	71–800
Total protein (g/l)	38	26–49
Uric acid (mmol/l)	498	100–500
Calcium (mmol/l)	2.9	1.9–2.4

Radiology (Fig. 2.72)

9. What is your diagnosis?

Final diagnosis

➤ Egg binding

Elevation in CK and AST is probably because of multiple injections. Calcium is usually higher in egg-laying birds. However 2.9 is rather low for a female with an egg.

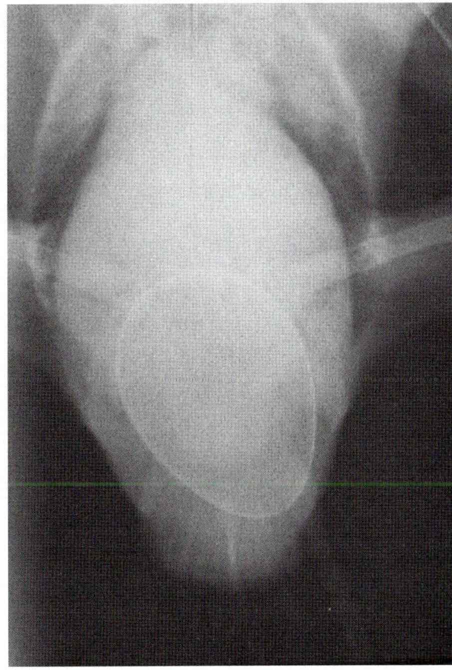

Fig. 2.72 Ventrodorsal radiograph of the cockatoo.

Q *10. What therapy would you recommend?*

Therapy

We started with calcium injections twice daily (calcium gluconolactobionate 10%, 2 ml/kg) and subcutaneous fluids in combination with a vitamin ADEC preparation. After the second injection, the egg was laid and the bird was sent home.

Discussion

Although the diagnosis "Chlamydophiliosis" was easy and very obvious, there can always be a second problem involved. In this case, the problem developed during therapy and could also be a side effect of the doxycycline therapy, as tetracyclines are known to bind calcium and this might also be a problem during therapy. The plasma calcium concentration of 2.9 mmol/l is very low for an egg-producing female, although it is higher than the normal range which is usually established for non-reproducing birds.

The pathogenesis of egg binding in a particular case can be multifactorial. The pubic bones are not fused in birds and pelvic deformities seldom play a role in dystocia. Common causes of egg binding are oviduct muscle dysfunction, like calcium metabolic disease or excessive egg production.

The most important consideration in initiating therapy for dystocia is to establish a physiological normal state. Attempts to remove the egg are secondary to stabilizing the patient. In minimally depressed patients, like this hen, the egg usually passes if the bird is provided with supplemental heat, injectable calcium, vitamin E, selenium, vitamin D3 and easy access to water and food. Particularly in species where males tend to be very aggressive during the breeding season, a lack of nutrients is a possible cause. Oxytocin injections are seldom necessary and can often make the situation worse.

Further reading

Harrison, G.J., Lightfoot, T.L., 2006. Clinical Avian Medicine. Spix Publishing, Inc., Palm Beach.

Hurley, V., 2008. The State of Australian Birds. Major Mitchell's Cockatoo: changing threats. Birds Australia, Carlton, Victoria.

Samour, J., 2008. Avian Medicine, second ed. Mosby Elsevier, London.

Case 2.29 *R. J. Doneley*

Clinical history

An 18-year-old male long-billed corella (*Cacatua tenuirostris*) was presented for a sore eye. The current owners had obtained the bird 4 years previously from friends. It was housed in an outdoor cage and fed on seed. Although exposed to wild birds, no other birds were housed with the patient.

Two weeks prior to presentation the owners had noticed the bird's right eye was swollen and there was a discharge from the right nare. No sneezing had been noted, but the bird now had difficulty in closing its beak and appeared to be having some trouble breathing. Despite this, the bird retained a good appetite.

Clinical examination

On presentation, the bird was in good body condition, weighing 637 g. Its feathering was normal, and adequate powder down was present. The beak was overgrown, especially on the right mandible. The preorbital diverticulum of the right infraorbital sinus was visibly distended and soft on palpation. The right eye was slightly exophthalmic (Fig. 2.73).

Blood was collected for in-house haematology and biochemistry.

Clinical diagnosis laboratory

The results of the clinical diagnosis laboratory assays are shown in Tables 2.67 and 2.68.

RBC, WBC and thrombocyte morphology

- Erythrocyte, leucocyte and thrombocyte morphology was normal

1. *What is your interpretation of the haematology and blood chemistry values?*

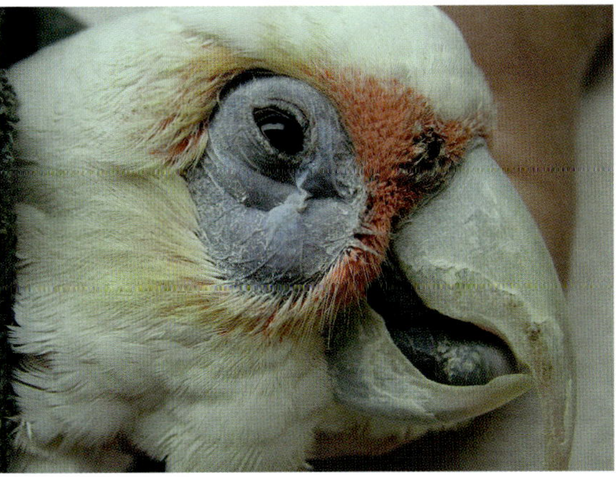

Fig. 2.73 The long-billed corella on presentation. Please note the clearly distended infraorbital sinus.

Table 2.67 Haematology values of the corella

Parameters	Results	Reference values
PCV (%)	52	43–55
Estimated WBC ($\times 10^9$/l)	14	6–14
Heterophils (%)	81	41–77
Lymphocytes (%)	14	22–57
Monocytes (%)	5	0–2
Eosinophils (%)	0	0–1
Basophils (%)	0	0–1

Table 2.68 Blood chemistry values of the corella

Analysis	Results	Reference values
Bile acids (μmol/l)	<35	12–96
Calcium (mmol/l)	2.39	2–3.49
CK (U/l)	770	123–875
AST (U/l)	176	100–350
Glucose (mmol/l)	21.4	14.21–19.98
Total protein (g/l)	38	27–44
Uric acid (μmol/l)	453	117.8–648.3

Results

- Haematology analysis showed low normal PCV. The WBC was slightly elevated with a monocytosis. Cellular morphology was normal
- Blood chemistry analysis was normal

Please evaluate the clinical history, Fig. 2.73, the results of the physical examination and clinical diagnosis laboratory tests.

2. List your differential diagnoses.

Differential diagnoses

- Chlamydiosis
- Sinusitis (bacterial or fungal)
- Mycobacteriosis
- Neoplasia

3. What would your next diagnostic step be?

Results

The bird was anaesthetized with isoflurane and oxygen via mask induction. A small amount of gelatinous material was obtained by fine needle aspirate and submitted for in-house cytology. A sample was submitted to the University of Sydney for culture.

A modified Wright-Giemsa stain (Diff Quik) and Gram stain showed erythrocytes and moderate numbers of an encapsulated yeast, all in a proteinaceous matrix. The culture confirmed the presence of *Cryptococcus gattii*.

Final diagnosis

- Cryptococcal sinusitis

 *4. List your therapeutic strategy.*

Therapy

- Fluconazole 10 mg/kg PO BID

Outcome

After 4 weeks of antifungal therapy the sinus distension was still present, although more clearly circumscribed. Under isoflurane anaesthesia, the sinus was opened and a large gel-like mass was removed from within the sinus by blunt and sharp dissection (Fig. 2.74a, b). The skin was closed with 5-0 polydioxanone suture and the bird discharged to continue the fluconazole.

A recheck 4 weeks later showed no recurrence of the sinus distension and the owner reported the bird had improved dramatically; it was again vocalizing, eating well and more active.

The fluconazole was continued for another 4 weeks. Subsequent rechecks over 2 years showed no recurrence.

Discussion

The yeast genus *Cryptococcus* is divided into two species (*C. neoformans* and *C. gattii*) based on distinct clinical manifestations and biological characteristics. *C. gattii*, formerly known as *C. bacillisporus* (and before that, *C. neoformans var gattii*), has previously been associated with upper respiratory tract infections in parrots in Australia. There is strong epidemiological evidence linking infections in animals (including people) and eucalyptus trees, especially the river red gum (*Eucalyptus camaldulensis*) and the forest red gum (*Eucalyptus tereticornis*). *C. gattii* has also been cultured from the air and the bark and bases of a variety of trees in the Pacific Northwest of North America. The role that trees play in the life cycle of *C gattii* is not clear, but its association with decaying wood is suggestive of an endophytic existence, in common with other wood-rot fungi. The primary mode of infection is most likely inhalation of the basidiospore stage or desiccated yeast cells from the environment. The association of *C. gattii* with woody

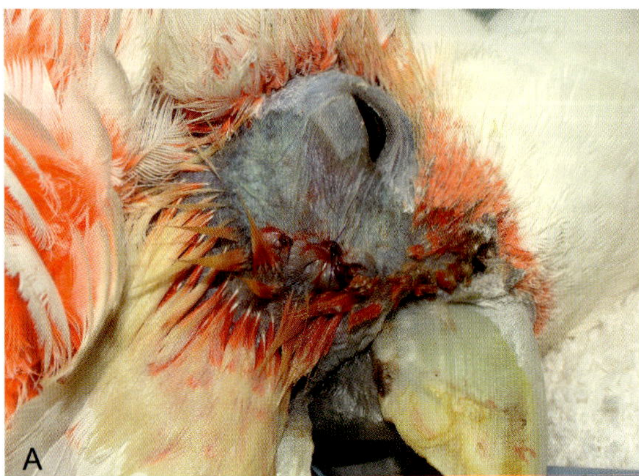

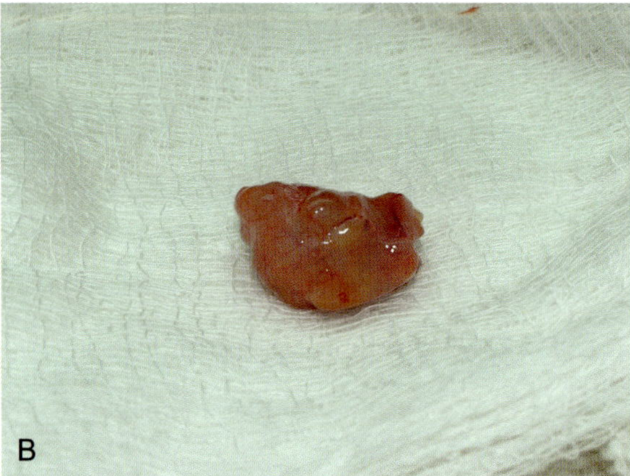

Fig. 2.74 (a) Long-billed corella under anaesthesia after surgery to remove a gelatinous mass from the infraorbital sinus; (b) gelatinous mass removed from the infraorbital sinus of the long-billed corella.

materials distinguishes this species from *C. neoformans*' niche in soil and pigeon droppings. The bird described in this case report lives in a semi-rural area of Australia and was housed outdoors. As such, its exposure to eucalyptus and other trees is high, making this the most likely source of infection.

In a previous review of avian cryptococcosis, *C. gattii* produced localized invasive disease of the upper respiratory tract of captive parrots in Australia, resulting in signs referable to mycotic rhinitis or to involvement of structures contiguous with the nasal cavity including the beak, sinuses, choana, retrobulbar space and palate. This contrasted with *C. neoformans* infections reported in birds in America and Europe, where the yeast typically penetrated the lower respiratory tract or disseminated widely to a variety of internal organs. These findings suggested different patterns of disease for the two species of *Cryptococcus*, with *C. gattii* apparently acting as a primary pathogen of immunocompetent hosts, while *C. neoformans* may act as an opportunistic infection of immunodeficient hosts. In both birds and cats, the primary infection site is thought to occur within the respiratory tract. It has been suggested that the upper respiratory tract may be particularly susceptible to initial colonization because of its lower temperature. In some cases, this initial colonization of the upper respiratory tract may lead to disseminated infection, with lesions in the lungs, air sacs, heart, liver, spleen, kidneys, intestines and central nervous system.

Diagnosis of cryptococcal sinusitis can be straightforward. A definitive diagnosis of cryptococcosis is defined as the culture and identification of the organism by a reputable laboratory. However, it is possible to obtain a high index of suspicion of cryptococcosis by demonstrating characteristic capsulate, narrow-necked budding yeasts in cytological smears or histology sections. In animal tissues, *C. gattii* exists as round, yeast-like organisms with a variably-sized polysaccharide capsule as its distinguishing feature. The capsule provides protection from environmental insults (e.g. desiccation) and the phagocytic response of the host.

Cytological examination can be performed on fine needle aspirates or crush preparations of biopsy samples. Romanowsky-type stains (Diff Quik, Giemsa and Wright's), new methylene blue and Gram's stain are all satisfactory for making a cytological diagnosis.

The organism can be easily cultured from aspirates, exudates, and biopsies. PCR testing of these samples is also available. The detection of cryptococcal capsular antigen by the latex agglutination procedure is the most widely utilized serological test and may be useful in a veterinary setting. Cultures of nasal washings from dogs, cats and koalas have shown that both *C. neoformans* and *C. gattii* can be carried asymptomatically in the upper respiratory tract and the same might be true for birds. Therefore, a diagnosis of cryptococcosis should be based on cytology in combination with culture or PCR, rather than culture or PCR of nasochoanal swabs or washes alone.

Treatment with the triazole antifungal drugs (fluconazole, itraconazole and voriconazole) has become common in avian medicine. They have a good safety profile, a broad spectrum of activity and are available in topical, oral and intravenous formulations. They exert their antifungal effect on the cell membrane of the yeast by inhibiting synthesis of the primary sterol of the fungal cell membrane, ergosterol. They are fungistatic at recommended doses, and many months of treatment is recommended.

Fluconazole is the least likely triazole to cause adverse side effects as it has a low affinity for mammalian cytochrome P-450 and is therefore less likely to result in adverse effects. Its availability as an oral suspension with good bioavailability makes it an attractive option for treating many species. Resistance of *C. gattii* to fluconazole has been reported, and sensitivity testing is recommended before commencing the long-term treatment necessary to treat successfully cryptococcal sinusitis.

Further reading

Burns, R.E., Mohr, F.C., 2010. Pathology in practice: severe chronic multifocal to coalescing granulomatous meningoencephalomyelitis, rhinitis and sinusitis, with intralesional yeasts consistent with *Cryptococcus* spp. J. Am. Vet. Med. Assoc. 236 (10), 1069–1070.

Malik, R., Krockenberger, M.B., Cross, G., et al., 2003. Avian cryptococcosis. Med. Mycol. 41 (2), 115–124.

Malik, R., Krockenberger, M., Martin, P., et al., 2002. Pathomechanisms of systemic fungal infection. In: Proceedings of the European College of Veterinary Internal Medicine. http://www.vin.com/Members/Proceedings/Proceedings.plw (accessed 04.09.10).

Malik, R., 2003. Feline cryptococcosis. In: Proceedings of the Annual Conference of the World Small Animal Veterinary Association. http://www.vin.com/Members/Proceedings/Proceedings.plx (accessed 04.09.10).

Pfeiffer, T.J., Ellis, D.H., 1992. Environmental isolation of *Cryptococcus neoformans* var. *gattii* from *Eucalyptus tereticornis*. Med. Mycol. 30 (5), 407–408.

Raidal, S.R., Butler, R., 2001. Chronic rhinosinusitis and rhamphothecal destruction in a Major Mitchell's cockatoo (*Cacatua leadbeateri*) due to *Cryptococcus neoformans* var *gattii*. J. Avian Med. Surg. 15 (2), 121–125.

Raso, T.F., Werther, K., Mirandas, E.T., et al., 2004. Cryptococcosis outbreak in psittacine birds in Brazil. Med. Mycol. 42, 355–362.

Springer, D.J., Chaturvedi, V., 2010. Projecting global occurrence of *Cryptococcus gattii*. Emerg. Infect. Dis. 16 (1), 14–29.

Sorrell, T.C., 2001. *Cryptococcus neoformans* variety *gattii*. Med. Mycol. 39 (2), 155–168.

Stewart, A.J., Salazar, T., 2005. Fungal infections of the respiratory tract. In: Proceedings of the European College of Veterinary Internal Medicine. http://www.vin.com/Members/Proceedings/Proceedings.plx (accessed 04.09.10).

Case 2.30 *B. Gartrell*

Clinical history

Lori, an 8-year-old male rainbow lorikeet, had been happy and healthy ever since his owner bought him as a newly weaned bird. He lived free range inside the house when the owner was at home and lived in an outdoor aviary when she was away at work (Fig. 2.75). His diet had been a good commercial lorikeet dry and wet mix (Wombaroo), supplemented with fresh blossoms from flowering gums, banksias and pohutakawa. Lori had fresh fruit daily and the owner was fanatical about hygiene.

In the last month, Lori's voice had altered becoming progressively hoarse and distorted. Otherwise Lori remained bright and active.

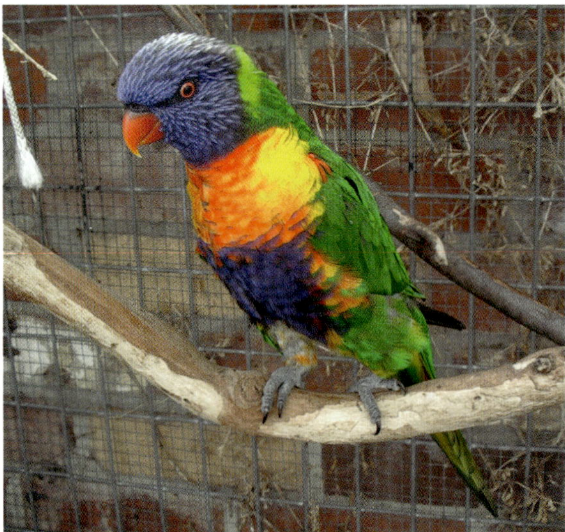

Fig. 2.75 Rainbow lorikeet.

Physical examination

Distance examination

On distance examination, Lori appeared normal in the cage, with no significant abnormalities detectable. His breathing was steady at 40 bpm and there was no noise or respiratory effort.

Physical examination

On initial physical examination, there were no significant findings. Lori weighed 125 g and was in good pectoral condition. On auscultation of the chest, there were no abnormal respiratory noises audible.

The faeces were liquid with large amounts of urine but microscopic examination of faecal smears showed no abnormalities.

Clinical diagnosis examination

Radiology (Fig. 2.76)

1. What is your interpretation of the radiographs in Fig. 2.76a, b?

Clinical diagnosis laboratory examination

Blood samples were collected for haematology and blood chemistry. A *Chlamydia* antigen test from a conjunctival swab was negative.

The results of the clinical diagnosis laboratory assays are shown in Table 2.69.

2. What is your interpretation of the haematology and blood chemistry values shown in Table 2.69?

3. In view of the clinical signs, would you conduct any further diagnostics?

Summary of diagnostic results

- There is leucocytosis due to a heterophilia and monocytosis
- There is a relative hyperglobulinaemia as shown by the albumin to globulin ratio
- The radiographs show a dorsal displacement of the intrathoracic trachea and syrinx on the lateral view and a lateral displacement on the ventrodorsal radiograph. Endoscopic evaluation of the trachea using a 2.7 mm diameter endoscope was unable to reach the syrinx. The upper trachea and air sacs showed no gross abnormalities. The lungs appeared congested (Fig. 2.77) and endoscopic biopsies were taken (Fig. 2.78)
- The cultures obtained at endoscopy grew no bacteria or fungi

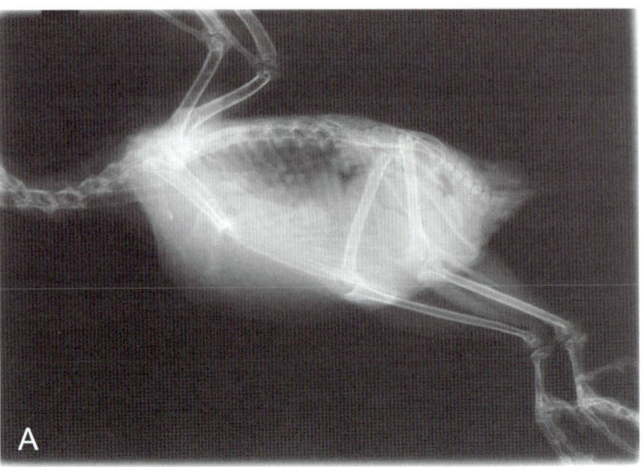

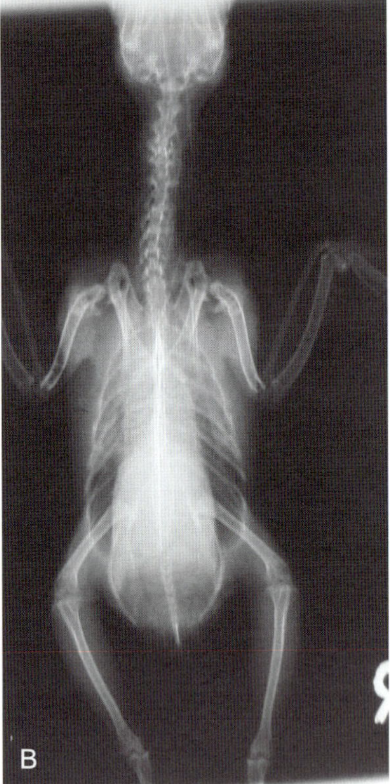

Fig. 2.76 (a) Lateral survey radiograph of an 8-year-old male rainbow lorikeet; (b) ventrodorsal survey radiograph of an 8-year-old male rainbow lorikeet.

Table 2.69 Haematology and serum biochemistry

Haematology			
Parameters	**Results**	**Absolute count**	**Reference range**
HCT	46		0.35–0.55
WBC (×10⁹/l)	27.6		3–15
	Diff		
Heterophils (%)	76	20.7	
Lymphocytes (%)	4	1.1	
Monocytes (%)	20	5.5	
Total protein (g/l)	23		22–50
Serum biochemistry			
Uric acid (μmol/l)	118		0–600
CK (IU/l)	435		120–875
AST (IU/l)	160		100–350
GGT	0		0–5
Total protein (g/l)	25		22–50
Albumin (g/l)	12		12–20
Globulin (g/l)	13		10–20
A:G ratio	1.1		1.4–3.3
Calcium	2.3		2.1–2.6
Glucose (μmol/l)	20		11–25
Sodium	144		139–159
Potassium	2.8		2.2–3.7
Chloride	125		95–144
Bile acids	50		20–70

➤ The histopathology reported that the biopsies contained a mix of ciliated epithelium, numerous foamy macrophages, necrotic inflammatory cells, and a low number of heterophils. Within one area of necrosis, there was a small piece of keratin suggesting a foreign body inflammation. No bacteria or fungi were evident in special stains

Please evaluate the clinical history, Fig. 2.76a, b, the results of the physical examination and clinical and laboratory diagnostic tests.

Q *4. List your differential diagnoses.*

Q *5. List your therapeutic strategy.*

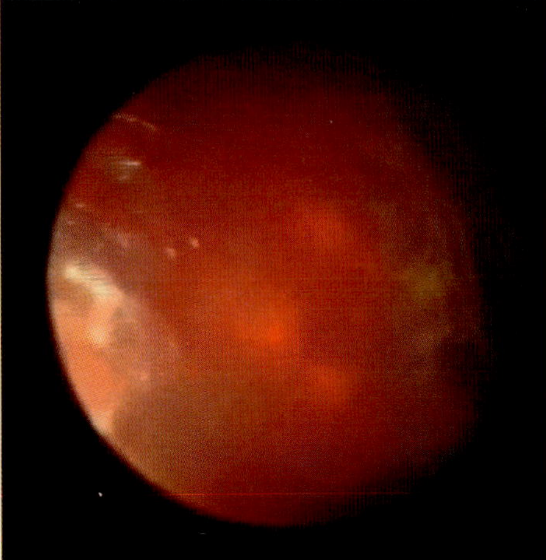

Fig. 2.77 At endoscopy examination the lungs appeared congested (Fig. 2.77) and biopsies were obtained (Fig. 2.78).

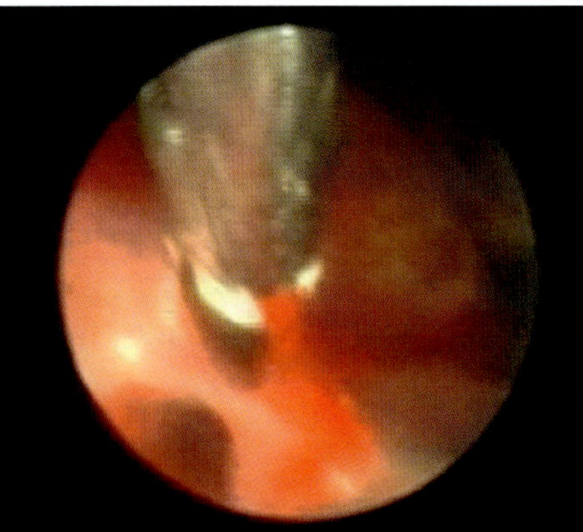

Fig. 2.78

Differential diagnoses

- Extraluminal tracheal foreign body
- Extraluminal granuloma including mycotic (*Aspergillus, Cryptococcus, Mucor* spp.), bacterial (*Salmonella, Nocardia, Staphylococcus*), mycobacterial granulomas
- Neoplasm

Therapy

In this case, the clinician opted to treat with:

- Nebulization 15 minutes BID of an F10: saline mix (1:200)
- Amoxicillin/clavulanate at 100 mg/kg BID PO

- Itraconazole 10 mg/kg BID PO
- Balanced electrolytes (lactated Ringer's solution) 100 ml/kg/day PO (5 ml BID PO).

The bird continued on the initial treatment for 7 days at which stage the owner expressed reluctance to continue with hospitalized therapy due to cost. The bird had remained bright but had not vocalized during its hospitalization. In this case, against the veterinarian's recommendations, the owners opted to withdraw all treatment. It was planned to monitor Lori closely for 14 days and reassess him by haematology at this time.

However, one week after discharge, Lori was presented in severe respiratory distress, with vomiting of bloody mucus and died before treatment could be instituted.

Post-mortem examination

On post-mortem examination, there was a large solitary granuloma at the base of the heart displacing the trachea dorsally. No other gross abnormalities were noted at post mortem.

Provisional post-mortem diagnosis

- Extraluminal tracheal granulomas

Post-mortem laboratory findings

- A heavy growth of *Aspergillus fumigatus* was isolated by fungal culture of the granuloma

Final diagnosis

- Extra-luminal syringeal granuloma due to *Aspergillus fumigatus*

Discussion

The history of a recent voice change should give the clinician a high index of suspicion for lower respiratory tract disease, especially involving the syrinx. There is a range of differential diagnoses for diseases of the lower respiratory tract but the most common cause is aspergillosis. If the size of the patient allows, then endoscopy of the trachea down to the syrinx or via the cervicocephalic air sac to examine for extraluminal masses is highly recommended. In smaller patients, such as this lorikeet, presumptive treatment for aspergillosis may be indicated, however, this involves weeks to months of intensive treatment. There is some controversy over the use of F10 as a nebulizing treatment for aspergillosis with some veterinarians preferring only to nebulize those drugs that can be given safely intravenously. In this case, the bird died due to a fatal haemorrhage. *Aspergillus fumigatus* is a haematophilic fungus and will often invade blood vessels resulting in thrombosis or haemorrhage.

Further reading

Beernaert, L.A., Pasmans, F., van Waeyenberghe, L., et al., 2010. Aspergillus infections in birds: a review. Avian Pathol. 39, 325–331.

Cray, C., Reavill, D., Romagnano, A., et al., 2009. Galactomannan assay and plasma protein electrophoresis findings in psittacine birds with aspergillosis. J. Avian Med. Surg. 23, 125–135.

Gugnani, H.C., 2003. Ecology and taxonomy of pathogenic aspergilli. Front. Biosci. 8, s346–s357.

Tell, L.A., 2005. Aspergillosis in mammals and birds: impact on veterinary medicine. Med. Mycol. 43, S71–S73.

Case 2.31 *M. Hochleithner*

Clinical history

A Jardine's parrot (*Poicephalus gulielmi*) of unknown gender and over 30 years old was presented because of a swelling "on the left eye" for the past 6 weeks (Fig. 2.79). During the past week, the bird started to rub the left side of the face on the walls of the cage and the perches. The bird was tame and kept alone and fed mainly on seeds but it also consumed some table food. The owners had had this bird for 30 years and never visited a veterinarian before.

Clinical examination

The bodyweight was 186 g and the behaviour was normal for a tame bird. The appearance of his feathers were low grade toneless, but considering its age and diet, this was interpreted as "normal".

1. How do you interpret the age of 30 years in a Jardine's parrot?

Although the information about maximum age in Jardine's parrots varies, most authors describe 40–50 years as the maximum age. However, 30 years for a bird kept alone and fed a seed diet seems to be old.

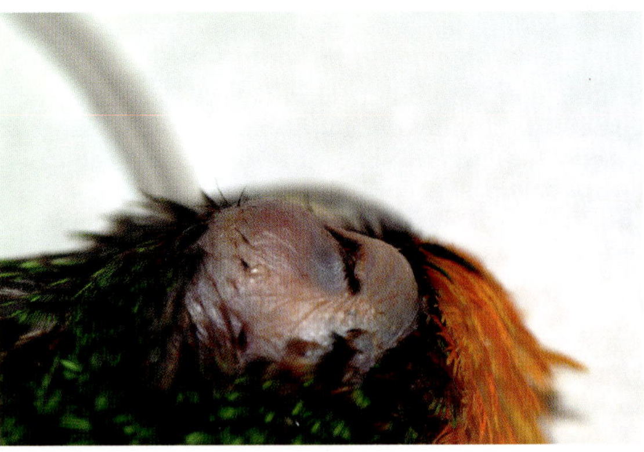

Fig. 2.79 Left side of the bird's face.

Q *2. Do you have a preliminary diagnosis and could you start a treatment?*

No. Although sinusitis could be the cause of such a swelling, without further diagnosis no therapy should be started.

Q *3. What would be the next diagnostic steps?*

Considering the advanced age of the bird, it would be recommended to subject the bird to a short anaesthesia using isoflurane and perform a thorough examination of the head. This is in most cases impossible if the bird is fully awake. Examination of the oropharynx is absolutely necessary if possible also using an endoscope.

- Inspection of the oral cavity showed that the choanal slit was deflected to the right side

Q *4. What further diagnostic steps could be performed?*

- Radiology
- Biopsy and cytology
- Fine needle aspiration
- Ultrasound
- Microbiology
- Haematology
- Blood chemistry
- Computed tomography

The owners decided that they only wanted to spend money for two further tests. What would you recommend?

Taking into consideration the age of the bird, a full blood panel and a whole body radiograph would be very useful. However, this would not give much information about the pathology process on the head. In practice, it is often very difficult to convince the owners about the necessary diagnostic procedures due to financial limitations. For this reason, we decided to perform a radiograph of the head and a fine needle aspiration.

Results (Fig. 2.80)

 *5. How do you interpret the radiographs?*

Radiology

- Diffused unilateral opacity of the left side including the sinuses

When palpating the swelling around the eye, it was suspected that the process was not sinusitis. Because haemorrhage can be a problem, especially in an old bird with "unknown" history and possible liver problems and coagulopathy, we decided not to access the sinus and perform a full biopsy. Therefore, a fine needle aspiration was performed using a 22g needle. The content of the needle after aspiration was then smeared onto four microscopic slides.

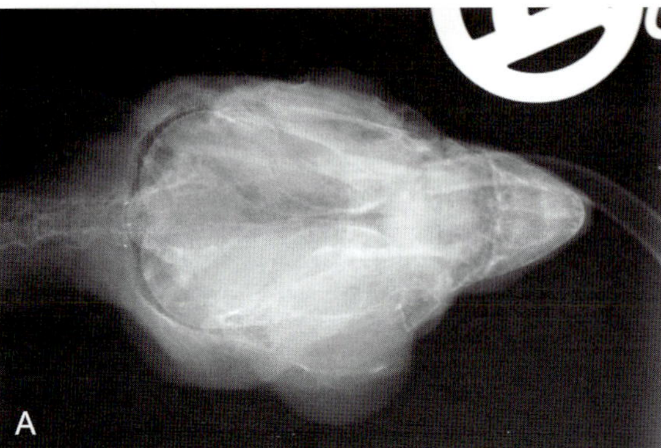

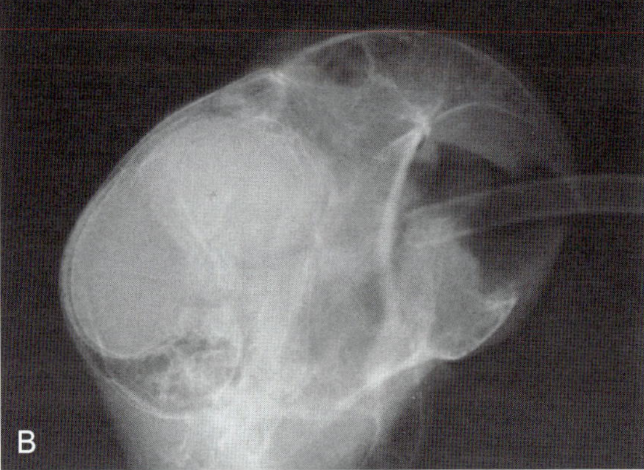

Fig. 2.80 (a) Ventrodorsal view of the head of the Jardine's parrot; (b) latero-lateral view of the head of the Jardine's parrot.

Q *6. How would you stain the slides?*

We used Diff Quik and acid-fast (Ziehl-Neelsen) stains.

Q *7. What is the reason for the acid-fast stain?*

Particularly in older birds, mycobacterial infections can be found. Granulomas can be seen in such patients and care has to be taken because of potential risk for humans.

Results

- Acid-fast stain: negative
- Diff Quik: high numbers of good differentiated lymphoid cells, monomorphic picture, few mitoses

Q *8. What is your diagnosis?*

Final diagnosis

➤ Lymphoma

 *9. What would you recommend to the owner?*

Because the bird started with rubbing the left side of the head 1 week ago, which we interpreted as signs of discomfort and there is no well-developed treatment regimen for avian lymphoma in psittacine birds, we recommended euthanasia in this bird. If the bird had not shown any signs of discomfort we would not have recommended euthanasia.

Discussion

Lymphomas (Fig. 2.81), especially in the oculonasal region have been described before (Harcourt-Brown 2009). This pathological condition is seen from time to time by veterinarians. However, it is very likely that many cases are misdiagnosed because sinusitis or aspergillus can look very similar. In this case, the mass was rather big and obvious. On histological examination of the organs, which we performed because of "scientific interest" as the owner did not want to spend money on a necropsy, lymphoid infiltrations could be found also in the thyroid and parathyroid. Even in cases where owners are not willing to cover the cost of a necropsy, it is advisable to carry out such examination as part of a continuing education programme.

Further reading

Harcourt-Brown, N., 2009. Oculonasal lymphoma in five parrots. Scientific Meeting, European College of Avian Medicine and Surgery, Antwerp.

Lightfoot, T.L., 2008. The geriatric psittacine patient. In: 80th Western Veterinary Conference, Las Vegas.

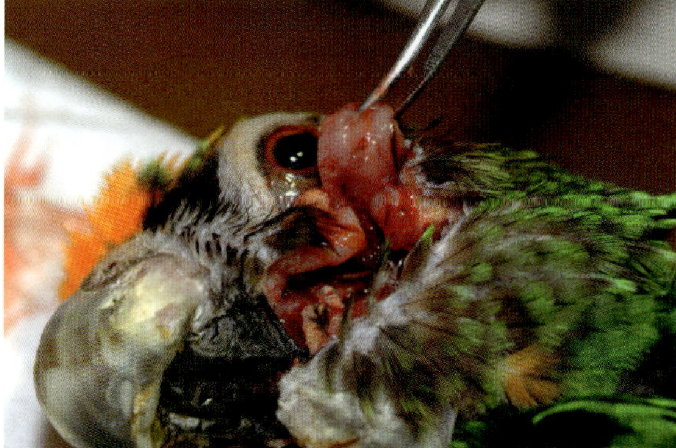

Fig. 2.81 Appearance of the lymphoma at post-mortem examination.

Case 2.32 *P. Sandmeier*

Clinical history

A 3-year-old female budgerigar (*Melopsittacus undulatus*) weighing 53 g was presented with the following clinical signs:

- Abdominal swelling
- Polyuria
- Slight depression
- Slight laborious breathing.

The budgerigar was kept as a pet together with a second budgerigar. The birds lived in a room of their own within the apartment and had continuous free flight within this room.

1. List your differential diagnoses for abdominal swelling in a budgerigar.

Differential diagnoses

- Ascites (neoplasia, liver disease, heart disease, coelomic bleeding)
- Egg binding
- Neoplasia within coelomic cavity
- Lipoma (subcutaneous fat)
- Adipositas (subcutaneous fat)
- Ovarian cyst
- Non-neoplastic organomegaly
- Abdominal hernia

Clinical examination

On presentation, the bird had a good body condition. Palpation of the coelomic cavity revealed a solid prominent swelling. Surprisingly, the budgerigar was only slightly depressed and respiratory distress was also only minimal. The crop appeared distended and could be palpated over the outside surface of the breast muscles. A total volume of 0.5 ml barium sulphate was administered directly into the crop and 60 minutes later survey radiographs were taken (Fig. 2.82a, b).

Radiology

2. What is your diagnosis based on interpretation of the radiographs in Fig. 2.82a, b.

Interpretation of radiographs and final diagnosis

- Egg binding with herniation of the ventral coelomic wall
- Division of crop with pendulous part over the ventral aspect of the breast muscles
- Delayed barium transit time
- Polyostotic hyperostosis of the long bones

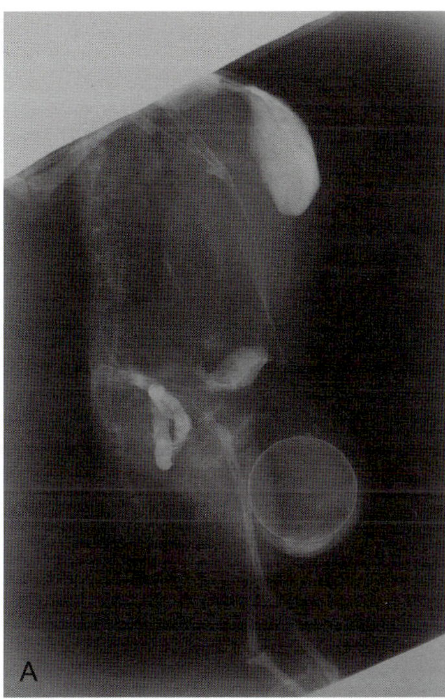

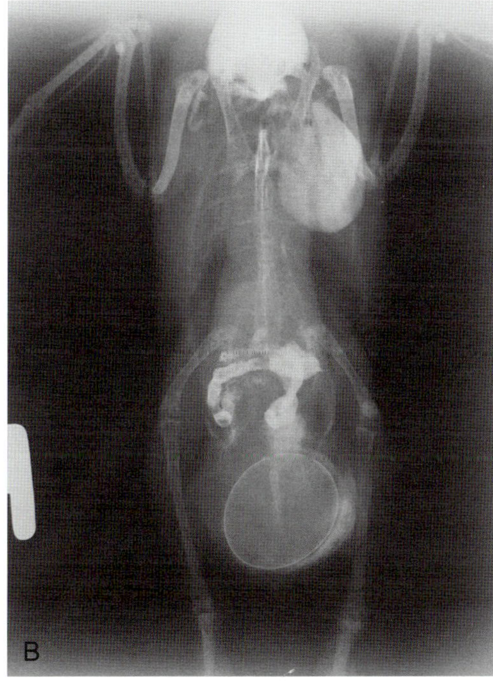

Fig. 2.82 (a) Lateral survey contrast radiograph of the budgerigar; (b) ventrodorsal survey contrast radiograph of the budgerigar.

3. Describe the pathogenesis of these clinical and radiographic findings?

Pathogenesis of clinical and radiographic findings

- Malnutrition, lack of exercise and pathology of the female endocrine system with probable increased secretion of oestrogen or other related hormones, leading to weakening of the musculature of the coelomic wall causing herniation, and weakening of the fibrous tissue of the crop wall causing an extended crop wall leading to a pendulous crop
- Hormonal status causing increased storage of calcium within the long bones leading to the increased bone density described as polyostotic hyperostosis
- Egg binding secondary to coelomic herniation
- Lack of acute symptoms of egg binding and cardiovascular compromise due to lack of intracoelomic pressure because of coelomic hernia
- Increased barium transit time due to increased volume of urogenital tract, displacing the intestines

4. List your therapeutic strategy.

Therapy (Table 2.70)

Table 2.70 Therapy

Leuprolide acetate (Lucrin®)	1000 µg/kg IM To regulate female hormone status and stop the production of a second egg, stop further weakening of abdominal and crop wall and positively influence the polyostotic hyperostosis
Vitamin ADEC	Vitamin A 20 000 IU/kg IM once In preparation for surgery
Vitamin B complex	Thiamine 30 mg/kg IM once In preparation for surgery
Fluids	Ringer's lactate 20 ml/kg SC In preparation for surgery
Butorphanol	4 mg/kg IM For pre-emptive analgesia
Coelomic surgery	Opening of the coelomic cavity using a ventral midline incision. Removal of egg through an incision of the salpinx. Routine closure including closure of the abdominal hernia
Assisted feeding	Parrot hand feeding formula, as soon as patient fully recovered from anaesthesia

Consider surgery of the pendulous crop after full recovery from coelomic surgery.

Discussion

Abdominal swelling is a common clinical presentation in budgerigars. This is frequently caused by pathology of the female reproductive system with increased secretion of oestrogen and related ovarian hormones. Clinical manifestations include weakening of fibrous and muscle tissue leading to herniation of the coelomic wall or distension of the crop wall, egg binding or polyostotic hyperostosis, although the only study on polyostotic hyperostosis could not support the hypothesis that this is caused by hyperoestrogenism. Occasionally, more than one of these clinical presentations can be combined as in this case. Malnutrition and lack of exercise are two important predisposing factors leading to the development of hormonal imbalances and the symptoms observed in this case.

Egg binding is normally a life-threatening situation that needs to be addressed immediately. This case was a combination of egg binding and abdominal hernia leading to a chronic condition, without cardiovascular compromise.

Important factors for intracoelomic surgery in small birds include all perioperative measures such as vitamin injections, fluid therapy, recovery in a humid, warm, protected environment and nutritional support.

Further reading

Bowles, H.L., 2006. Evaluating and treating the reproductive system. In: Harrison, G.J., Lightfoot, T.L. (Eds.), Clinical Avian Medicine. Spix Publishing, Inc., Palm Beach, pp. 519–539.

Baumgartner, R., Hatt, J.M., Dobeli, M., et al., 1995. Endocrinologic and pathologic findings in birds with polyostotic hyperostosis. J. Avian Med. Surg. 9, 251–254.

Sandmeier, P., Baumgartner, R., Isenbügel, E., 2008. Wellensittiche (Budgerigars). In: Gabrisch, K., Zwart, P. (Eds.), Krankheiten der Heimtiere. Schlütersche, pp. 437–490.

Case 2.33 *P. Coutteel, G. Dorrestein*

Clinical history

At the end of the breeding season, a canary breeder with 100 pairs requested a visit to his aviary (Fig. 2.83) because the young birds were progressively getting lethargic and dying.

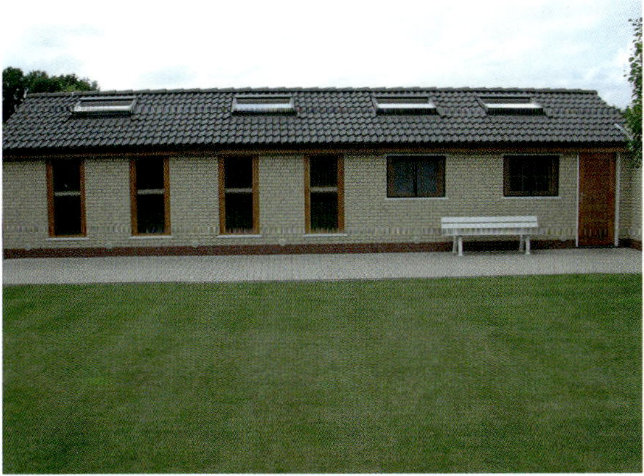

Fig. 2.83 General view of the facility housing 100 pairs of canaries.

The breeding season had not been that good this year. The first round was much better than the second one, so he decided to continue breeding with the pairs that had not raised a second clutch.

In the end the results were four youngsters per couple, so 400 young birds.

Inspection of the aviary

The young birds were kept in a building separate from the breeding room and were living together in groups of approximately 50 birds (Fig. 2.84a, b). They had access to food and drinking water and soft food *ad libitum*. At the bottom there was a special wood substrate. There was abundant natural light through windows fitted with mosquito netting.

The aviaries appeared well designed, but were built using wood making disinfection or treating red mites difficult during the hot summer months. There were some young birds 2 months old sitting on the ground showing ruffled feathers and looking lethargic. They were taken into the practice for further examination together with a couple of parents which had not produced fertile eggs.

The breeder also mentioned that he euthanased some young birds with central nervous problems. These affected fledglings were temporarily losing balance, shaking their heads and could not fly. The adult birds appeared normal but sometimes, especially in the evening, there were clicking noises.

Q ***1. List possible infectious agents and parasites or circumstances that could cause these problems.***

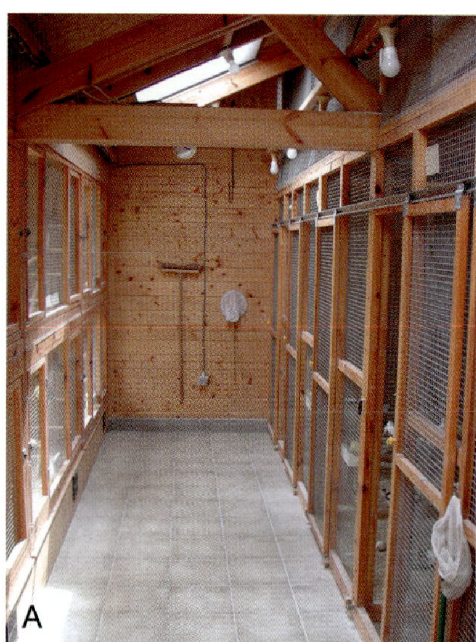

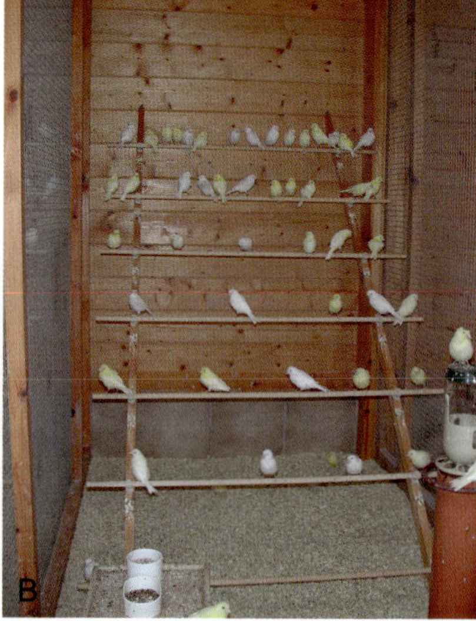

Fig. 2.84 (a and b) Internal view of the aviaries housing the young birds.

Possible infectious agents (Table 2.71)

Table 2.71 Possible infectious agents

Bacterial	Parasitic	Viral	Fungal	Other
E. coli	Trichomoniasis	Polyomavirus	*Macrorhabdus*	Intoxication
Klebsiella	Coccidiosis	Circovirus		Husbandry
Chlamydophila	Atoxoplasmosis			
Pseudomonas	Red mite			

Clinical examination of the affected birds

The *adult birds* were checked physically without finding any abnormalities. One of the birds was producing a clicking noise during clinical examination. A wet mount of the crop was taken but found negative for trichomoniasis. Examination of wet mount and stained smear of faeces and crop contents failed to show the presence of endoparasites, yeast or bacteria.

The body condition of the *young birds* was below the average as they showed low pectoral muscle volume. The skin looked dehydrated. Feathers of wing and tail were normally developed. When blowing apart the feathers on the abdomen, a red swollen duodenal loop and a slightly enlarged liver were visible through the bird's skin as a black spot.

 *2. What further tests would you recommend performing?*

Clinical diagnosis laboratory examination

Post-mortem examination findings of the young birds (Fig. 2.85a, b) were as follows:

- Cachexia
- Splenomegaly
- Enlarged liver
- Pale foci on the liver
- Lung and kidney normal
- Not anaemic
- In bird no. 2 (Fig. 2.85b), an extended duodenal loop with focal haemorrhages due to fasting and hypoglycaemia causing haemorrhagic diathesis was found.

 *3. What other fast tests would you perform to come up with a diagnosis?*

Cytology (Fig. 2.86a–d)

 *4. All smears were stained with Hemacolor, what are your findings?*

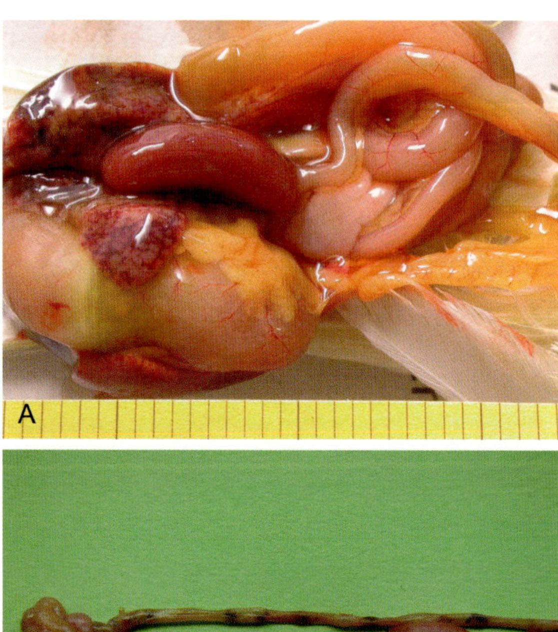

Fig. 2.85 (a and b) Necropsy of young birds.

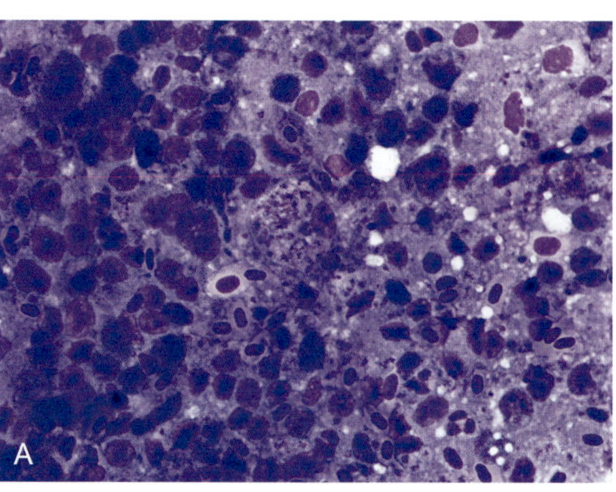

Fig. 2.86 (a–d) Cytology preparations of the intestinal mucosa, lung, spleen and liver.

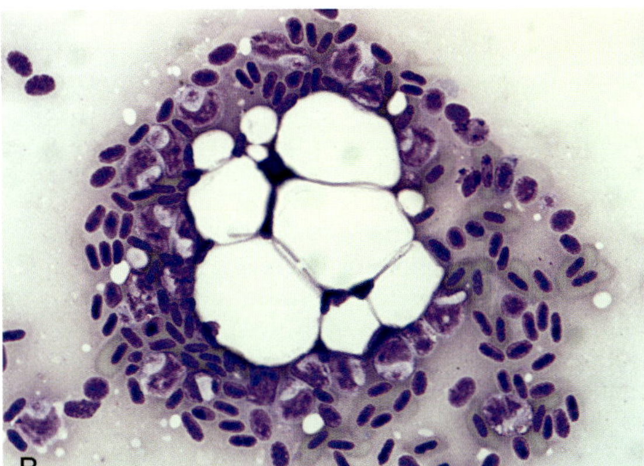

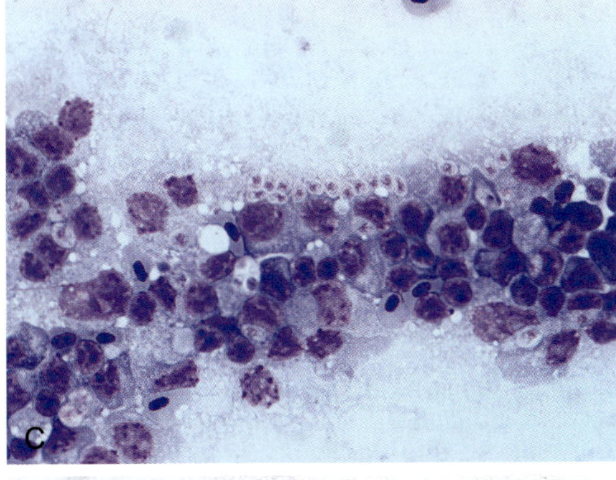

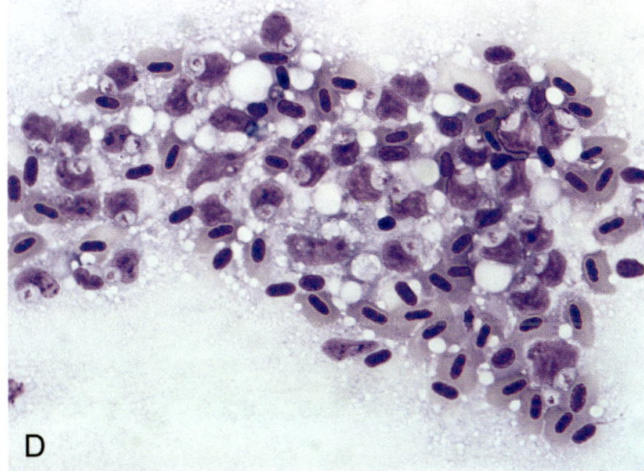

Fig. 2.86—cont'd

Cytology findings

- Fig. 2.86 (a) A smear of the intestinal mucosa scraping from the haemorrhagic site. In the middle you see a schizont with many merozoites as a developing stage of *Isospora serini*, the causative coccidium for atoxoplasmosis. In other cells, protozoal stages with a morphology typical of atoxoplasma trophozoites can be seen
- Fig. 2.86 (b) Impression smear of the lung revealed many trophozoites of atoxoplasma in mononuclear cells. Maybe these were responsible for the clicking noises
- Fig. 2.86 (c) Free atoxoplasma trophozoites in the impressions of the spleen
- Fig. 2.86 (d) Protozoal trophozoites in monocytes in the liver. In the cytoplasm, the parasitic stages cause an indented nucleus (moon-shaped) giving the infected cells a characteristic appearance. Also macrophages may contain atoxoplasma merozoites or trophozoites

Further clinical laboratory diagnosis

Bacteriology

- Moderate infection of *E. coli* which is believed to be secondary

Histopathology (courtesy of NOIVBD – Gerry Dorrestein)

The histopathology was characterized by a large number of parasitized round nuclear cells (mainly monocytes) and macrophages. These cells contained one or more trophozoites in the cytoplasm, causing the typical indent as can be seen in the cytology. Microscopically, there was an infiltration of the intestinal lamina propria by mononuclear cells that contained intracytoplasmic protozoa. These can be single trophozoites or meronts (the asexual cycle). This is also the location where the typical intestinal coccidial stage is developing in the epithelial cells, producing the low number of oocysts that are shed to complete the sexual cycle.

The parasitized cells tend to attach themselves to the endothelium of blood vessels and sinusoids in all organs. This can lead to reduced circulation in the afferent area. When this is the case in the liver, necrosis can be the result of the veno-occlusion effect. In the lungs, these cells are easily recognized as a "rosary" on the surface of the endothelium of the larger vessels (Figs 2.87 and 2.88). In the brain, this can block small blood vessels leading to nervous symptoms.

- Fig. 2.88 (a) Lung: the main changes visible are the lining of the vessels by the parasitized cells. In the right detail, this is seen as a "rosary" on the endothelium of the blood vessel
- Fig. 2.88 (b) The myocardium with lining of the vessels by parasitized cells
- Fig. 2.88 (c) The liver with infiltration of round nuclear cells and veno-occlusion

Diagnosis

Diagnosis of atoxoplasmosis has always been via necropsy followed by cytology and histopathology.

Identification of *atoxoplasma* oocysts in a faecal sample is difficult because they look very similar to those of *Isospora* spp. and are only sporadically shed by infected birds.

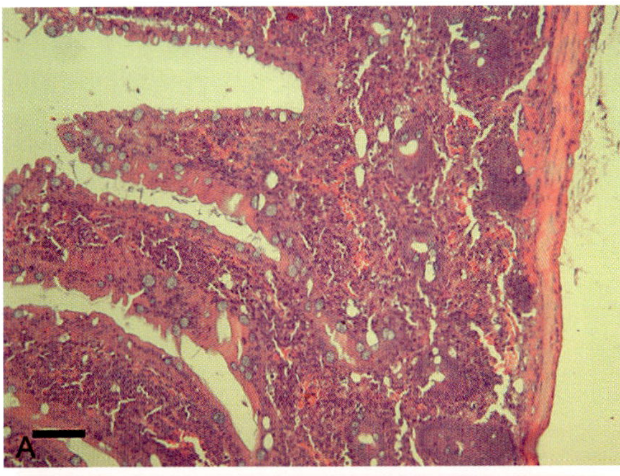

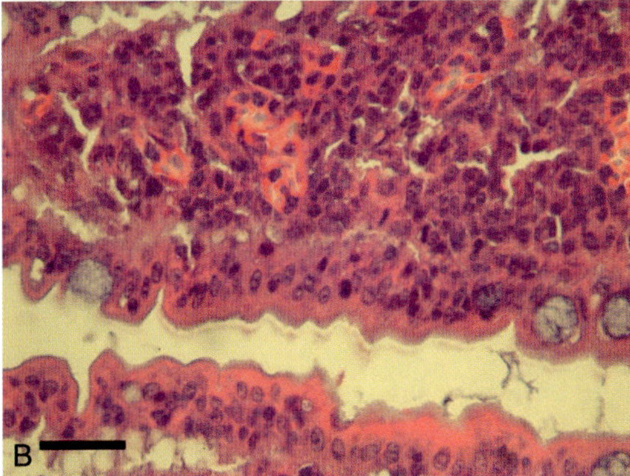

Fig. 2.87 (a and b) Histology of the duodenum showing infiltration of many round nuclear cells in the lamina propria. HE bar 50 resp 20 μm.

Diagnosis can also be made on a living bird using a peripheral blood smear examination stained with Wright's, Giemsa or Diff-Quik. Examination of buffy coat smears increases the likelihood of finding organisms as intracytoplasmic merozoites in monocytes cause an indented nucleus.

Therapy

Effective treatment for atoxoplasmosis is not possible at the moment. Mild infections may even stimulate the immune system and prevent systemic atoxoplasmosis.

- Sulphonamides administered to adults before the breeding season and again during moult period to all birds have been suggested to reduce chick morbidity. However, these treatment protocols cannot completely clear a bird of *Atoxoplasma* spp. infection
- ESB3 30% (Sulphachlorpyrazine) inhibits the intestinal stages of the parasite life cycle and has been shown to reduce or clear oocyst shedding for as long as it is regularly administered

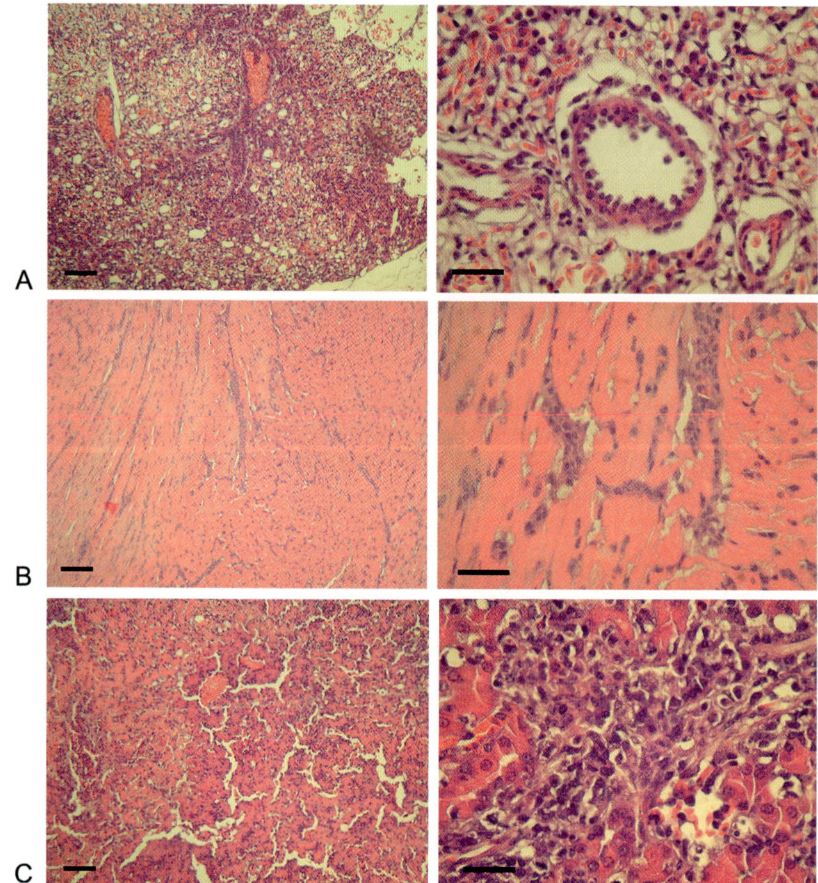

Fig. 2.88 (a–c) Histopathological changes due to Atoxoplasmosis in a canary. HE Bar left 50 μm, right 20 μm.

- Baycox® (Toltrazuril) and Appertex® (Diclazuril) may reduce the life cycle but cannot be given continuously.

The recommended treatment adopted by the authors is the following scheme in the drinking water (with no bathing water available):

- Baycox 2.5% 2 ml per litre for 2 days
- ESB3 30% 2 g per litre for 5 days
- Cosumix Plus 2 g per litre for 5 days
- Vitamins and probiotics for 5 days + bathing water

Baycox® 2.5% (Bayer) = toltrazuril, ESB3® 30% (Novartis) = sulphachlorpyrazine, Cosumix Plus® (Novartis) = sulphachlorpyridazine sodium and trimethoprim.

- Perfect hygiene to reduce faecal contamination
- Avoid stress and overpopulation.

Prevention

Effective prophylaxis for atoxoplasmosis is hard to reach. Adult breeding birds can look perfectly healthy and breed. Oocysts are passed in the faeces beginning nine to ten days post-infection and continue to pass for months. Reduction of faecal–oral transmission can be achieved by cleaning cages frequently and trying to avoid any contact with possibly infected droppings. Also frequently changing the drinking and bathing water can help to minimize faecal contamination. After a positive diagnosis with symptoms, a preventative treatment is suggested during the next breeding season with sulphonamides added in the soft food during the whole breeding period.

Discussion

- Mortality rates for atoxoplasmosis can vary between 20 and 80% in young passerines
- Adult birds are shedding oocysts and may lack clinical signs
- Oocysts are very stable in the environment and are not inactivated by most disinfectants as they can persist for long periods of time in the soil
- Elimination of the parasite from aviaries is difficult
- Patency of infection lasts up to 8 months due to the long life of macrophages in birds which are a pool of merozoites
- Atoxoplasma is especially virulent due to the damage to intestinal epithelium with haemorrhages to liver, spleen and myocardium in young birds
- Atoxoplasma enter the blood stream via the vasculature of the intestinal wall and invade mononuclear leukocytes, undergo asexual division in circulating and tissue lymphocytes, monocytes and macrophages, as well as in intestinal epithelial cells
- Clicking respiratory noises and central nervous symptoms are believed to be associated with the atoxoplasma cycle in the bloodstream

Acknowledgement

I would like to thank Peter Wencel very much, not only for the cytological pictures but also for the drive to prove that cytology is a major diagnostic tool in our private avian practice.

Further reading

Ball, S.J., Brown, M.A., Daszak, P., et al., 1998. *Atoxoplasma* (Apicomplexa: Eimeriorina: Atoxoplasmatidae) in the greenfinch (*Carduelis chloris*). J. Parasitol. 84, 813–817.

Box, E.D., 1970. *Atoxoplasma* associated with an isosporan oocyst in canaries. J. Protozool. 17, 391–396.

Box, E.D., 1975. Exogenous stages of *Isospora serini* (Aragao) and *Isospora canaria* sp. in the canary (*Serinus canaria linnaeus*). J. Protozool. 22, 165–169.

Box, E.D., 1981. *Isospora* as an extraintestinal parasite of passerine birds. J. Protozool. 28, 244–246.

Davies, R.R., 2008. Passerine birds going light. In: Chitty, J., Lierz, M. (Eds.), BSAVA Manual of Raptors, Pigeons and Passerine Birds. British Small Animal Veterinary Association, Gloucester, pp. 365–369.

Greiner, E.C., Ritchie, B.W., 1994. Parasites. In: Ritchie, B.W., Harrison, G.J., Harrison, L.R. (Eds.), Avian Medicine: Principles and Application. Wingers Publishing Inc., Lake Worth, pp. 1007–1029.

Levine, H., 1982. The genus *Atoxoplasma* (Protozoa, Apicomplexa). J. Parasitol. 68, 719–723.

Little, S.E., Kelley, L.S., Norton., et al., 2001, Developing diagnostic tools to further our understanding of Atoxoplasma species. In: Proceedings of the Association of Avian Veterinarians. pp. 157–159.

MacWhirter, P., 1994. Passeriformes. In: Ritchie, B.W., Harrison, G.J., Harrison, L.R. (Eds.), Avian Medicine: Principles and Application. Wingers Publishing Inc., Lake Worth, pp. 1172–1199.

McNamee, P., et al., 1995. Clinical and pathological changes associated with *Atoxoplasma* in a captive bullfinch (*Pyrrhula pyrrhula*). Vet. Rec. 136, 221–222.

Partington, C.J., 1989. Atoxoplasmosis in Bali mynahs. J. Zoo Wildl. Med. 20, 328–335.

Quiroga, M.I., Aleman, N., Vazquez, S., et al., 2000. Diagnosis of atoxoplasmosis in a canary (*Serinus canaria*) by histopathologic and ultrastructural examination. Avian Dis. 44, 465–469.

Sandmeier, P., Coutteel, P., 2006. Passerines. In: Harrison, G.J., Lightfoot, T.L. (Eds.), Clinical Avian Medicine. Spix publishing Inc., Lake Worth, pp. 879–913.

Swayne, D.E., Getzy, D., Slemons, R.D., et al., 1991. Coccidiosis as a cause of transmural lymphocytic enteritis and mortality in captive Nashville warblers (*Vermivora ruficapilla*). J. Wildl. Dis. 27, 615–620.

Case 2.34 *P. Coutteel, G. Dorrestein*

Clinical history

A breeder of Lady Gouldian finches (*Erythrura gouldiae*, formerly *Chloebia gouldiae*) was facing a 30% mortality only with his young birds. In the same facility there were also ceres amadines (*Aidemosyna modesta*), long-tailed finches (*Poephila acuticauda*) and diamond firetails (*Emblema guttata*), but they were breeding normally and showing no clinical signs (Fig. 2.89).

The young Gouldian finches reached the age of 1 month and then started to lose weight and were dying (Fig. 2.90). After 2 months he had lost 100 youngsters, all about the same age.

Inspection of the aviary

- The breeding facility was a closed building and completely artificially lighted and heated
- The spectrum of the lamps was 6500 Kelvin and were changed every year
- The frequency of the fluorescent lamps was 50 Hz
- The room temperature was stable and approximately 20 °C

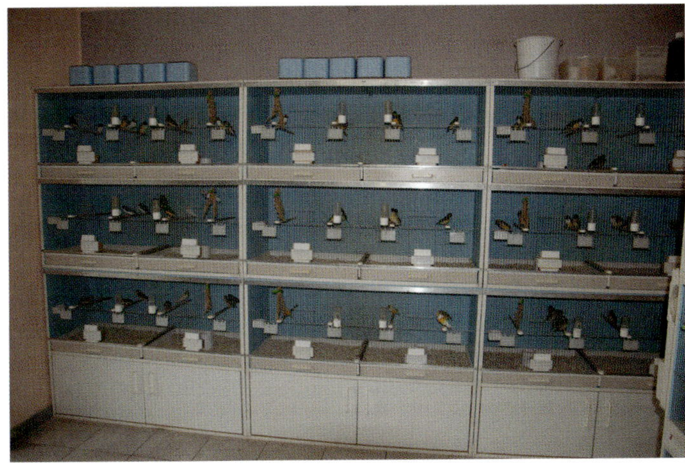

Fig. 2.89 General view of the aviary housing the birds in this case.

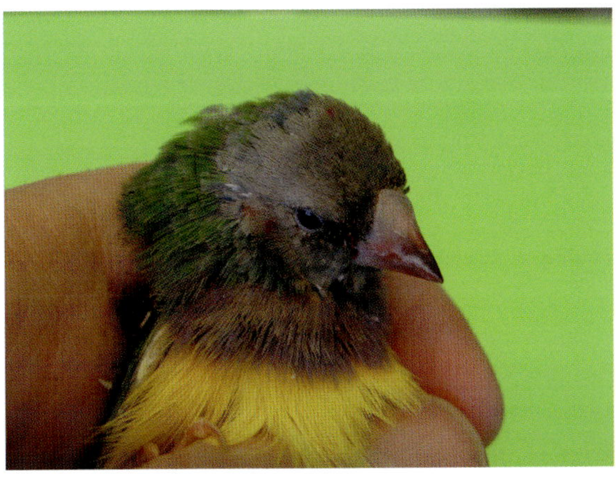

Fig. 2.90 An affected young bird.

- They had a light regime of 15 hours a day
- Seed mixture for small exotics (large white millets)
- Oyster shells, grit and cuttlebone were not always available
- Soft food was only administered when they were raising youngsters

Society finches (*Lonchura striata domestica*) were used as foster parents. The chicks fledged at approximately 21–24 days and stayed out with the parents for an additional 2–3 weeks.

Q *1. List possible infectious agents and parasites or circumstances that could cause these problems.*

Possible infectious agents (Table 2.72)

Table 2.72 Possible infectious agents

Bacterial	Parasitic	Viral	Fungal	Other
E. coli	Cochlosomosis	Polyoma	*Macrorhabdus*	Intoxication
Campylobacter	Coccidiosis	Cytomegalo	*Candida albicans*	Husbandry
Chlamydophila	Atoxoplasmosis			Food
Pseudomonas	Red mite			

Clinical examination of the affected birds

- Age of affected young birds: 30–35 days
- Sleeping a lot, sitting on the bottom
- Visible liver
- Cachectic
- Delayed moult on the head
- Faeces were yellowish, voluminous and containing undigested seeds (Fig. 2.91).
- Birds were dying because of malabsorption and lack of energy
- Treatment with enrofloxacin (Baytril 10% 2 ml per litre) for 5 days was not successful

 *2. What further tests would you recommend to perform?*

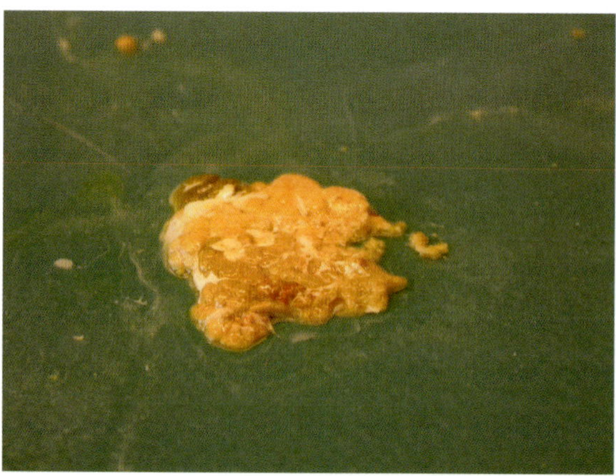

Fig. 2.91 Faeces of an affected bird.

Clinical diagnosis support

Crop swab

- Negative

Faeces examination

- Collected pool sample from young birds: microscopic with polarized lighting much undigested starch was found but no presence of parasites, nor oocysts
- Examination of a fresh stool revealed the presence of many motile flagellates. The movement was corresponding to *Cochlosoma* spp. trophozoites

Bacteriology

- Two rods per field (1000×)
- Presence of yeast
- Negative for *Salmonella, Yersinia, Shigella* and *Campylobacter*

Post-mortem examination (Fig. 2.92)

The following observations were made during the post-mortem examination:

- Cachexia
- Spleen: orange/yellow and small
- Liver, lung and kidney normal
- Crop and proventriculus empty
- Distended duodenal loop with haemorrhagic content due to starvation (blood leakage of the villous atrophy).

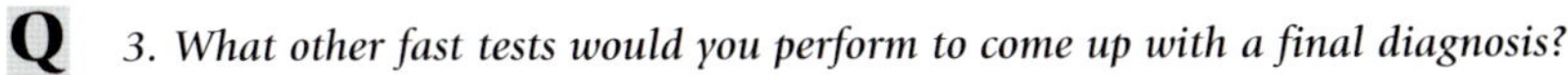

Q *3. What other fast tests would you perform to come up with a final diagnosis?*

A fast stain of an air-dried faecal smear was examined in a wet mount and the presence of *Campylobacter* was detected.

Cytology

- Liver: vacuolization and anisokaryosis
- Spleen: erythropoiesis, in between cells many vacuoles
- Crop: nothing special
- Lung and kidney: nothing special
- Ventriculus: some yeast, some bacteria
- Duodenum (Fig. 2.93): many *Campylobacter* spp. and some cocci
- Rectum: some cocci and rods and few *Campylobacter* spp.

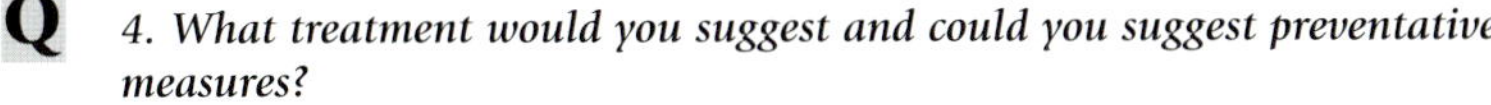

Q *4. What treatment would you suggest and could you suggest preventative measures?*

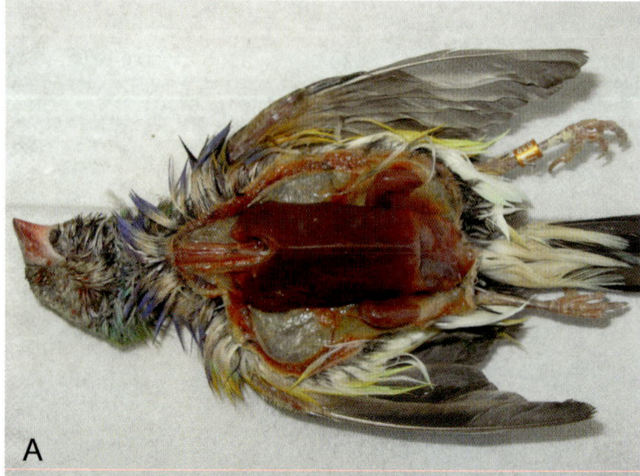

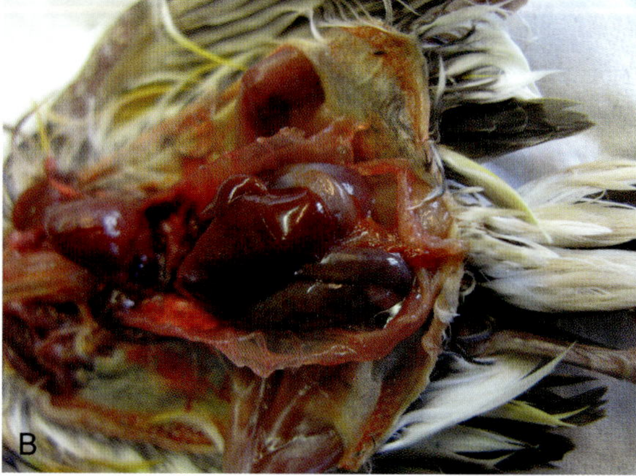

Fig. 2.92 (a and b) Post-mortem examination of an affected bird.

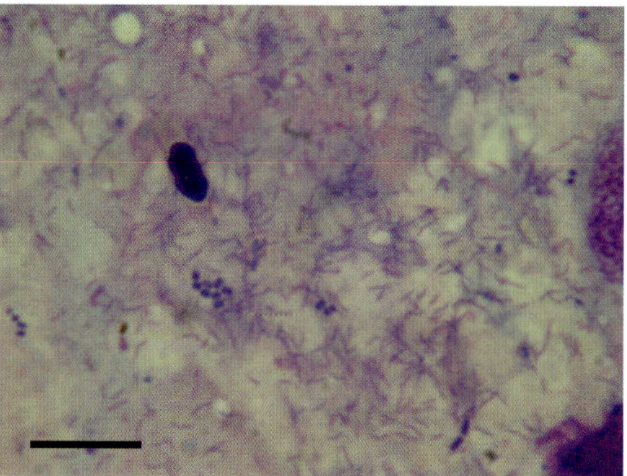

Fig. 2.93 Cytology preparation of the duodenum (courtesy of Gerry Dorrestein).

Conclusion

- *Campylobacter* and *Cochlosoma* spp.

Therapy

- Erythromycin + ronidazole + electrolytes
- In drinking water for 10–14 days
- The soft food should also be moistened with this medicated drinking water

Prevention

Foster parents (society finches) should be treated before and during the breeding season for at least 10 days because they are often asymptomatic carriers of *Campylobacter* and *Cochlosoma*. Macrolides are preferred to enrofloxacin.

Discussion

- Negative bacteriology due to the already given medication and the difficulties encountered to grow *Campylobacter* can mask your diagnosis (need of selective culture media and special conditions)
- Fresh stool or a living bird is needed to check for *Cochlosoma*
- Often more diseases are present at the same time causing problems at the same age
- Young Gouldians are very fragile until their final moult
- Other species in the same room can show no clinical signs (species-specific diseases)
- Artificial lighting is very important. Low frequency light causes flickering and can lead to a stress situation with a drop in immunity. High frequency lamps are preferable
- Insufficient iodine in the diet often results in a loss of feathers around the head. A potassium iodine source should be available every day

Tips for detecting *Cochlosoma* spp. in a wet faecal smear

The smear should be examined in a certain way to be sure about the presence or absence of *Cochlosoma*:

- The faeces should be fresh – dead flagellates will not move
- The smear has to be thin, therefore it is good to use a coverslip and prepare a monolayer of faeces
- The diaphragm should be almost completely closed because of the need of good contrast to see the small moving organisms
- Do not examine too fast, take the time needed to scan properly.

Further reading

Filippich, L.J., O'Donoghue, P.J., 1997. *Cochlosoma* infections in finches. Aust. Vet. J. 75 (8), 561–563.

Sandmeier, P., Coutteel, P., 2006. Passerines. In: Harrison, G.J., Lightfoot, T.L. (Eds.), Clinical Avian Medicine. Spix publishing Inc., Palm Beach, pp. 879–913.

Schmidt, R.E., Reavill, D.R., Phalen, D.N., 2008. Pathology of pet and aviary birds. Iowa State Press, Ames.

Case 2.35 *P. Coutteel, G. Dorrestein*

Clinical history

Three 12-day-old yellowhammer fledglings were presented as representatives for a one hundred individual flock of young birds bred in this season (from two clutches) (Fig. 2.94). This breeder of buntings had cases of sudden deaths in youngsters, especially from the second clutch, with mortality reaching 15% of the fledglings. No specific signs of disease were reported. No mortality in adults.

Hatchlings were parent raised and after a period of 7 days switched to hand feeding with a mixture formula of 20% Kaytee Exact® and 80% commercial turkey food. They were fed every two hours with the same syringe used for all young birds in the aviary. Water used for soft food preparation was medicated with Ronidazole 200 mg per litre. The owner was not aware of the presence of any medication in the turkey feed.

Clinical examination

During clinical examination, two fledglings were in good condition, showing interest in their surroundings and were begging for food; one died shortly before examination.

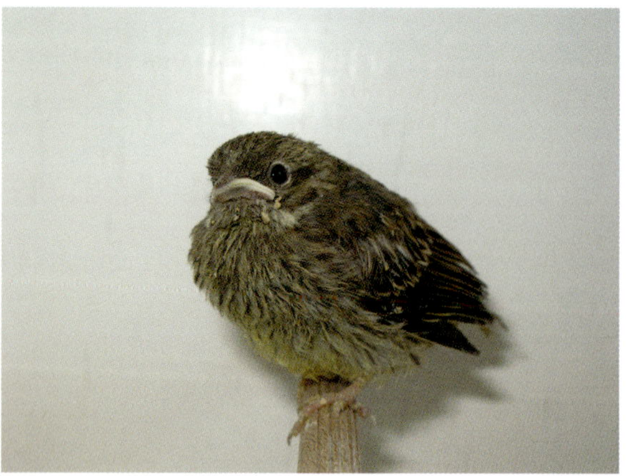

Fig. 2.94 Yellowhammer (*Emberiza citrinella*).

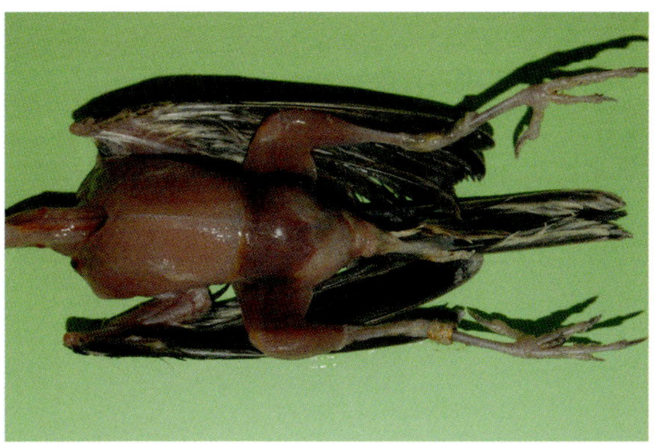

Fig. 2.95 Post-mortem examination of a young yellowhammer.

Wet mount examination of a faecal smear showed no presence of endoparasites, coccidian oocysts nor the presence of *Macrorhabdus*.

The turkey food "Aveve Kruimel voor kalkoenkuikens Nr. 67" contained 25.5% proteins. Also added to this food were Diclazuril 100 mg per kg and copper (II) sulphate 15 mg per kg.

Q *1. What abnormalities can you see in this bird (Fig. 2.95)?*

- Excellent body condition, but no fat tissue
- Pale pectoral muscles
- Distended abdomen with enlarged liver
- Enlarged gall bladder visible through the abdominal wall (Fig. 2.95)

 *2. What parasitic, bacterial and viral diseases can occur in young passerines presented with these symptoms? What are the characteristics and diagnostic possibilities in these?*

Parasitic, bacterial, fungal and viral diseases (Table 2.73)

Table 2.73 Parasitic, bacterial, fungal and viral diseases

Parasitic	Bacterial	Fungal	Viral
Atoxoplasma	*Salmonella* spp.	*Macrorhabdus*	Circovirus
Coccidiosis	*Yersinia* spp.	*Candida* spp.	Polyomavirus
Flagellates	*E. coli*		Herpesvirus
Bloodsucking mites	*Campylobacter* spp.		

Post-mortem examination

A comprehensive post-mortem examination was carried out (Fig. 2.96a, b).

Q *3. List the findings of the post-mortem examination shown in the pictures*

- Enlarged liver
- Congested gall bladder
- Enlarged, pale spleen
- Severe congestion of the lungs
- Pale pectoral muscles
- No dehydration

Q *4. What further steps would you consider to take to come up with the diagnosis?*

Clinical laboratory diagnosis

During necropsy, samples for cytology, bacteriology and histopathology were taken.

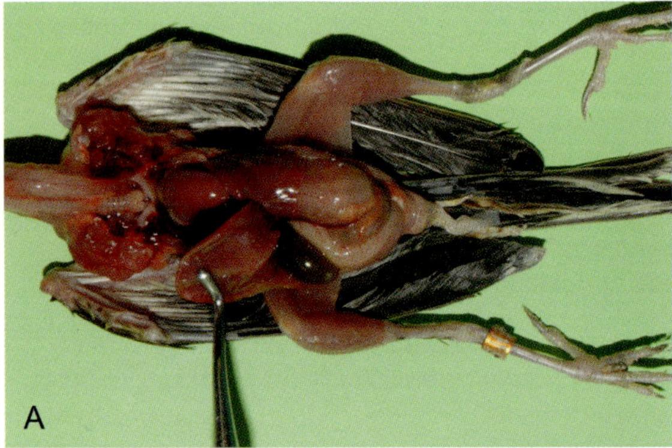

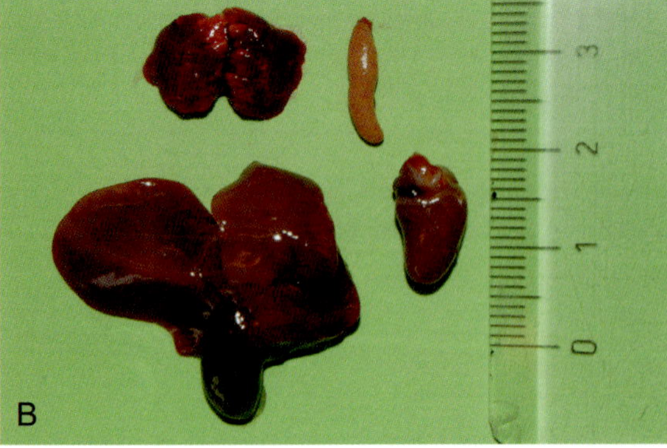

Fig. 2.96 (a and b) Post-mortem examination of a young yellowhammer.

Cytology

Smears made from crop swab, intestinal contents, bile, together with touch preparations of sampled organs and bone marrow from tibiotarsus were air dried and stained with Hemacolor® (Merck HX956294, Darmastadt, Germany) for rapid cytological testing (Fig. 2.97a, b).

The results of examination of both wet mounts and Hemacolor®-stained, air-dried smears of crop contents, bile and faeces showed no abnormalities in morphology of epithelial cells, but the presence of large numbers of bacteria and yeast cells.

The cytological examination of touch preparations of liver, spleen, lung and bone marrow smears revealed large numbers of rod-shaped bacteria with a morphology typical for *Enterobacteriaceae*, phagocytized by macrophages and present between the cells of all sampled organs. The largest amount of bacteria was found in liver, bone marrow, spleen and lung, respectively. The presence of bacteria in bone marrow and in the macrophages confirmed that death was caused by bacterial septicaemia.

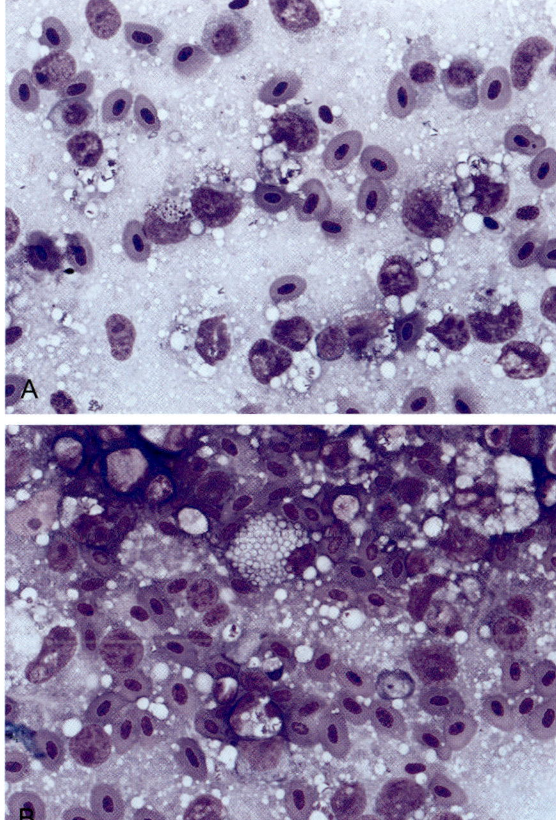

Fig. 2.97 (a) Cytology preparation showing phagocytes and inclusions; (b) Mott cell in the liver.

Q *5. Present your therapeutic strategy based on the above findings.*

Preliminary treatment

The treatment of the flock based on the necropsy findings and cytology was:

- A combination of chloramphenicol and furaltadone HCl + nystatin
- All medication was administered with the hand-feeding formula and given every two hours
- Stop treatment with ronidazole because of the potential toxicity especially for growing youngsters. The indicated dose of ronidazole for adult birds is 100 mg per litre of drinking water!
- Thorough disinfection of the hand-feeding boxes and hygiene of the syringes.

Further clinical laboratory diagnosis

Bacteriology (AML laboratory (002/0.08.47543))

- Gram-positive rods found in liver
- *Micrococcus* spp. sensitive to chloramphenicol

Histopathology (Fig. 2.98 a–f)

(a) Lungs very compact (HE 10× bar 50 μm); (b) lung with several pale nuclei (HE 50× bar 20 μm); (c) kidney with large pale nuclei in the mesangium and (d) in a tubulus lumen a large Gram-positive bacterial growth; (e) myocardium with few large pale nuclei and bacterial growth; (f) liver with large pale nuclei.

The selected formalin-fixed organs were processed routinely and thin slides were cut and stained with hemaluin-eosin (HE) and Gram stain for demonstrating bacteria.

The findings were:

The lungs (a) were very compact and large areas were not containing air. In the respiratory tissue, several enlarged nuclei were seen with nuclear wall hyperchromatosis (b). The architecture of the kidneys was normal (c and d). Distributed through the kidney in glomeruli and tubuli, colonization by Gram-positive bacteria could be seen. In the mesangium of the glomeruli, enlarged nuclei were seen with nuclear wall hyperchromatosis (c). (e) In the myocardium, the enlarged nuclei were present as well as bacterial colonization of blood caplillaries. (f) In the liver, in the sinusoids also enlarged "clear" nuclei were seen and also bacterial colonization and some hepatocellular necrosis.

Conclusion: high suspicion of a polyomavirus infection based on the presence of the enlarged "clear" nuclei with nuclear wall hyperchromatosis as a result of inclusion body formation. The bacterial sepsis is considered to be an agonal secondary infection based on the presence of bacteria in macrophages and the absence of other inflammatory reactions of the host.

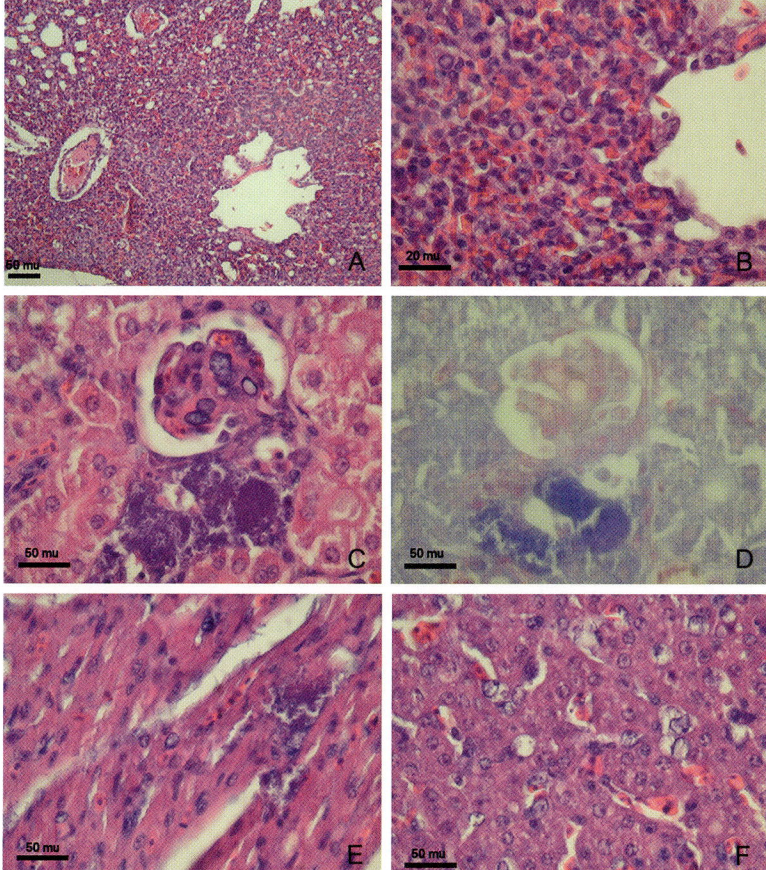

Fig. 2.98 (a–f) Histopathology of the yellowhammer (PA-10-0713).

Viral examination (NOIVBD (PA-10-0713/2))

Since fresh tissue was not available at the moment the histological examination was done; paraffin cut material was sent for PCR testing to a routine molecular diagnostic laboratory. The results were negative for polyomavirus.

Because the histopathology was strongly suggestive for polyomavirus and the existence of a finch polyomavirus was already shown by the Virology Institute of the University of Leipzig (Wittig et al., 2007), paraffin material was also sent to Professor Vahlenkamp in Leipzig.

The polyomavirus consensus PCR was positive and sequencing resulted in 98% finch polyomavirus (V121/10).

Conclusion

Presented birds were diagnosed with bacterial infection of the lower respiratory tract, kidney, liver and heart resulting in a septicaemia. Organisms found during cytological examination were revealed to be rod-shaped bacteria of *Enterobacteriaceae* morphology. Organs were sampled for bacteriology and histopathology and were sent to laboratories for further testing. Initial results of bacteriology culture together with antimicrobial susceptibility testing should be available in 24 hours, histopathology in 7–10 days, viral testing one more week. A broad spectrum antimicrobial treatment combined with nystatin was proposed on the basis of necropsy and cytology findings. After 1 week no more birds died. The final diagnosis of polyomavirus was confirmed. Only young birds died at a typical age. Mortality problems started with an overpopulation with the second clutch.

Discussion

The two other young birds, presented for examination, died suddenly a few hours later. The owner treated all other young birds with the prescribed medication, and mortality stopped at the level of 20%.

Small passerines and especially fledglings constitute a challenge for a practitioner, not only because of the variety of possible diseases with many different clinical presentations, but also with the size of the patients.

The shortcomings concerned with collecting samples from living birds for further testing resulting from the size of the bird cannot be overemphasized. In cases where the health of the flock is more important than of an individual, the best possible results are obtained with culling birds showing clinical signs of disease and examining them thoroughly.

However, in cases of very valuable single birds, the practitioner is limited with the small size and fragility of the patient. Even so, a drop of a centrifuged 0.2 µl of capillary blood may be enough to come up with a diagnosis. Quick stains (e.g. Hemacolor®) are an indispensable tool for fast evaluation of smears and preparations and, even when dealing with bacteria in a clinical specimen, this stain gives very valuable information about the presence, numbers and shape of the bacteria and the presence of yeasts (including *Macrorhabdus*). Also a good knowledge of the normal appearance of blood and organ cells is necessary to achieve good results with diseases of passerines. One must not forget about the differences between passerines and other bird groups and be aware that some diseases are true problems only at a certain age.

Acknowledgement

I would like to thank Peter Wencel, not only for the cytological pictures but also for the drive to prove that cytology is a major diagnostic tool in our private avian practice and in the pathology laboratory.

Further reading

Dorrestein, G.M., 2009. Passerines. In: Tully, T.N., Dorrestein, G.M., Jones, A.K. (Eds.), Handbook of Avian Medicine, second ed. Saunders Elsevier, Edinburgh, pp. 169–208.

Johne, R., Müller, H., 2007. Polyomaviruses of birds: etiologic agents of inflammatory diseases in a tumor virus family. J. Virol. 81 (21), 11554–11559.

Wittig, W., Hoffman, K., Müller, H., et al., 2007. Detection of DNA of the finch polyomavirus in diseased bird species of the order Passeriformes. Berl. Munch. Tierarztl. Wochenschr. 120, 113–119.

CHAPTER

3 Reptiles

Case 3.1 *D. Fischer, M. Lierz*

Clinical history

A 3-year-old, 93 cm-long royal python (*Python regius*), weighing 2239 g, was presented with the following clinical signs of 10 days' duration:

- Fast growing swelling in the first third of the body on the left side.

The snake was bred in an American snake farm and bought in a pet shop. Since then it was kept in a 120 cm × 50 cm × 60 cm sized, glass terrarium, lined with coco humus. A 70 watts spotlight was installed as the only light and heat source, which generated a constant temperature of 30 °C during the day. The nocturnal temperature declined to 23 °C and the air humidity was consistently over 60%. UV radiation was absent. The snake received rodents as food.

Physical examination

The snake was presented with a good body condition and an unimpaired general health. The mucous membranes of the oral cavity and pharynx appeared unsuspicious and pink coloured. In the cranial third of the body, approximately. 8 cm caudal to the occiput, an 8 cm long and 3 cm wide, tough-elastic, non-moveable swelling was present (Fig. 3.1). Nothing abnormal was detectable on the rest of the snake's body by adspection and palpation. The righting reflex and the cloacal tone were normal. Survey radiographs were taken (Fig. 3.2) and ultrasonographic examination of the neck region was performed. In addition, a sonographically-controlled fine needle biopsy of the mass was taken.

Clinical diagnosis examination

Radiology

Radiographs were taken in dorsoventral and latero-lateral planes (see Fig. 3.2).

Ultrasonographical examination

Ultrasonographic examination was done with a linear probe and a frequency of 10 MHz. The neck region around the swelling and the distension itself were scanned.

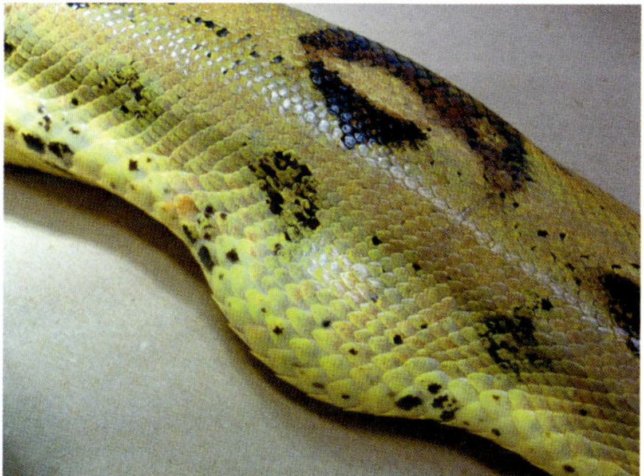

Fig. 3.1 In the cranial third of the body of a royal python (*Python regius*), an 8 cm long and 3 cm wide, tough, elastic, non-moveable swelling was palpable.

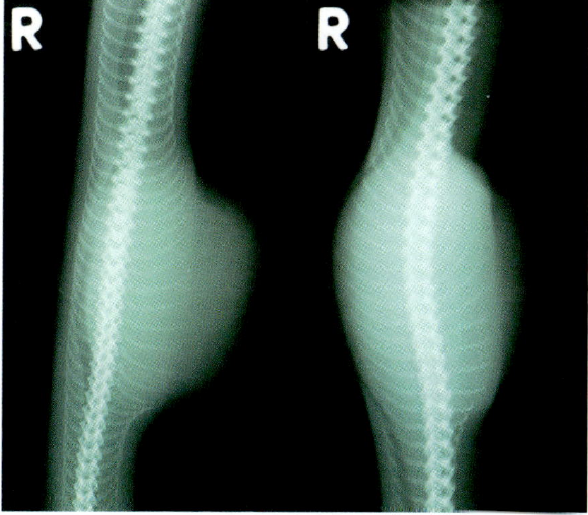

Fig. 3.2 Radiographs of the ball python in the dorsoventral and latero-lateral planes. The swelling appeared as a homogeneous radiopaque mass similar to soft tissue.

Fine needle aspiration

A sonography-guided fine needle biopsy was unsuccessful, as it was impossible to aspirate material from the swelling using a 23 G needle.

1. What is your interpretation of the clinical picture Fig. 3.1 and the radiograph in Fig. 3.2?

Results

- On radiographs, the distension appeared homogeneous, radiopaque, similar to soft tissues. Other organs, as assessable, appeared normal
- Ultrasonographic examination and colour Doppler sonography revealed the swelling as a homogeneous, strongly vascularized, 8 cm long and 3 cm wide mass. There were no clear borders to other surrounding tissue layers visible

Please evaluate the clinical history, Figs 3.1 and 3.2, the results of the physical examination and clinical diagnosis laboratory tests.

Q *2. List your differential diagnoses.*

Q *3. List your therapeutic strategy.*

Differential diagnoses for swellings/distensions in snakes

- Abscess following bacterial or mycotic infection, mechanical trauma, injuries caused by companions or food animals
- Granuloma (e.g. fungal, *Mycobacteria* spp.)
- Obstipation, coprostasis, caused by mismanagement or parasitic infection (e.g. *Cryptosporidia* spp.)
- Urolithiasis
- Gravidity, dystocy
- Neoplasia, spontaneous or caused by viral agents (e.g. retrovirus, C-type oncornavirus)
- Bone deformations following bacterial infections (e.g. *Salmonella* spp.) or caused by metabolic disorders
- Recent food uptake, especially in an environment too cold for the animal
- Recent subcutaneous injection

Therapy

The snake was hospitalized to perform surgical removal of the mass. Previous to surgery the snake received premedication (Table 3.1).

After anaesthesia and analgesia, the skin around the swelling was disinfected with an alcoholic antiseptic. Incision of the skin was made between the second and third row of lateral scales and underlying muscle layers separated by blunt dissection. The

Table 3.1 Therapy

Tiletamin/zolazepam	5 mg/kg IM
Isoflurane	3% inhalant mix with oxygen to maintain inhalation anaesthesia
Carprofen	4 mg/kg IM
Fluids	Ringer's lactate 20 ml/kg SC BID

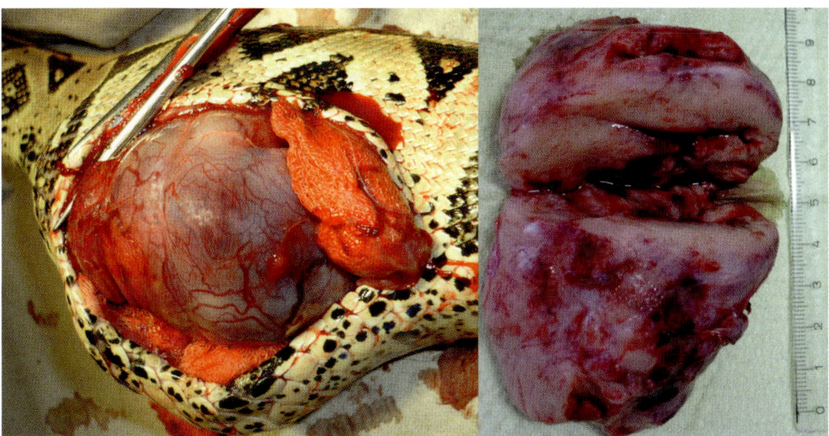

Fig. 3.3 Left: skin incision between the second and third row of lateral scales and separation of underlying muscle layers by blunt dissection make the mass visible inside the oesophagus. Right: section of the greasy-mushy, strongly vascularized mass after surgical removal.

mass (Fig. 3.3) was localized inside the oesophagus, which was incised to a length of 10 cm. The mucous membranes of the oesophagus were extensively infiltrated by the growth, so that a complete removal would have been impossible. As an extirpation was assumed to be connected with huge bleeding and tissue damage the animal was euthanized during surgery. Afterwards the greasy-mushy, strongly vascularized mass (Fig. 3.3) was removed and sent for histopathological examination.

Histopathological diagnosis

The removed mass was histopathologically identified as a lymphoma. The malignant neoplasia included parts of necrosis and purulent-necrotic inflammation.

Discussion

Swellings or distensions of different causes are common findings in reptiles. A thorough diagnostic including imaging (radiography and/or ultrasound), cytology and/or histopathology is needed to reveal the cause. Sometimes these findings are neoplastic in origin. Most diagnoses are based on histopathological examinations following necropsies or biopsies. Classifications of the growths are done according to the WHO classification scheme of mammalian tumours. Current case reports and retrospective studies mentioned an increasing number of neoplasms diagnosed in reptiles over the last years. Among the reptiles, high tumour prevalence (12.4–15% in zoological collections) was described in snakes compared to a lower prevalence in lizards, tortoises and crocodiles. The ophidian genera *Colubridae* (colubrids), *Crotalidae* (pit vipers) and *Viperidae* (vipers) were more often affected than the genus *Boidae* (boids). Neoplasms in serpents were found frequently in liver, skin and the gastrointestinal tract. Epithelial tumours were diagnosed more often than mesenchymal tumours, and malignant neoplasms (54–80%) more often than benign neoplasms. Metastases were found in liver, pancreas, heart, spleen and lung. Besides mast cell tumours, lymphomas, seminomas and adenomas, a great variety of malignant neoplasms have been described in snakes (e.g. undifferentiated sarcomas of soft tissues, melanomas, carcinomas, spindle cell sarcomas, adenocarcinomas, haemangiosarcomas, sertoli cell tumours, malignant histiocytomas, fibrosarcomas and lymphosarcomas).

The diagnosed lymphoma is a cancer of lymphoid cells of the immune system. Lymphoid neoplasms are the most commonly reported tumours in snakes beside haematopoietic neoplasms. In retrospective studies, it seems to be most common in vipers, particularly cobras and urutus. Lymphoid tumours in reptiles are often multicentric and have blast morphology (only occasionally plasmacytoid or histiocytic morphology). The oral manifestations of lymphomas are often admixed with inflammation, like in the described ball python. Malignant lymphomas or lymphosarcomas are frequently accompanied by leukaemia and metastases. In this case, it was not possible to exclude a metastasis as the owner refused a complete necropsy of the python, but palpation and radiography gave no hint of this.

For therapy of cancers, there are only a few oncologic strategies reported in reptiles. Besides the surgical removal of neoplastic material, corticosteroids (prednisolone) and cytostatics (cyclophosphamide, chlorambucil, melphalan or doxorubicin) have been used occasionally for chemotherapy. The use of chemotherapeutics is controversial because their effectiveness and their tolerance differ a lot between species and between individuals.

Further reading

Catao-Dias, J.L., Nichols, D.K., 1999. Neoplasia in snakes at the National Zoological Park, Washington, DC (1978–1997). J. Comp. Pathol. 120, 89–95.

Fry, F.L., 1994. Diagnosis and surgical treatment of reptilian neoplasms with a compilation of cases 1966–1993. In Vivo 8, 885–892.

Maulden, G.N., Done, L.B., 2006. Oncology. In: Mader, D.R. (Ed.), Reptile Medicine and Surgery, second ed. Saunders Elsevier, St Louis, pp. 299–322.

Ramsay, E.C., Munson, L., Lowenstin, L., et al., 1996. A retrospective study of neoplasia in a collection of captive snakes. J. Zoo Wildl. Med. 27, 28–34.

Sykes, J.M., Trupkievicz, J.G., 2006. Reptile neoplasia at the Philadelphia Zoological Garden 1990–2002. J. Zoo Wildl. Med. 37 (1), 11–19.

Case 3.2 *J-M. Hatt*

Clinical history

A female Pearl island boa (*Boa constrictor sabogae*) weighing 1220 g was presented with the clinical signs of depression and intermittent anorexia. Due to the anorexia, the owner observed a reduced weight and growth. Since the animal was wild-caught, the exact age was unknown.

The animal had lived with the owner for 6 months. It was kept in a terrarium with temperatures of 28–34 °C during the day and 22–26 °C during the night. Relative humidity was 70–85%. The diet consisted of dead mice.

Clinical examination

On presentation, the animal was alert and had a body condition of 2/5. Adspection and palpation did not reveal any abnormal clinical signs.

Radiography (Fig. 3.4a, b)

1. What is your interpretation of the radiographic image in Fig. 3.4a, b?

Clinical diagnosis laboratory

The results of the clinical diagnosis laboratory assays are shown in Tables 3.2 and 3.3.

RBC and WBC morphology

- Some anisocytosis in the RBC

Faecal examination

- Ova of *Strongyloides* spp. and *Rhabdias* spp.

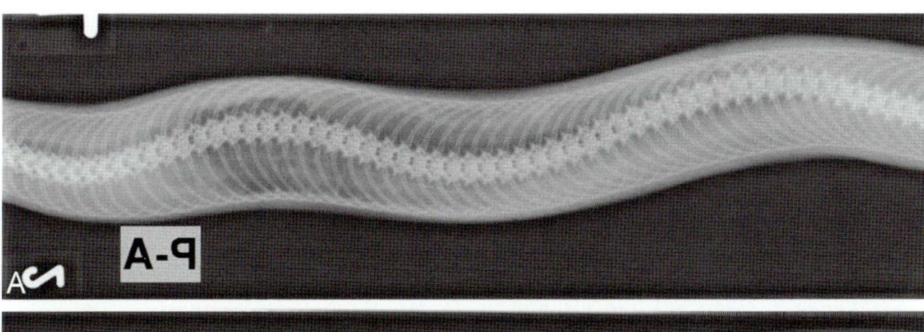

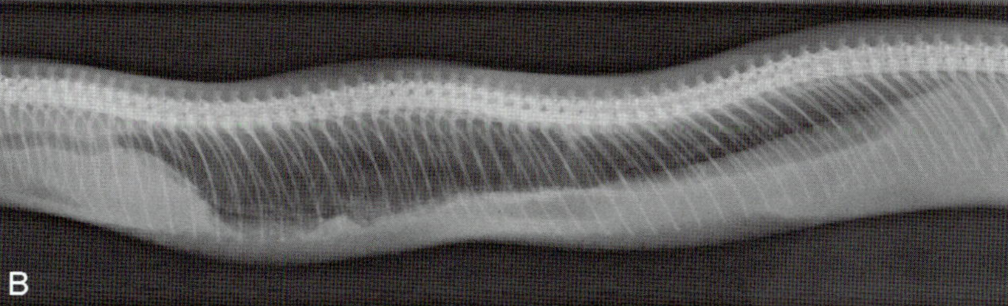

Fig. 3.4 (a) Dorsoventral radiographic image of the lung of the boa constrictor; (b) latero-lateral radiographic image of the lung of the boa constrictor.

Table 3.2 Haematology values of the boa constrictor

Parameters	Results (absolute)	Results (%)	Reference values
Hb (g/dl)	8.0		9.0±2.1
Hct (l/l)	0.28		0.28±0.06
Erythrocytes (×10⁶/µl)	0.7		0.7±0.39
MCHC (g/dl)	29		32±3.6
MCH (pg)	111		134±40.5
MCV (fl)	389		392±116.8
WBC (×10⁹/l)	23.0		8.0±4.8
Heterophils (×10⁹/l)	6.2	27.0	2.4±1.95
Azurophils (×10⁹/l)	7.3	31.5	1.6±1.39
Lymphocytes (×10⁹/l)	8.5	37.0	3.7±3.20
Monocytes (×10⁹/l)	0.2	1.0	0.7±1.12
Eosinophils (×10⁹/l)	0.7	3.0	0.2±0.26
Basophils (×10⁹/l)	0.1	0.5	0.4±0.46

Table 3.3 Blood chemistry values of the boa constrictor

Analysis	Results	Reference values
Calcium (mmol/l)	3.8	4.0±0.90
GOT (U/l)	3	32±45
Phosphorus (mmol/l)	0.82	1.5±0.65
Total protein (g/l)	84	70±13
Uric acid (µmol/l)	275	292±220

Reference values: ISIS Physiological Reference Values, 2002.

Q *2. What is your interpretation of the haematology and blood chemistry values shown in Tables 3.2 and 3.3, and the faecal examination findings?*

Results

- Radiography revealed a worm-like structure in the lung, lung consistency was increased and the margins were not clearly defined. The intrapulmonary bronchus was visible
- Haematology revealed a moderate leucocytosis, with azurophilia and heterophilia
- Parasitology indicated an infestation with nematodes

Please evaluate the clinical history, Fig. 3.4a, b and the results of the physical examination and clinical laboratory diagnostic tests.

 *3. List your differential diagnoses.*

Differential diagnoses

- Endoparasitosis larva migrans of *Strongyloides* spp. or *Rhabdias* spp. in the lung
- Pentastomid infestation
- Pneumonia of bacterial or viral origin
- Foreign body in the respiratory tract

 *4. What would be your next diagnostic steps to ascertain the diagnosis?*

Further diagnostic steps

- Endoscopic examination of the lung
- Computed tomography of the lung
- Magnetic resonance imaging of the lung

In this case, endoscopic examination of the right lung was chosen. General anaesthesia was induced with butorphanol (1 mg/kg IM) followed by propofol (5 mg/kg IV), subsequently the animal was intubated and anaesthesia was maintained with isoflurane and intermittent positive pressure ventilation.

The images obtained are shown in Figs 3.5 and 3.6.

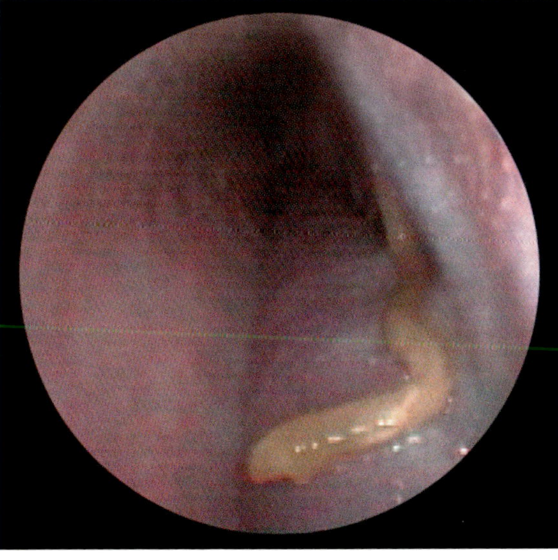

Fig. 3.5 Endoscopy of the right lung of the boa constrictor revealing a worm-like structure which was diagnosed as pentastomid.

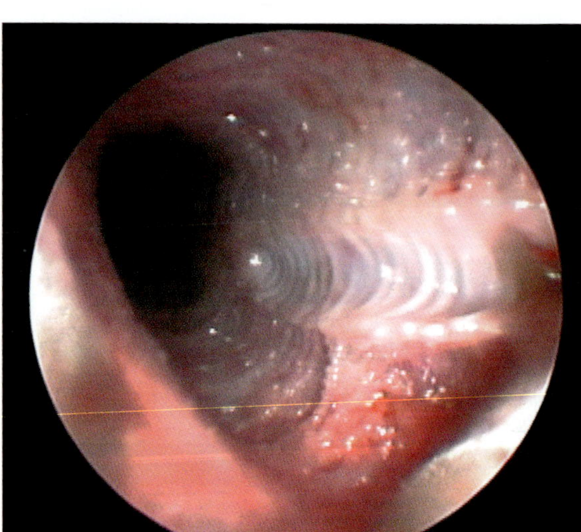

Fig. 3.6 Endoscopy of the right lung of the boa constrictor revealing moderate haemorrhagic inflammation. On the right side, the intrapulmonary bronchus can be recognized.

5. What would be your therapeutic approach?

Therapy (Table 3.4)

Table 3.4 Therapy

Fenbendazole	50 mg/kg PO SID × 5 days
Removal of pentastomidae	Minimally invasive by endoscopy, removal of 4 pentastomids
Fluids	Lactated Ringer's solution 20 ml/kg SC
Enrofloxacin	10 mg/kg IM SID × 5 days post-surgery

Final diagnosis

- Endoparasitosis with intestinal infestation with *Rhabdias* spp. and *Strongyloides* spp. and pulmonary infestation with Pentastomidae (*Porocephalus clavatus*)

Discussion

Pentastomidae are well-known parasites of reptiles, especially snakes. Typically, these parasites invade the lungs. The disease can be asymptomatic, but respiratory signs and even death have been noted. In this case, leucocytosis with azurophilia was observed. Increase of azurophils in reptiles is seen as a sign of inflammation, especially granulomatous inflammation. In the present case, significant inflammation was noted in the lung. Other clinical laboratory findings may include anaemia, eosinophilia and hypoproteinaemia.

Penstostomids usually have an indirect life cycle, but direct life cycles have also been found in certain species. Intermediate hosts typically include mammals such as rodents or primates. The latter also indicates a possible zoonotic risk of pentastomids. Due to the importance of an intermediate host, pentastomids are more frequently found in wild-caught reptiles, than in captive-bred animals. Treatment is controversial. The use of antiparasitic drugs, such as avermectins or levamisole, may kill the parasites. The risk that dead parasites in the lung may cause inflammation or obstruction of the trachea cannot be neglected. In the present case, endoscopic exploration of the right lung with mechanical removal of the parasites was successfully used. Postoperatively, the snake developed well and no complications were observed. The choice to investigate the right lung only was made on the basis that most snakes and boids, in particular, have a well-developed right lung, whereas the left lung is vestigial.

Further reading

Chinnadurai, S., DeVoe, R., 2009. Selected infectious diseases of reptiles. Vet. Clin. North Am. Exot. Anim. Pract. 12, 583–596.

Foldenauer, U., Pantchev, N., Simova-Curd, S., et al., 2008. Pentastomidenbefall bei Abgottschlangen (*Boa constrictor*). Diagnostik und endoskopische Parasitenentfernung. Tierärztliche Praxis 36, 443–449.

Greiner, E., Mader, D.R., 2006. Parasitology. In: Mader, D.R. (Ed.), Reptile Medicine and Surgery. Saunders Elsevier, St Louis, pp. 360–364.

Jacobsen, E., 2007. Parasites and parasitic diseases of reptiles. In: Jacobsen, E. (Ed.), Infectious Diseases and Pathology of Reptiles. Taylor & Francis Group, Boca Raton, pp. 590–593.

Schumacher, J., 2003. Reptile respiratory medicine. Vet. Clin. North Am. Exot. Anim. Pract. 6, 213–231.

Case 3.3 *D. Kaiser*

Clinical history

A 3-year-old female garter snake (*Thamnophis* spp.) was presented with the following clinical signs of 7 days' duration:

- Inappetence
- Tissue protruding from the cloaca.

The snake had changed ownership recently due to the inability of the previous owner to provide adequate husbandry. The snake had been treated with metronidazole for the past 7 days without improving.

Clinical examination

On presentation, the snake was in bad general condition (Figs 3.7 and 3.8). A moveable bulge cranial to the cloaca was palpable. A bluish tissue with a central lumen and a peripheral blind sac was detected by using a probe.

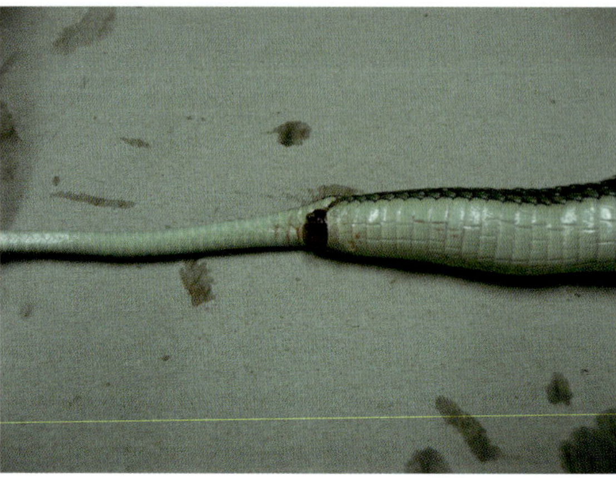

Fig. 3.7 Picture of the cloacal region of the snake.

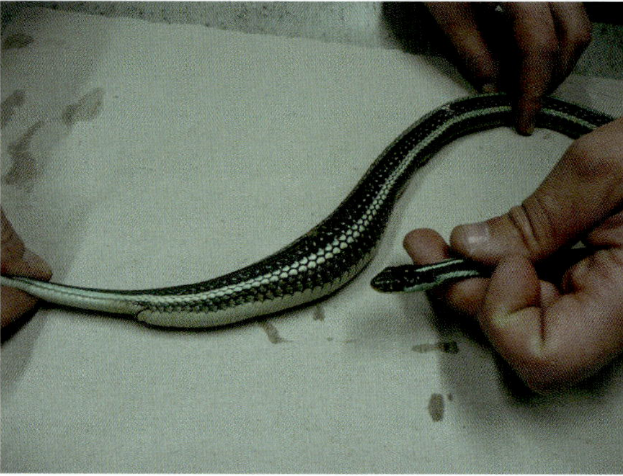

Fig. 3.8 Picture of the bulge in the caudal quarter of the garter snake.

Q *1. What is your interpretation of the clinical examination and Figs 3.7 and 3.8?*

- Cloacal prolapse or intestinal prolapse?

Q *2. What are your differential diagnoses? List your diagnostic plan.*

Differential diagnoses

- Egg retention
- Faecolith
- Intestinal foreign body
- Intussusception
- Endoparasitism

Clinical diagnosis examination

- Radiography
- Ultrasonography
- Faecal flotation and wet smear

Results

- Radiography showed a soft tissue dense swelling
- Faecal examination showed negative result for the presence of endoparasites in native smear preparations and flotation

Therapy

It was decided to lavage the cloaca and the colon through the rectum with lubricant solution and massage the bulge caudally. A large amount of kidney beans were passed out (Fig. 3.9) but the massage induced intestinal prolapse (Fig. 3.10). This was corrected by placing transverse cloacal sutures (Fig. 3.11, Table. 3.5).

Final diagnosis

- Constipation with foreign bodies

Discussion

Prolapse of the cloaca is generally the result of tenesmus. Constipation, bacterial enteritis and parasitic enteritis have been implicated. Constipation may be the result of environmental factors, such as excessively small enclosures inhibiting sufficient

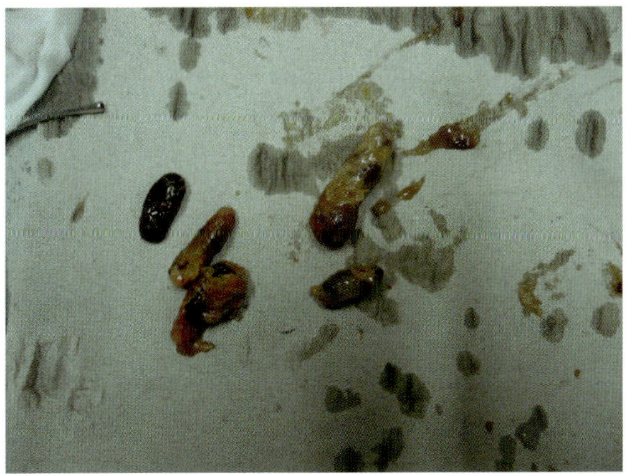

Fig. 3.9 Kidney beans were retrieved out of the intestines.

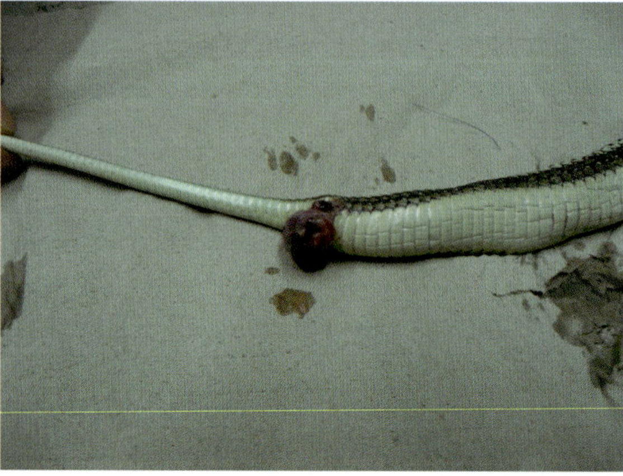

Fig. 3.10 Prolapsed intestine.

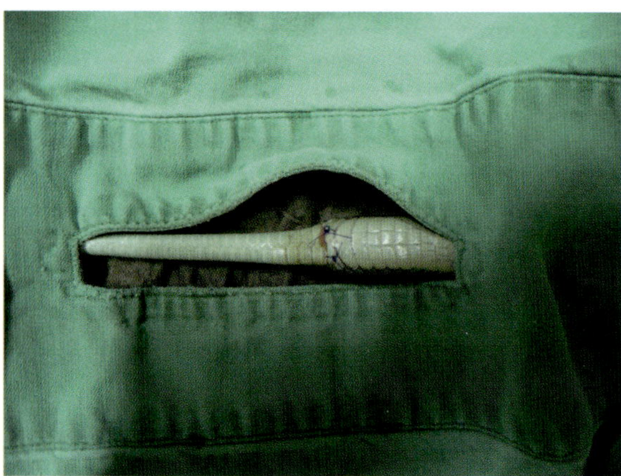

Fig. 3.11 Transverse cloacal sutures.

Table 3.5 Therapy

Enrofloxacin 2.5%	5–10 mg/kg IM SID for 10 days
Meloxicam	0.1–0.2 mg/kg SID SC

exercise to stimulate normal defecation. Determination of the cause of tenesmus and treatment of this, in conjunction with management of the prolapse, are important. In the acute phase, the prolapsed tissue is easily reduced and can be managed with either purse-string or transverse cloacal sutures. On questioning, the owner did not know the origin of the kidney beans. The snake was re-examined 6 weeks after surgery for suture removal and was presented in good health.

Further reading

Gabrisch, K., Zwart, P., Schlangen, P., 2008. In: Zwart, P., Sassenburg, L. (Eds.), Krankheiten der Heimtiere, seventh ed. Schlütersche Verlagsgesellschaft GmbH & Co, Hannover, pp. 739–794.

Girling, S.J., Raiti, P., 2004. BSAVA Manual of Reptiles, second ed. British Small Animal Veterinary Association, Gloucester, pp. 210–229.

Mader, D.R., 2006. Reptile Medicine and Surgery, second ed. Saunders Elsevier, St Louis, pp. 675–682, 751–755.

Case 3.4 *D. Kaiser*

Clinical history

A 6-year-old female African egg-eating snake (*Dasypeltis medici*) weighing 110 g was presented with the following clinical signs:

- Inappetence
- Opisthotonus.

Clinical examination

On presentation, the snake had a good body condition. It behaved motionless even when stimulated to move. The righting reflex was absent (Fig. 3.12). The palpation of the body was normal.

 ***1. What are your differential diagnoses? List your diagnostic plan.***

Differential diagnoses

- Myelitis (bacterial or viral)
- Inclusion body disease (IBD)

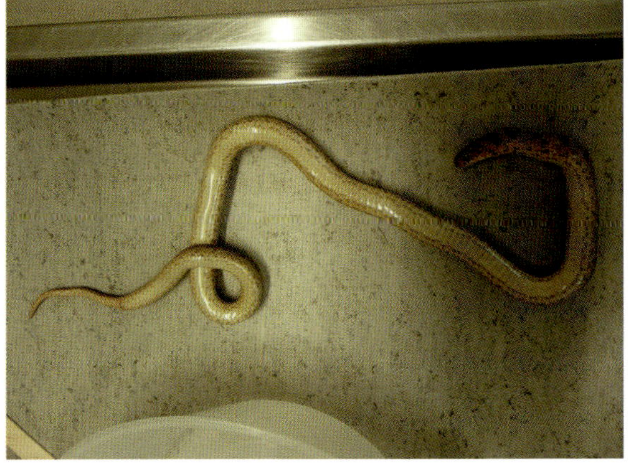

Fig. 3.12 Absent righting reflex of the egg-eating snake.

- ➤ Hypoglycaemia
- ➤ Systemic disease (hepatoencephalopathy)
- ➤ Death feigning
- ➤ Trance-like state

Clinical diagnosis laboratory

The results of the clinical diagnosis laboratory assays were as follows:

- Paramyxovirus-antibody titre was negative
- In blood smears no intracytoplasmic inclusion bodies were found, which cannot exclude IBD (retrovirus).

The size of the snake was a limiting factor for further investigation. Blood collection was done by heart punction and the blood volume was so small that careful consideration was given to the type of diagnostic test to choose. Also biopsies of the liver and pancreas to examine IBD or cerebrospinal fluid analysis could not be made due to the size. Radiographs were assumed not to bring any further information. Ultrasonography, computed tomography and magnetic resonance imaging were not considered useful or practical.

2. List your therapeutic strategy.

Therapy (Table 3.6)

Table 3.6 Therapy

Enrofloxacin 2.5%	5–10 mg/kg IM SID for 10 days
Serumproteins	Bioserin® (Paraimmunityinducer) 1 ml/kg TID PO for 7 days
Vitamin B-complex	Thiamine 30 mg/kg IM once
Fluids	10–25 ml/kg; 1/3 Ringer's lactate + 1/3 0.9% NaCl solution + 1/3 Glc 5%

Within 5 days the snake's general health got worse and so the decision was taken to euthanase it and to perform a thorough post-mortem examination.

Post-mortem findings

Histology

- ➤ Liver: a single histiocytic granuloma. There was a mild diffuse congestion. An infiltration of heterophil granulocytes in the sinusoids was found. Ziehl-Neelsen staining showed acid-fast organisms in the middle of the granuloma
- ➤ Heart: mild degeneration of the myocytes
- ➤ Brain: mild gliosis and vacuolization of the white and grey brain substance (demyelination)

Microbiology

➤ Bacteriological examination of the coelomic cavity was sterile

Summary: the main lesion was vacuolar degeneration in the brain. It appears to be related to demyelination which is related to a non-infectious cause. Histological examination showed that there were no inclusion bodies in the organs and therefore it is not IBD. In addition, the single, acid-fast positive granuloma indicates a mycobacterial infection.

 *3. What are your differential diagnoses now?*

Final diagnosis

➤ Hepatic encephalopathy
➤ Mycobacteriosis

Discussion

Hepatic encephalopathy may cause CNS signs in reptiles, such as convulsions. Chronic liver disease is associated with weakness, weight loss and anorexia.

Further reading

Mader, D.R., 2006. Reptile Medicine and Surgery, second ed. Saunders Elsevier, St Louis, pp. 239–250, 675–682, 852–887.

Gabrisch, K., Zwart, P., Schlangen, P., 2008. In: Zwart, P., Sassenburg, L. (Eds.), Krankheiten der Heimtiere, seventh ed. Schlütersche Verlagsgesellschaft GmbH & Co, Hannover, pp. 739–794.

Girling, S.J., Raiti, P., 2004. BSAVA Manual of Reptiles, second ed. British Small Animal Veterinary Association, Gloucester, pp. 273–288.

Case 3.5 *A. Montesinos*

Clinical history

A 10-year-old female green iguana (*Iguana iguana*) weighing 2800 g was presented with the following clinical signs of one week's duration:

- Anorexia
- Swollen abdomen
- Lack of production of stools.

The iguana was purchased when it was a hatchling and was kept in a large terrarium with adequate temperature gradient and adequate supplement of UV light. The diet of the lizard was based on fresh vegetables, commercial reptile food and insects.

Physical examination

On presentation, the iguana had a body condition of 2/5 and had thick saliva in the mouth and sunken eyes. Dehydration of 8% was estimated. Abdominal and rectal palpation showed ascites, gas-filled intestines and normal size kidneys.

Clinical diagnosis examination

Whole body radiographs were taken and blood samples were collected for haematology, blood chemistry and plasma protein electrophoresis.

Radiology (Fig. 3.13a, b)

1. What is your interpretation of the radiographs of Fig. 3.13a, b?

Clinical diagnosis laboratory examination

The results of the clinical diagnosis laboratory assays are shown in Tables 3.7–3.9.

RBC, WBC and thrombocyte morphology

- Toxic heterophils +++, activated monocytes +++, activated lymphocytes +++
- Irregular population of red blood cells

2. What is your interpretation of the haematology, blood chemistry, and protein electrophoresis values shown in Tables 3.7–3.9?

Results

- Radiographic findings included increased radiodensity on the whole abdomen, compatible with the presence of fluid in the coelom
- Haematology analysis showed low RBC and low Hct, high WBC with slight toxic heterophilia
- Blood chemistry analysis showed elevated bile acids, GGT and total proteins. There was also low sodium
- Plasma protein electrophoresis showed low total protein and low albumin and increased A:G ratio

Please evaluate the clinical history, Fig. 3.13a, b, the results of the physical examination and clinical diagnostic tests.

3. List your differential diagnoses.

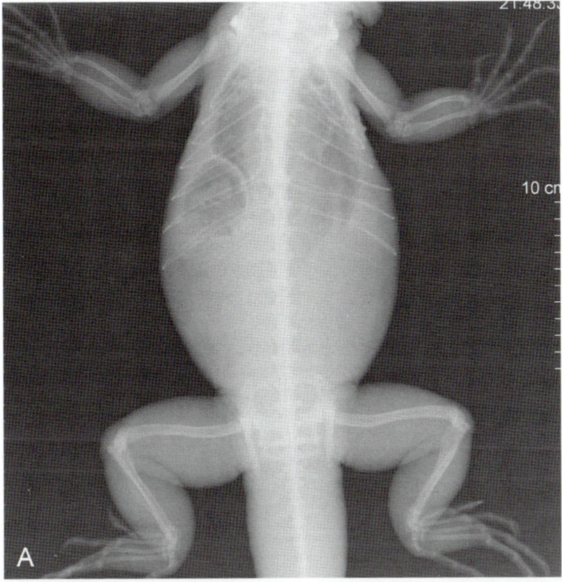

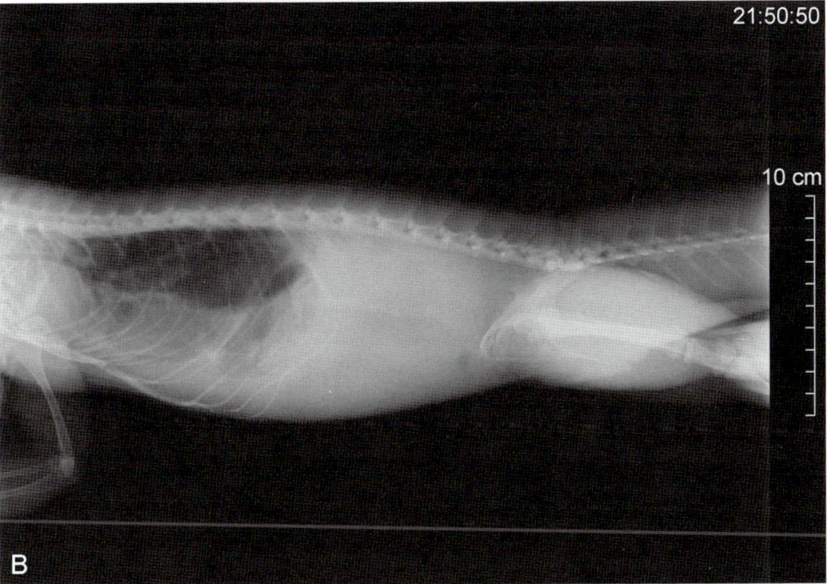

Fig. 3.13 (a) Ventrodorsal survey radiograph of a 10-year-old iguana with abdominal distension; (b) lateral survey radiograph of a 10-year-old iguana with abdominal distension.

Table 3.7 Haematology values of the green iguana

Parameters	Results (absolute)	Results (%)	Reference values
RBC ($\times10^{12}$/l)	0.76		1–1.9
Hb (g/dl)	4.2		6–10
Hct (l/l)	0.23	23	0.25–0.38
MCV (fl)	302		165–305
MCH (pg)	55.2		48–78
MCHC (g/dl)	18.2		20–38
WBC ($\times10^{9}$/l)	20		3–10
Heterophils ($\times10^{9}$/l)	12.6	63	30–52%
Lymphocytes ($\times10^{9}$/l)	2.6	13	40–55 %
Azurophils ($\times10^{9}$/l)	4	20	0–3 %
Eosinophils ($\times10^{9}$/l)	0	0	0–2 %
Basophils ($\times10^{9}$/l)	0.8	4	0–5 %
Monocytes ($\times10^{9}$/l)l	0	0	0–1%

Table 3.8 Blood chemistry values of the green iguana

Analysis	Results	Reference values
Albumin (g/l)	20	21–28
ALKP (U/l)	192.8	50–290
Bile acids (μmol/l)	43.1	2–17
Calcium (mg/dl)	11.4	8.8–14
Cholesterol (mg/dl)	99	104–333
CK (U/l)	399	200–700
GGT (U/l)	7	<0.1
GOT (U/l)	65	5–52
Glucose (mg/dl)	189	169–288
Phosphorus (mg/dl)	2.3	3–5
Potassium (mmol/l)	2.7	2–5
Sodium (mmol/l)	142	158–183
Total protein (g/l)	74	50–78
Triglycerides (mg/dl)	47	53–691
Uric acid (mg/dl)	0.8	2–10

Table 3.9 Plasma protein electrophoresis of the green iguana

Parameters	Fractions (%)	Concentration (g/l)
Total protein	100	74
Pre-albumin	6.62	4.9
Albumin	20.4	15.1
Alpha 1 globulins	0.02	2
Alpha 2 globulins	1.62	12
Beta globulins	18.91	14
Gamma globulins	35.13	26
A:G ratio	0.76	0.76

 *4. List your diagnostic strategy and possible diagnostic test.*

Differential diagnoses

- Hepatopathy due to generalized infection
- Cardiac disease with ascites

Diagnostic plan

More imaging techniques were necessary to discover the origin of the fluid-filled abdomen. The owner agreed to make an ultrasound study of the lizard.

Echography (Figs 3.14–3.17)

 *5. What is your interpretation of the ultrasound images of Figs 3.14–3.17?*

Results of the ultrasound study

- There was free fluid in the coelom of the lizard
- Liver was enlarged and echogeneity of this organ is decreased being an image compatible with liver pathologies, such as cirrhosis or fibrosis
- The image and size of the gallbladder is abnormal, being huge and fluid-filled
- The spleen is enlarged and with ultrasound image compatible with active infection
- Normal size and echogenicity of the kidneys

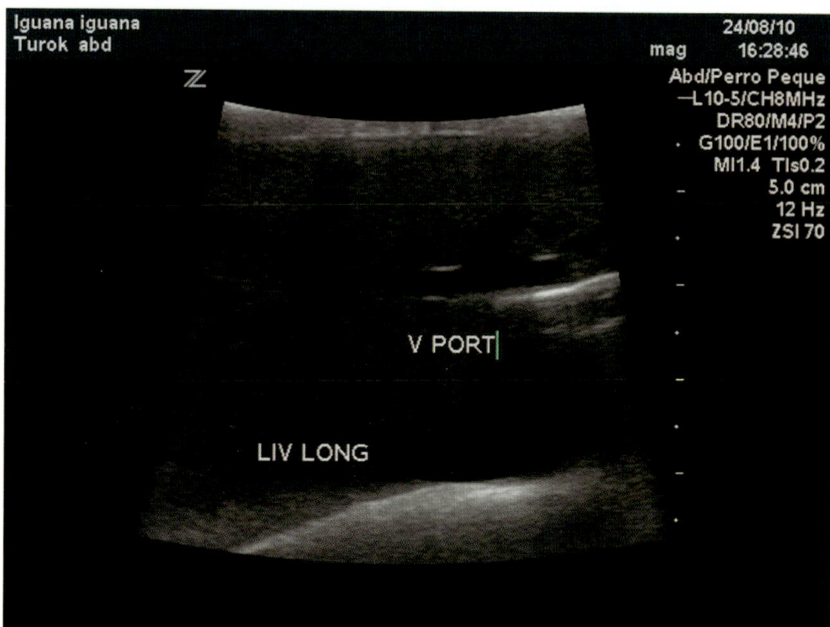

Fig. 3.14 Ultrasound view of the congested liver and portal vein of the green iguana.

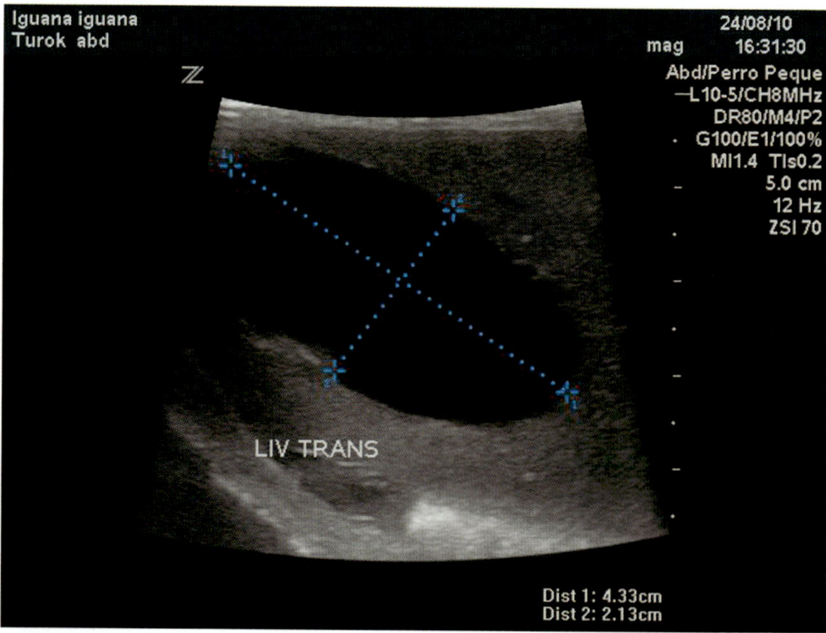

Fig. 3.15 Ultrasound view of the gall bladder of the green iguana notably distended. Measurements of this organ were taken.

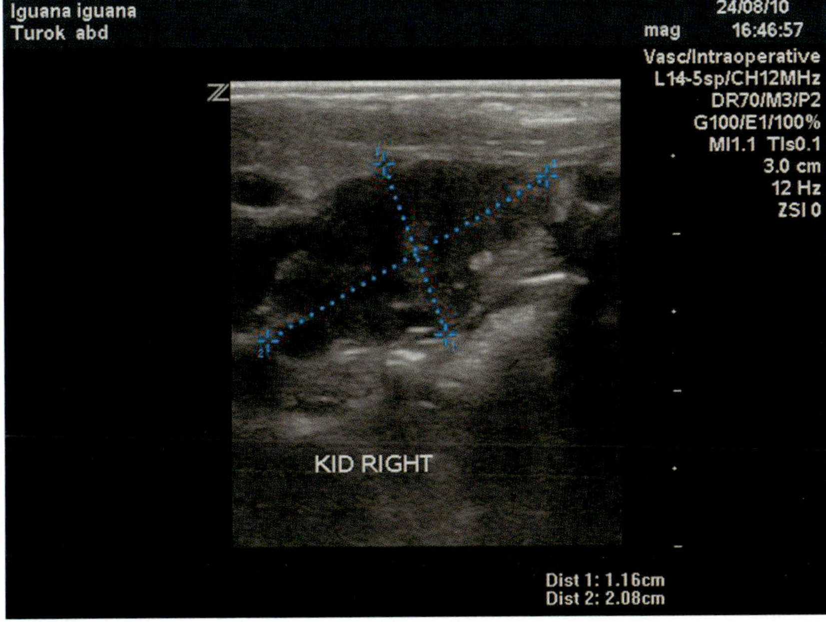

Fig. 3.16 Ultrasound view of the right kidney of the green iguana.

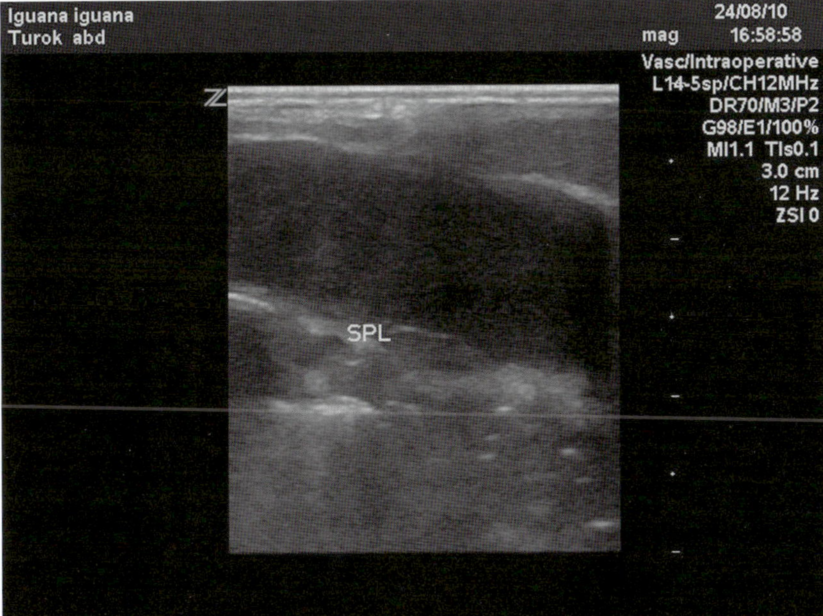

Fig. 3.17 Ultrasound view of the spleen of the iguana.

Therapy

Because the iguana blood results were strongly suggestive of a generalized infection, a treatment with a broad spectrum antibiotic was started and exploratory laparotomy was suggested to the owners to get a definitive diagnosis. After an IO catheter was positioned in the right femur, fluid therapy was started in order to correct the ionic imbalances discovered in the iguana (Table 3.10).

Surgery

The iguana was anaesthetized with an induction dose of alfaxolone 10 mg/kg. Rectal temperature, haemoglobin saturation, blood pressure and end tidal CO_2 concentration were monitored during the surgical procedure (Fig. 3.18). After paramedial incision, 100 ml of ascitic fluid was eliminated from the coelomic cavity (Fig. 3.19). The ascetic fluid contained lower glucose levels than peripheral blood suggesting active infectious peritonitis. Four structures compatible with neoplasia masses or bacterial granulomas were found attached to the intestinal meso and to the mesovary; the four structures were surgically removed (Fig. 3.20). An exceedingly enlarged gallbladder containing 50 ml of bile was found during the exploratory laparotomy (Fig. 3.21). The bile was removed using a 60 ml syringe and total cholecystectomy was carried out (Fig. 3.22). The liver lobe surrounding the gall bladder was resected as well in the same surgical procedure (Fig. 3.23). The laparotomy was closed using routinely described techniques and the lizard recovered from anaesthesia uneventfully.

Biopsy findings

The four structures found in the lizard coelom were bacterial granulomas containing coccobacilli. The liver had chronic advanced cirrhosis, severe biliary hyperplasia and moderate multifocal fibrosis and moderate lipidosis and was an air sac carcinoma. Histopathology of the gall bladder showed severe diffuse necrosis of the mucosal layer, oedema and perilesional thrombosis.

Final diagnosis

- Coelom bacterial granulomas possibly from intestinal origin
- Ascendant gall bladder infection with necrosis of the mucosal layer
- Liver cirrhosis, liver fibrosis and liver lipidosis

Table 3.10 Therapy

Ceftazidime 100 mg/ml	200 mg/kg IM one dose every 2 days, 3 weeks
Butorphanol 10 mg/ml	1 mg/kg IM SID 1 week
Fluids	Saline plus KCl 2 ml/kg/day IO IRC

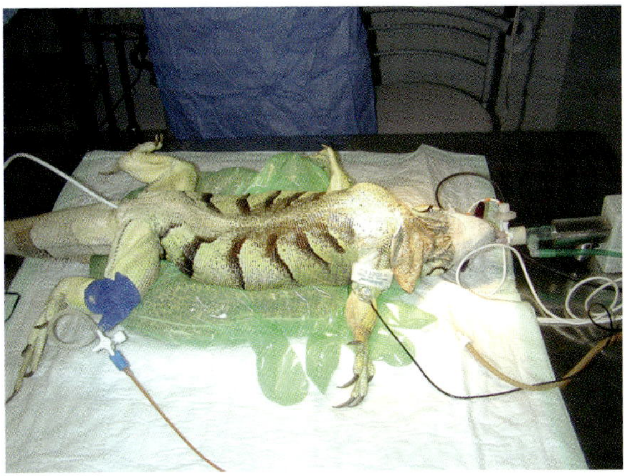

Fig. 3.18 View of the iguana totally monitored prior to the surgical laparotomy. Blood pressure, haemoglobin saturation, rectal temperature and end tidal CO_2 were monitored during the surgical procedure.

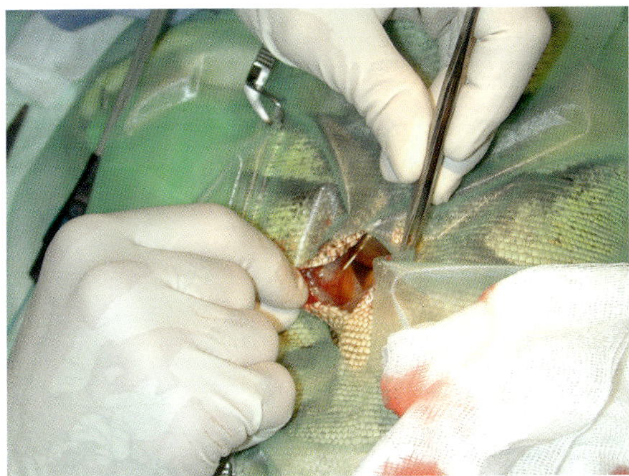

Fig. 3.19 More than 100 ml of free fluid was removed from the coelomic cavity of the green iguana.

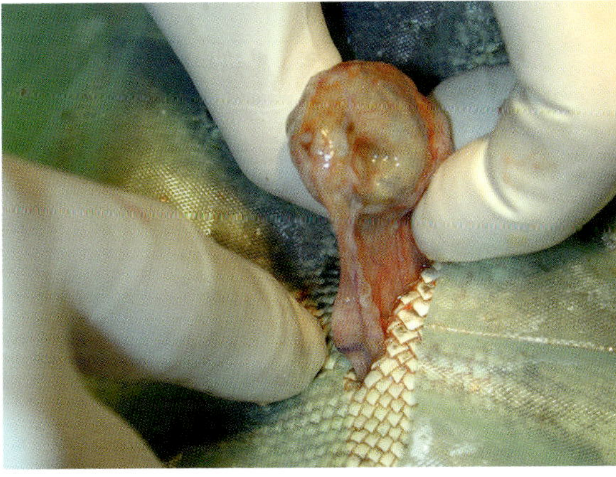

Fig. 3.20 Four structures resembling neoplasia or bacterial granulomas were found attached to the intestine and ovarian mesos. The four structures were removed during the surgery and submitted for histopathological analysis.

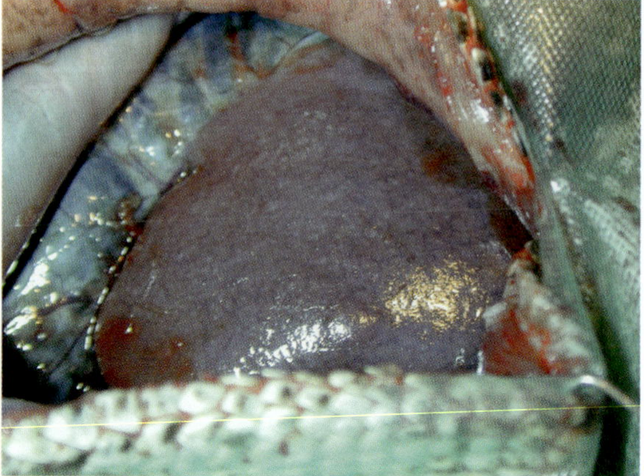

Fig. 3.21 Intraoperative view of the liver. The organ was pale and firm. On the left part of the image the gall bladder appears distended.

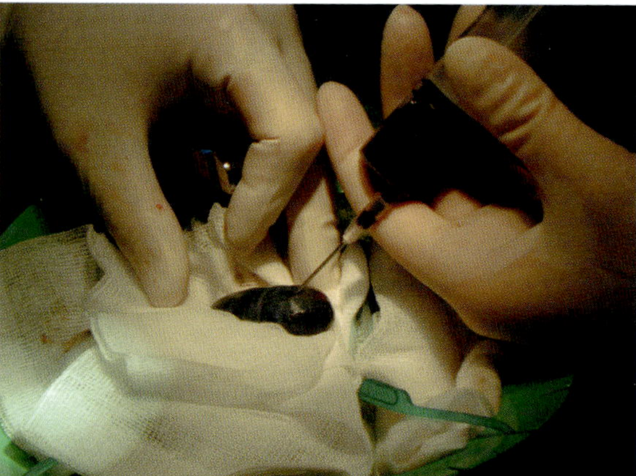

Fig. 3.22 More than 50 ml of bile were extracted from the gall bladder using a 60 ml syringe.

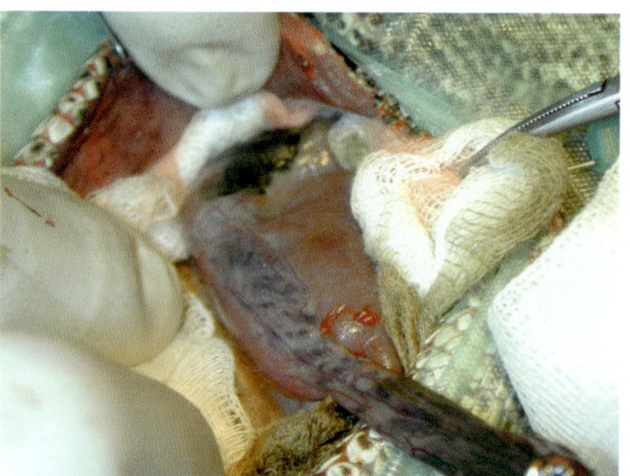

Fig. 3.23 The empty gall bladder and the attached liver lobe were removed surgically using standard procedures.

Follow up

After 4 days of hospitalization, the iguana was sent home with antibiotic treatment for 2 weeks. Fourteen days after surgery the iguana was rechecked, including physical examination, blood analysis and ultrasound exam. There was still a raised WBC count and a small volume of intracoelomic fluid but the health status of the lizard was much improved. Posterior revaluation of the iguana 45 days and 3 months after surgery showed decreasing numbers of WBC to normality and decreased intracoelomic fluid. Bile acids were normal 2 weeks after surgery.

Discussion

Liver disease in iguanas has rarely been described in reptilian literature. Description of necropsies and specific infectious diseases such as viral infections have been reported but not from a practitioner's point of view. This case describes the approach to liver disease in this iguana from a logical sequence of clinical procedures followed for other species. The author has not found any other report about cholecystectomy and liver lobe resection for green iguana in the scientific literature.

Further reading

Harr, K.E., Allegan, R., Dennos, P.M., et al., 2001. Morphologic and cytochemical characteristics of blood cells and haematological and biochemical referents ranges in green iguanas (*Iguana iguana*). J. Am. Vet. Med. Assoc. 218 (6), 915–921.

Hernandez-Divers, S.J., 2005. Diagnostic techniques. In: Mader, D.R. (Ed.), Reptile Medicine and Surgery, second ed. Saunders Elsevier, St Louis, pp. 490–532.

Hernandez-Divers, S.J., Cooper, J.E., 2005. Hepatic lipidosis. In: Mader, D.R. (Ed.), Reptile Medicine and Surgery, second ed. Saunders Elsevier, St Louis, pp. 806–813.

Hernandez-Divers, S.J., 2006. Preliminary evaluation of pre-and prandial 3a-hydroxy bile acids in the green iguana *Iguana iguana*. J.Herp. Med. Surg. 16 (4), 106–110.

Holland, M.F., Hernandez-Divers, S., Paul, F.M., 2008. Ultrasonographic appearance of the coelomic cavity in healthy green iguanas. J. Am. Vet. Med. Assoc. 233 (4), 590–596.

Wagner, R.A., Wetzel, R., 1999. Tissue and plasma enzyme activities in juvenile green iguanas (*Iguana iguana*). Am. J. Vet. Res. 60 (2), 201 203.

Case 3.6 *J-M. Hatt*

Clinical history

A 4-year-old, female green iguana (*Iguana iguana*) weighing 1900 g was presented with the clinical sign of anorexia.

The animal had lived for two years with the owner and was kept in a vivarium with five adult animals. The diet consisted of a mixture of leafy green vegetables and fruits. The iguana had undergone an elective ovariohysterectomy a year earlier and had since shown intermittent phases of anorexia, which were treated with antibiotics and ranitidine (histamine H2-receptor antagonist).

Clinical examination

On presentation, the animal was alert and had a body condition of 3/5. Survey radiographs were carried out and blood samples were collected for haematology and blood chemistry. A faecal sample was collected to examine for the presence of endoparasites.

Radiology (Fig. 3.24)

1. What is your interpretation of the radiographs in Fig. 3.24a, b

Clinical diagnosis laboratory

The results of the clinical diagnosis laboratory assays are shown in Tables 3.11 and 3.12.

RBC and WBC morphology

- Nothing abnormal detected

2. What is your interpretation of the haematology and blood chemistry values shown in Tables 3.11 and 3.12?

Results

- Faecal examination showed negative result for the presence of endoparasites
- Radiographic findings included generalized loss of detail in the coelomic cavity most likely due to fluid accumulation. Bone density appeared

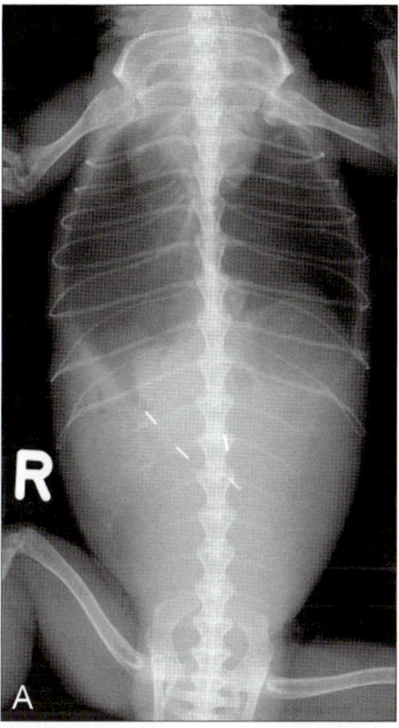

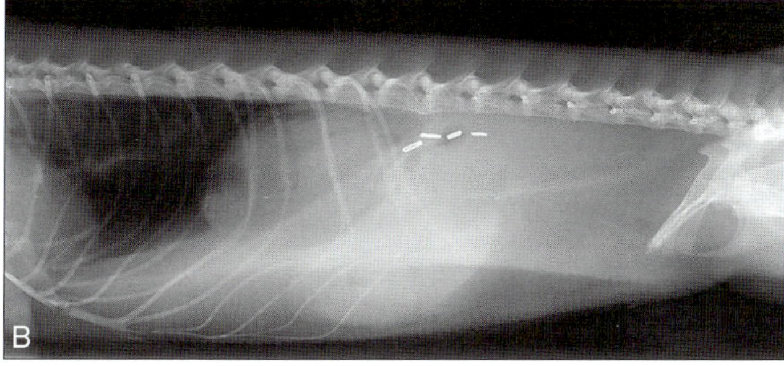

Fig. 3.24 (a) Dorsoventral survey radiograph of the green iguana; (b) lateral survey radiograph of the green iguana.

normal due to well-delineated cortices. Four metal dense structures in the mid-dorsal coelom were identified as the staples of the ovariohysterectomy.

➤ Haematology analyses showed mild anaemia

Please evaluate the clinical history, Fig. 3.24a, b, the results of the physical examination and clinical diagnosis laboratory tests.

Q *3. List your differential diagnoses.*

Q *4. List your further diagnostic investigations.*

Table 3.11 Haematology values of the green iguana

Parameters	Results (absolute)	Results (%)	Reference values
Hb (g/dl)	7.9		9.7±2.2
Hct (l/l)	0.27		0.4±0.07
MCHC (g/dl)	29		28.2±0.53
WBC (×10^9/l)	6.9		11.1±6.53
Heterophils (×10^9/l)	5.3	78	4.6±3.34
Lymphocytes (×10^9/l)	1.3	19	5.1±4.45
Monocytes (×10^9/l)	0.1	2	0.5±0.53
Azurophils (×10^9/l)	0.1	2	1.1±0.88
Basophils (×10^9/l)	0.03	0.5	0.4±0.43

Table 3.12 Blood chemistry values of the green iguana

Analysis	Results	Reference values
Bile acids (μmol/l)	25	<60
Calcium (mmol/l)	3.3	3.1±0.65
Creatine kinase (U/l)	305	1947±2058
GOT (U/l)	37	46±58
Phosphorus (mmol/l)	1.05	2.4±1.20
Total protein (g/l)	62	62±12
Uric acid (μmol/l)	108	150±70

Reference values for bile acids: Divers SJ (2000) Reptilian liver and gastrointestinal testing. In: Fudge AM, ed. Laboratory Medicine Avian and Exotic Pets, WB Saunders Co, Philadelphia, pp. 205–209; all other values ISIS Physiological Reference Values, 2002.

Differential diagnoses

- Coelomitis
- Ascites
- Neoplasia

Further diagnostic investigations

- Ultrasonography
- Coelioscopy
- Coelomic fluid collection (with cytology and microbiology, including antibiotic resistance testing)

In the ultrasound examination, hyperechogenic coelomic fluid was seen and 2 ml were collected (Table 3.13). The liver appeared of homogeneous consistency.

Cytology of coelomic fluid (Figs 3.25 and 3.26)

Microbiology

The haemolytic *Escherichia coli* found in the coelomic fluid were tested for antibiotic resistance (Table 3.14).

5. What is your interpretation of the results of the additional testing and what is the most likely diagnosis?

Table 3.13 Coelomic fluid values

Analysis	Results
Transparency	Clear
Colour	Yellow-orange
Cells	300/µl
Specific gravity	1032N
Protein	48 g/l

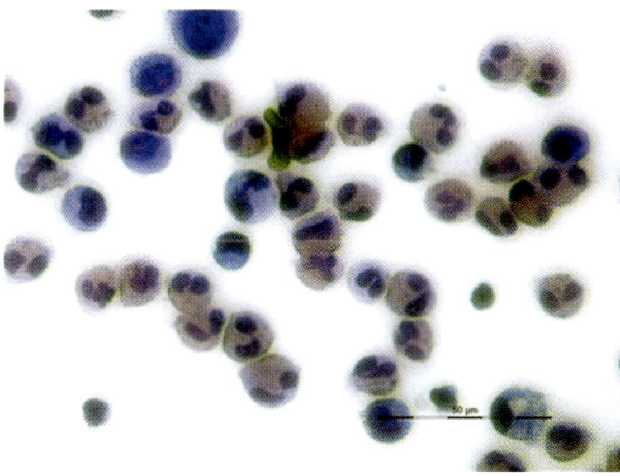

Fig. 3.25 Cytology of coelomic fluid from the green iguana (Diff Quik stain) 400x.

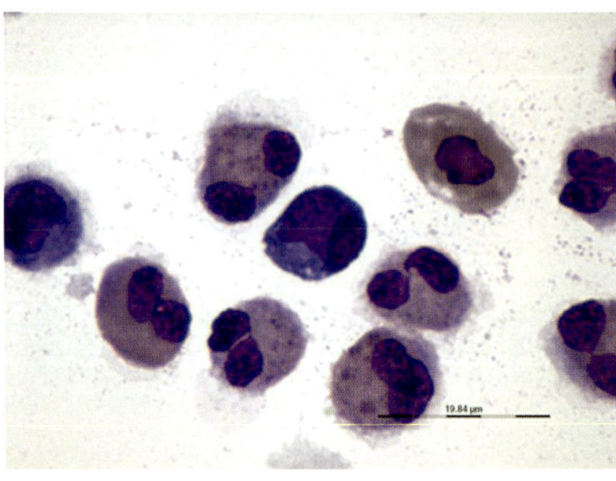

Fig. 3.26 Cytology of coelomic fluid from the green iguana (Diff Quik stain) 1000×.

Table 3.14 Antibiotic resistance testing

Antibiotic	Results
Penicillin	Resistant
Ampicillin	Susceptible
Amoxicillin	Susceptible
Amoxicillin + clavulanic acid	Susceptible
Cephalosporins	Susceptible
Sulphonamide + trimethoprim	Intermediate
Tetracycline	Intermediate
Clindamycin	Resistant
Enrofloxacin	Intermediate
Marbofloxacin	Intermediate
Cefovecine	Intermediate

➤ The coelomic fluid was a modified transudate, with granulocytes and lymphocytes, leading to the diagnosis of coelomitis.

Q *6. How would you treat this condition?*

Therapy (Table 3.15, Figs 3.27 and 3.28)

Final diagnosis

➤ Chronic coelomitis due to *E. coli*

Table 3.15 Therapy

Meloxicam	0.1 mg/kg PO SID × 2 weeks
Enrofloxacin	10 mg/kg PO SID × 2 weeks
Doxycycline	50 mg/kg I COELOM q 72h × 3 weeks
Sucralfat	250 mg/kg PO SID
Cimetidine	4 mg/kg PO SID
Fluids	Saline solution 40 ml/kg SC SID
Intracoelomic catheter placement	16 Ch (5.3 mm × 182 mm) trochar catheter (Mallinckrodt® Medical, Athlone, Ireland) for active drainage and flushing for 10 days
Forced feeding	Mixture Critical Care™ for herbivores and water, 30–40 ml SID

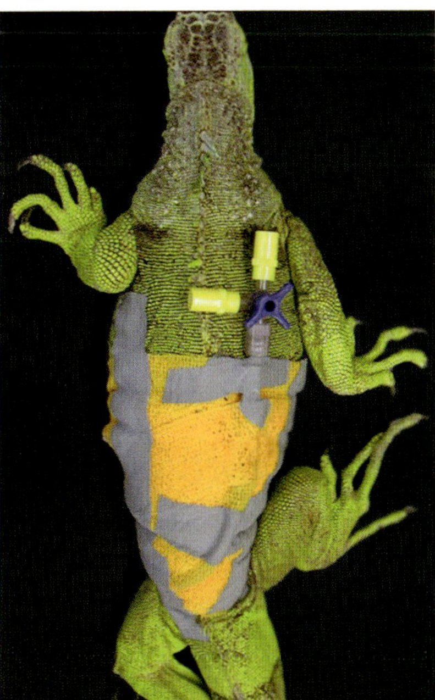

Fig. 3.27 Green iguana with intracoelomic catheter placement.

Discussion

Coelomitis is not uncommon in reptiles and lizards in general. Causes are pre- or postovulatory stasis, yolk coelomitis, sepsis or post-surgical complications. The last is the most likely cause in the present case. The duration of 12 months with intermittent anorexia emphasizes the slow progression of disease that is not surprising in reptiles. For the successful treatment of this case aggressive therapy including regular flushing of the coelomic cavity was needed.

Fig. 3.28 Radiographic image of the green iguana with intracoelomic catheter.

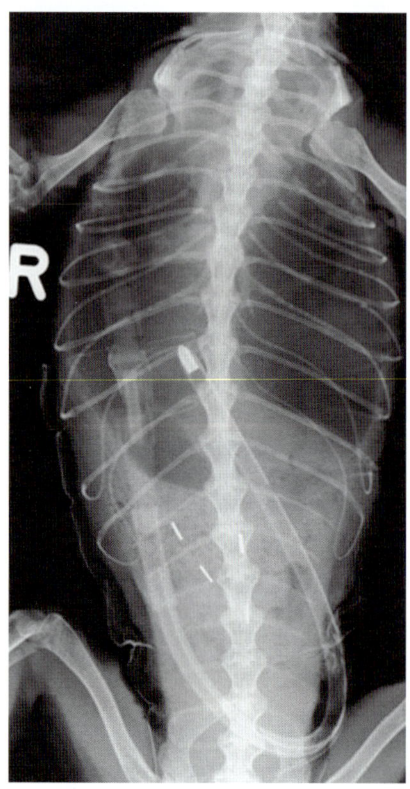

Further reading

Mader, D.R., 2006. Reptile Medicine and Surgery, second ed. Saunders Elsevier, St Louis.

Stacy, B.A., Howard, L., Kinkaid, J., et al., 2008. Yolk coelomitis in Fiji Island banded iguanas (*Brachylophus fasciatus*). J. Zoo Wildl. Med. 39, 161–169.

Zerbe, P., Gull, J., Steinmetz, H.W., et al., 2010. Placement of a permanent coelomic catheter for the treatment of chronic coelomitis in a green iguana (*Iguana iguana*). Proceedings of the International Conference of Diseases of Zoo and Wild Animals 314–315.

Case 3.7 *M. Hochleithner*

Clinical history

Two female leopard geckos (*Eublepharis macularius*) were presented for examination with the history of one individual (gecko no. 3) within a terrarium, in a group of three, having died without any obvious clinical signs 2 days previously. The owner had 26 geckos in total kept in eight different terrariums.

The surviving geckos were both females, but had never laid eggs. The age was unknown. Both geckos had been with the owner for over 1 year. The owner did not keep the body of the dead gecko. However, he requested a medical check up since gecko no. 1 had not been eating well for the past 10 days and the owner wanted to be sure there was no infectious disease involved.

Physical examination

Both geckos were active. Gecko no. 1 weighed 50 g, with a body condition of 4/5. Two hard moveable structures about 8 mm diameter could be palpated within the abdomen. Gecko no. 2 weighed 42 g, with a body condition of 5/5 and no clinical signs.

The hard structures in gecko no. 1 were shown to the owner. He gave the approval for further investigations but within a restricted budget. The owner declined any further investigations for gecko no. 2.

1. What diagnostic tests can and/or should be considered?

Please remember that the primary cause of the consultation was the death of gecko no. 3 in the terrarium.

Clinical diagnosis examination

- Radiology
- Ultrasound
- Computed tomography

Clinical diagnosis laboratory examination

- Faecal examination for parasites including flotation
- PCR for cryptosporidia
- Bacteriological examination including *Salmonella*
- Haematology and blood chemistry

2. What are the advantages and disadvantages of each diagnostic test applicable to this case?

- *Radiology*: good information about mineralization of bones and possible fractures, high density foreign body could be observed. Soft tissue within abdomen might be difficult to identify. Does not provide information concerning any possible infectious agent within the herpetology collection

- *Ultrasound*: good information on soft tissue and organs within abdomen including kidneys if enlarged. Does not provide information concerning any possible infectious agent within the collection. Examiner has to have experience with reptiles!
- *Faecal examination for parasites including flotation*: endoparasites are often a problem within a herpetology collection. However, these are very seldom a matter of major concern. A faecal smear can provide instant results and easily show that there is a hygiene problem in the collection if large numbers of parasitic forms are found. Cryptosporidia can easily be missed. Careful with some species as pseudoparasites can be found from the animals used as food!
- *PCR for Cryptosporidia*: specific information about Cryptosporidia which is often a problem in geckos
- *Bacteriological examination of faeces and maybe a swab from the throat to examine for the presence of* Salmonella: *Salmonella* can often also be found in healthy reptiles. Faeces and throat swabs are difficult to interpret
- *Haematology*: depending on the experience of the laboratory doing the differential, good information can be collected from morphology of blood cells, possible blood parasites, suspected infection and/or anaemia
- *Blood chemistry*: although reference ranges are often not specific and often very broad, information about the individual animal can be obtained, especially about kidney function (Ca, P, uric acid)
- *Computed tomography*: best method to identify the hard structure within the abdomen and also size of kidneys. Expensive and anaesthesia often necessary

3. What would be the next diagnostic step when only one or two procedures are allowed by the owner?

A faecal parasitological examination and ultrasound to identify the structures within the abdomen were recommended.

Results

Parasitology

- *Oxyuris* spp. ++
- *Nyctoderus*: +

4. How would you interpret that result?

Oxyuris spp. is a very common finding. *Nyctoderus* is a ciliated protozoon which is also found in free-living geckos. It is believed to be non-pathogenic. With this examination, Cryptosporidia can be missed easily!

Ultrasound

At least four (in one single image) longitudinal hyperechoic structures (the approximate size was 1.5 cm long and 0.8 cm in diameter) with a slightly irregular hypoechoic pattern. In one of the structures layers and a small hyperechoic wall could be visualized on the surface of each structure. They were arranged from cranial to caudally behind and beside each other and could not be pushed apart (Figs 3.29–3.33).

Q *5. Interpretation of the result?*

Suspected post-ovulatory egg binding with multi-ovulation (normally leopard geckos only lay two eggs with a size approximately 2.5 cm length and 1 cm diameter). Usually, the shape of the follicles prior to ovulation is round, after ovulation the shape changes to elongated and the egg shell is formed.

Q *6. What would you recommend for gecko no. 2 and the rest of the geckos at home? Can you postulate from the information provided so far the cause of death of gecko no. 3?*

Q *7. What kind of therapy would you recommend for gecko no. 1?*

Therapy

- Deworming with fenbendazole 25 mg/kg q 7days, four times
- With the diagnostic procedures performed, it was not possible to identify the cause of death of gecko no. 3
- It is very important to emphasize to the owner that any dead animal should always be examined post mortem
- As per the interpretation of the ultrasound, post-ovulatory egg binding was suspected in gecko no. 1. The initial therapy consisted of the administration of calcium gluconolactobionate 10%, 20 mg/kg SC and orally for 5 days followed by one injection SC of oxytocin 10 IU/kg.

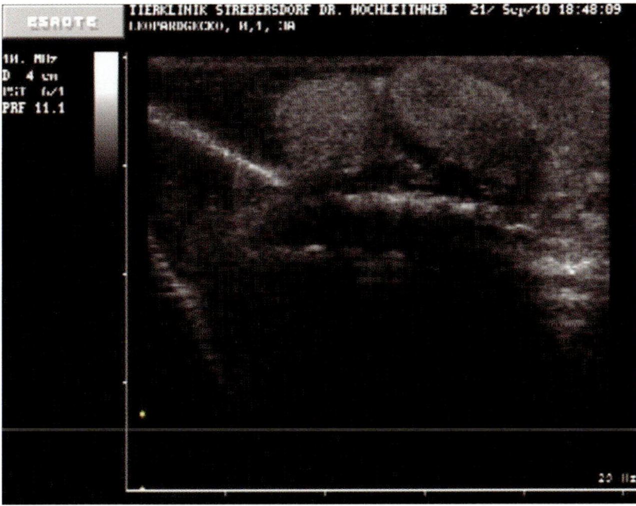

Figs 3.29 to 3.33. In ultrasound scanning, it is always essential to have at least two views such as in radiography – longitudinal and transversal views. Compare the pictures of gecko no. 1 with normal eggs. However, as a moving imaging technique, the counting of, for example, eggs or young has to be done very carefully.

(Continued)

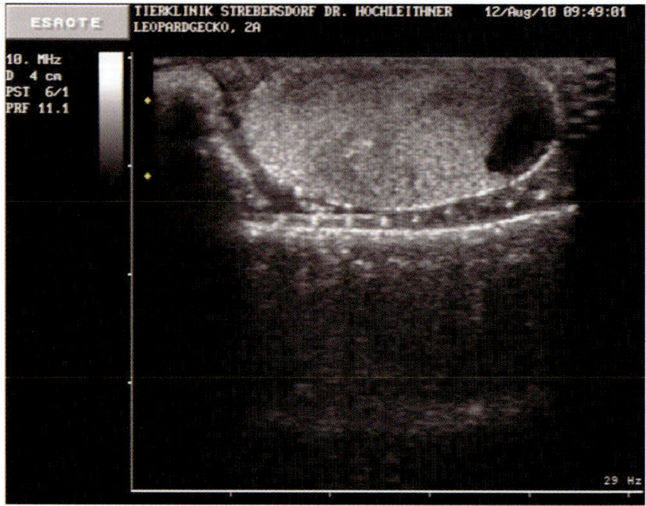

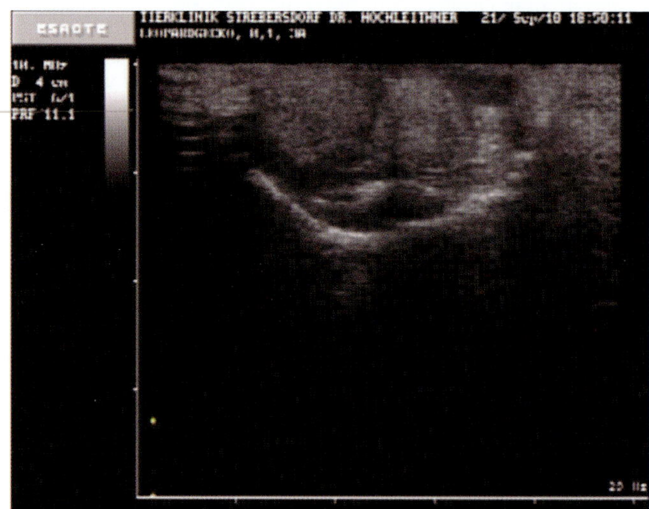

Figs 3.29 to 3.33—cont'd

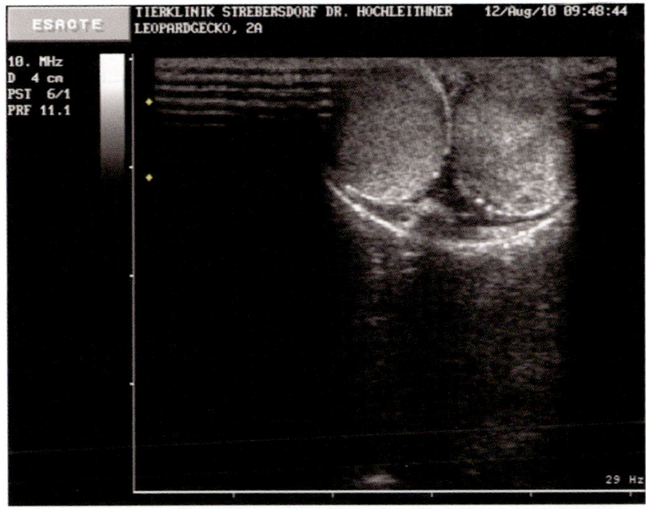

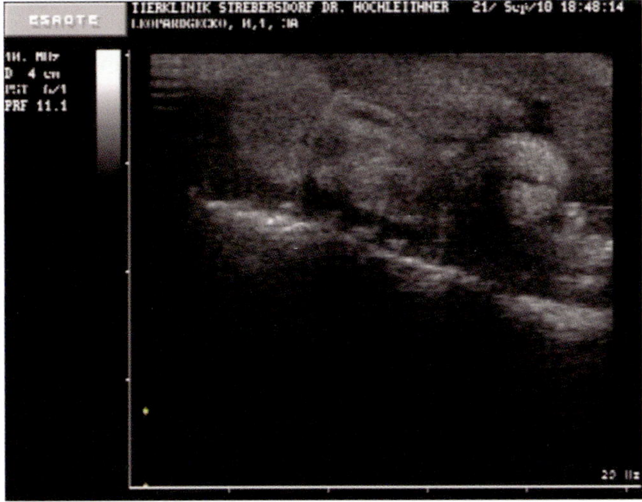

Figs 3.29 to 3.33—cont'd

Q *8. How quickly should this therapy be successful?*

Most cases of egg binding are due to lack of calcium; therefore oxytocin without calcium often does not help. After oxytocin injection, the eggs are usually laid within 24 hours.

There was no effect after treatment for 7 days and the ultrasound investigation showed no significant change. The gecko had stopped feeding totally 8 days before. The decision was made to remove the eggs surgically (Figs 3.34 and 3.35).

Q *9. How do you interpret this surgical in situ?*

This is clearly not a post-ovulatory egg binding. The structure that could be palpated is on the ovary, however, normal follicles are never hard and usually cannot be palpated.

Q ***10. Would you perform further investigation after both ovaries are surgically removed? The gecko developed normally post-surgically.***

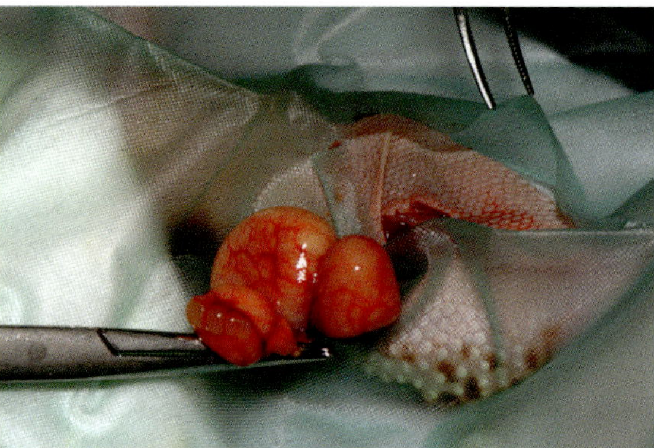

Fig. 3.34 The ovary is clearly visible in connection with the two large follicles.

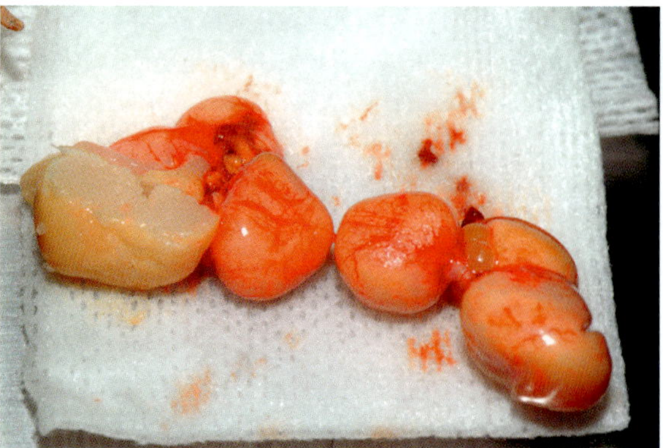

Fig. 3.35 Postoperative. The follicles have a hard (cooked-like) appearance.

The reason for this ovary condition has not been described scientifically, however, it is sometimes seen in geckos by different reptile specialists. Former histological examinations of the hard follicles have indicated a bacterial infection which was also confirmed, in this case, by isolating *E. coli* from the centre of both removed ovaries.

Discussion

Many conditions in different species of reptiles are not yet fully understood. The financial limitations of many owners very often limit the number of diagnostic investigations in private practice, however, good documentation and discussion with other veterinarians can help understand many of these problems.

The ovary in geckos moves freely within the coelomic cavity, therefore, the location and palpation are not hints to differentiate between pre- and post-ovulatory egg binding. Normally, they lay two eggs with a size of more than 2.5 cm of length and approximately 1 cm diameter. Cases with three to four smaller eggs have been seen but are not normal!

Usually, the shape of the follicles prior to ovulation is from round hypoechoic to hyperechoic depending on the stage of the ovulation. After ovulation, the shape changes to elongated and the egg shell is formed. These are the best parameters to differentiate between the different stages of egg binding. In this particular case, the follicles showed the oval shape with hyperechoic wall but the multilayered structure due to the infection with *E. coli* was misinterpreted by ultrasound. In pre-ovulatory egg binding, calcium and oxytocin have no therapeutic effect and surgery is the therapy of choice when the gecko stops eating and there are no signs that the follicle is reabsorbed (ultrasound).

Surgical removal of the ovaries together with hysterectomy can be performed easily in geckos and sutures are removed after 6–8 weeks.

Ovarian infections with *E. coli* in association with changes in the structure of some follicles are pathological findings previously observed in geckos by the author. This should be considered as part of the differential diagnosis when palpating hard structures within the abdomen in geckos. Caution should be exercised with the interpretation of the ultrasound result in such cases.

Further reading

Beck, W., 2006. Praktische Parasitologie bei Heimtieren. Schlätersche, Hannover.
Carpenter, J.W., 2005. Exotic Animal Formulary. Saunders Elsevier, St Louis.
Mader, D.R., 2006. Reptile Medicine and Surgery, second ed. Saunders Elsevier, St Louis.

Case 3.8 *J. Samour, J. Naldo*

Clinical history

A subadult male spiny-tailed lizard (*Uromastyx aegyptia*) was brought into a veterinary clinic for examination with a history of lameness for the past two to three weeks. The lizard was kept in a large indoor room together with one adult male and five adult females and maintained as part of a private herpetological collection. Environmental conditions within the room, including overall temperature, spot temperature, relative humidity and photoperiod, were fully controlled. The diet consisted primarily of chopped alfalfa, mixed fruit and mixed vegetables together with a commercially available mineral/vitamin preparation for reptiles.

Physical examination

The lizard was in a relatively good bodily condition with a score of 4/5 and a bodyweight of 625 g. On examination, it was noticed the lizard was in the last stage of completing its seasonal ecdysis with only two incomplete rings of the old skin remaining around the base and the middle of the tail. Nothing abnormal was detected on physical examination with the exception of a mild swelling around the left elbow joint. No ectoparasites were observed.

Clinical diagnosis examination

Survey radiographs were obtained in the ventrodorsal and latero-lateral positions while the lizard was under anaesthesia with a mixture of isoflurane and oxygen delivered via a face mask (Fig. 3.36).

1. Can you observe any abnormality in the lizard shown in Fig. 3.36?

Radiology (Fig. 3.37)

2. What is your interpretation of the radiology view shown in Fig. 3.37?

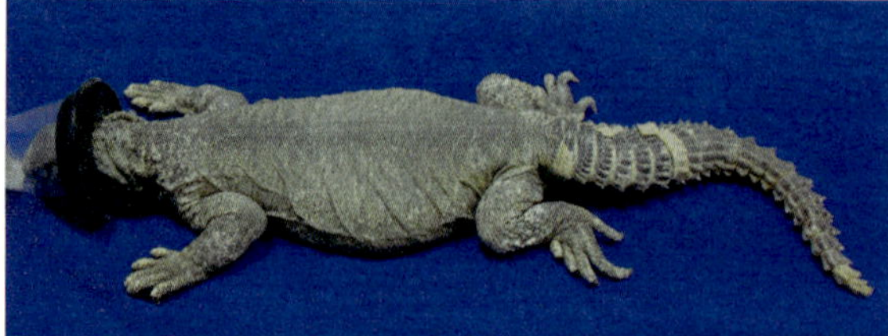

Fig. 3.36 Spiny-tailed lizard under anaesthesia with a mixture of isoflurane and oxygen during the physical examination procedure.

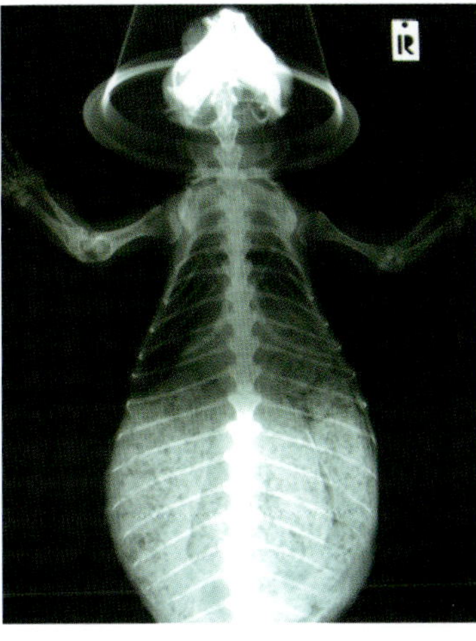

Fig. 3.37 Ventrodorsal view of the spiny-tailed lizard showing the cranial and middle area of the body. A second image was obtained from the distal area including the full tail.

Clinical diagnosis laboratory examination

Blood samples were collected for haematology and blood chemistry analyses from the ventral coccygeal vein using a 23 gauge × 1 inch disposable needle and a 3 ml disposable syringe. A faecal sample was obtained from the transport box and examined for the presence of endoparasites.

Tables 3.16 and 3.17 show the results obtained in the haematology and blood chemistry analyses.

 *3. What is your evaluation of the haematology and blood chemistry results?*

Summary of diagnosis results

- On radiology examination, the lizard showed mild osteomyelitis and arthritis of the left elbow joint
- Haematology analyses revealed a slightly lower RBC and haemoglobin, while the WBC showed moderate elevation with mild to moderate heterophilia, lymphocytosis and monocytosis and the fibrinogen was mildly elevated compared with the mean value, but within the normal range of values published for this species. Examination of the blood film revealed the presence of two different species of haemoparasites temporarily identified as possible new species of *Hepatozoon* and *Karyolysus*
- All the blood chemistry results were within the normal ranges of values published for this species
- The faecal examination did not reveal the presence of any endoparasite

Final diagnosis

- Osteomyelitis
- Arthritis

Table 3.16 Haematology values of the spiny-tailed lizard

Parameters	Absolute value	Normal range	Percentage value	Normal range
RBC (×10¹²/l)	0.75	0.78±0.05* (0.33–4.1)		
Hb (g/dl)	9.9	9.93±0.26 (3.3–17.4)		
Hct (l/l)	30.0	29.70±0.74 (4.9–44.5)		
MCV (fl)	400.0	415.47±9.34 (119.5–614)		
MCH (pg)	132.0	133.65±3.46 (1.2–203.5)		
MCHC (g/dl)	33.0	32.55±0.38 (22.2–41.3)		
WBC (×10⁹/l)	6.6	3.10±0.17 (1.0–8.1)		
Heterophils (×10⁹/l)	4.01	2.00±0.12 (0.59–5.36)	61	64.44±1.43 (35.0–81.0)
Lymphocytes (×10⁹/l)	2.18	0.99±0.08 (0.27–4.05)	33	32.08±1.34 (17.0–60.0)
Monocytes (×10⁹/l)	0.26	0.04±0.01 (0.0–0.5)	4	1.30±0.22 (0.0–14.0)
Eosinophils (×10⁹/l)	0	0.04±0.01 (0.0–0.2)		1.32±0.19 (0.0–8.0)
Basophils (×10⁹/l)	0.13	0.03±0.01 (0.0–0.33)	2	0.79±0.11 (0.0–4.0)
Fibrinogen (g/l)	2.5	1.80±0.13 (0.0–6.0)		
Thrombocytes (×10⁹/l)	15	9.58±0.94 (2.9–22.9)		

**Mean ± standard error of mean (minimum–maximum).*

4. Can you propose a therapeutic plan for the lizard in view of the clinical laboratory findings and the final diagnosis?

Therapy

Different treatments options were discussed with the owner and a conservative approach was selected. A cast made of thermoplastic tape was applied around the affected limb and the lizard sent home with a course of cephalexin at the dose rate of 25 mg/kg PO BID for 2 weeks and meloxicam at the dose rate of 0.2 mg/kg PO SID also for 2 weeks. The cast was removed 3 weeks later after which time the swelling and the lameness had been resolved and the lizard was able to move without any apparent discomfort.

Table 3.17 Blood chemistry values of the spiny-tailed lizard

Analyses	Results	Reference values
Albumin (g/dl)	2.1	2.02±0.05* (1.2–3.1)
ALKP (U/l)	45.3	30.81±3.23 (5.9–139.3)
BUN (mg/dl)	0.16	0.56±0.08 (0.0–3.0)
Calcium (mg/dl)	9.65	9.88±0.18 (7.2–13.2)
Cholesterol (mg/dl)	292.0	160.66±7.21 (64.0–295.0)
Creatinine (mg/dl)	2.1	0.40±0.04 (0.1–3.0)
CK (U/l)	180.6	1778.36±234.75 (141.1–10016.0)
GGT (U/l)	3.0	0.79±0.12 (0.0–5.0)
GOT (U/l)	86.9	73.06±4.59 (28.5–172.0)
GPT (U/l)	3.3	11.0±0.78 (2.4–34.8)
Glucose (mg/dl)	226.7	200.35±6.04 (67.7–355.6)
LDH (U/l)	32.0	209.61±24.89 (22.0–899.0)
Magnesium (mg/dl)	3.8	3.48±0.14 (2.1–10.2)
Total protein (mg/dl)	5.0	4.03±0.11 (2.6–7.4)
Uric acid (mg/dl)	5.8	2.94±0.18 (0.3–7.3)

**Mean±standard error of mean (minimum–maximum).*

Discussion

The lizard was suffering from a mild case of osteomyelitis and arthritis on the left elbow joint. This very likely occurred during a territorial fight with a companion, probably the larger male, or it was sustained as a result of other trauma. The ideal treatment plan for this condition would have been the application of transarticular fixation using an external skeletal fixator consisting of positive-profile threaded pins and an external connector using a short acrylic bar. This would have been left for a minimum of 3 weeks together with a week or two of antibiotic therapy.

Further reading

Mader, D.R., 2006. Reptile Medicine and Surgery, second ed. Saunders Elsevier, St Louis.
Naldo, J.L., Libanan, N.L., Samour, J.H., 2009. Health assessment of a spiny tailed lizard (*Uromastyx* spp.) population in Abu Dhabi, United Arab Emirates. J. Zoo Wildl. Med. 40 (3), 445–452.
Samour, J.H., Risley, D., March, T., et al., 1984. Blood sampling techniques in reptiles. Vet. Rec. 114, 472–476.

Case 3.9 *D. Kaiser*

Clinical history

A 5-year-old Indian star tortoise (*Geochelone elegans*) weighing 267 g was presented with the following clinical signs:

- Anorexia
- Weight loss.

Clinical examination

On presentation, the tortoise felt empty when picked up and on palpation of the prefemoral fossae they felt hollow. The plastron and carapace were well formed and hard. The beak was normal. The eyes were clear and without discharge, examination of the oral cavity was not possible and the ears and tympanic membranes were unremarkable.

1. What are your differential diagnoses and can you propose a diagnostic work-up plan?

Differential diagnoses

- Gastrointestinal obstruction or parasites
- Liver disease
- Respiratory disease (e.g. pneumonia, upper respiratory tract infection, rhinitis)
- Urogenital disease (e.g. egg retention, renal failure)

Clinical diagnosis examination

Diagnostic work up was done in the following order: faecal analyses, nasal flush, blood samples for blood chemistry and finally dorsoventral and craniocaudal radiographs.

Clinical diagnosis laboratory

The results of the clinical diagnosis laboratory assays are shown in Table 3.18.

Table 3.18 Blood chemistry values of the Indian star tortoise

Analysis	Results	Reference values
AP (U/l)	53	36–156
AST (U/l)	8	7–102
LDH (U/l)	664	12–95
CK (U/l)	851	<1000
Uric acid (μmol/l)	41	113–653
BUN (mmol/l)	103	58–140
Creatinine	21	<35.4
Glucose (mmol/l)	13.8	6.7–22
Potassium (mmol/l)	5	4.5–5
Phosphorus (mmol/l)	2	1.7–3.3
Total protein (g/l)	4	49–76

Because it is challenging taking blood samples from tortoises of this size, these were taken by venepuncture of the subcarapacial vein.

Results

- Faecal examination showed negative result for the presence of endoparasites in native smear preparations and flotation
- Nasal flushes were negative for *Mycoplasma* spp.
- Blood chemistry analysis showed elevated levels of LDH and reduced levels of total protein and uric acid

Q *2. What is your interpretation of the coprological examination, the nasal flush and the blood chemistry values shown in Table 3.18?*

- Elevated LDH because of muscle atrophy or organ failure
- Decreased total protein because of malabsorption, protein-losing enteropathy and anorexia
- Decreased uric acid because of anorexia or polyuria

Radiology (Fig. 3.38)

Q *3. What is your interpretation of the radiographs in Fig. 3.38a, b?*

Radiographic findings

- Radiographic findings were pulmonary infiltrates in the right pulmonary field

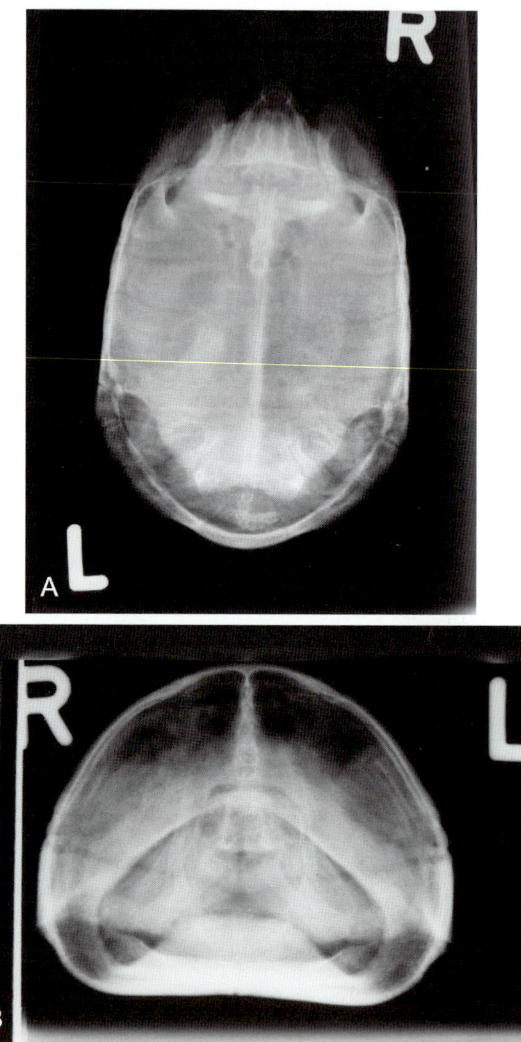

Fig. 3.38 (a) Dorsoventral survey radiograph of the 5-year-old Indian star tortoise; (b) craniocaudal survey radiograph of the 5-year-old Indian star tortoise.

Q *4. List your differential diagnoses again.*

Differential diagnoses

- Pneumonia

Table 3.19 Therapy

Enrofloxacin 2.5%	5–10 mg/kg IM SID for 10 days
Serum proteins	Bioserin® (Paraimmunityinducer) 1 ml/kg TID PO for 7 days
Nebulization	F10 SC™ 0.1 ml + normal saline 25 ml for 30 min BID for 20 days

5. List your therapeutic strategy.

Therapy (Table 3.19)

Discussion

Pneumonia is common in chelonians and can be due to different aetiologies including Trematodes, Coccidia, *Aspergillus* spp., *Candida* spp., herpesvirus, iridovirus, *Mycobacteria*, *Chlamydophila* and *Mycoplasma*. Underlying causes may include poor husbandry (especially low environmental temperatures and poor sanitation), underlying disease (e.g. gut parasite burdens, viral disease, hypovitaminosis A) and inhalation of water. The small size and limited accessibility of Indian star tortoises often limit the possibility of further diagnostics such as CBC, tracheoscopy or broncheal wash. The tortoise made an uneventful recovery and has been without any symptoms for the past 6 months. Follow-up radiographs were not made.

Further reading

Gabrisch, K., Zwart, P., 2008. Schildkröten. In: Zwart, P., Sassenburg, L. (Eds.), Krankheiten der Heimtiere, seventh ed. Schlütersche Verlagsgesellschaft GmbH & Co, Hannover, pp. 653–738.

Girling, S.J., Raiti, P., 2004. BSAVA Manual of Reptiles, second ed. British Small Animal Veterinary Association, Gloucester.

Kölle, P., 2009. Die Schildkröte. Enke Verlag, Stuttgart.

Mader, D.R., 2006. Reptile Medicine and Surgery, second ed. Saunders Elsevier, St Louis.

Case 3.10 *M. Lierz, D. Fischer*

Clinical history

An 8-year-old, female Chinese soft shell turtle (*Trionyx sinensis* seu *Pelodiscus sinensis*) was presented with the following clinical signs of 3 weeks' duration:

- Numerous pustules and ulcerated lesions across plastron, carapaces and adjacent skin
- Inappetence
- Weakness.

For reasons of animal welfare, the turtle was taken away from the owner by the authorities as the husbandry conditions were evaluated as insufficient. The turtle was housed in a 90 cm × 45 cm × 45 cm sized glass tank without access to a land area. The water quality was poor, as there was no filtering system installed inside the tank. The temperature inside the water was kept at 25 °C continuously. The turtle was fed on small live fish, crabs and commercial pellet food.

Physical examination

On presentation, the turtle was of average to good body condition with an admission weight of 1854 g. It was calm but alert and responsive. The whole body surface was covered with multifocal pustules. Every single dark, greenish-yellow pustule had a target-like surface with a firm margin and a smooth, friable and convex curved centre (Fig. 3.39).

Clinical diagnosis examination

Survey radiographs were taken in ventrodorsal and craniocaudal positions. Swabs from throat, cloaca and two skin lesions were submitted for microbiological and virological examination. Blood was taken for haematocrit analysis, basic haematology and blood chemistry. One skin lesion was sampled for histology using a biopsy swage. While taking the biopsy, it was visible that the superficial skin lesions involved deeper areas of subcutaneous soft tissue underneath so that every lesion was like a delimited, solid, cylindrical clot surrounded by unvaried skin (see Fig. 3.39).

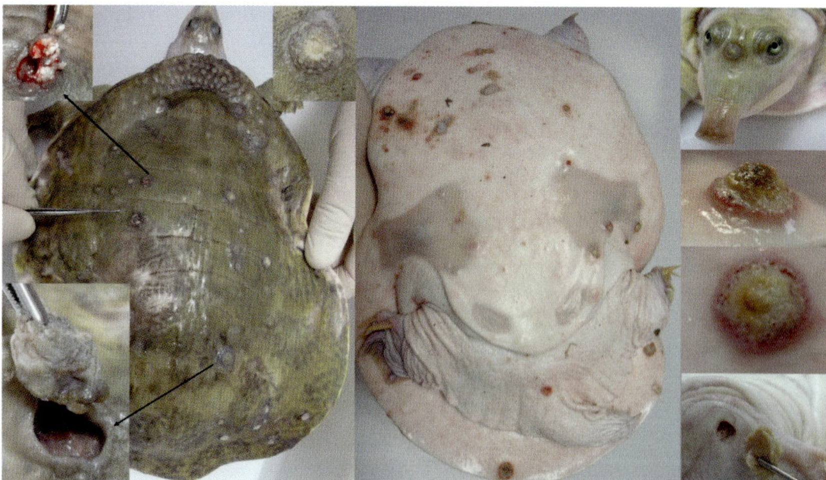

Fig. 3.39 Chinese soft shell turtle (*Trionyx sinensis* seu *Pelodiscus sinensis*) with numerous pustules and ulcerated lesions across plastron, carapaces and adjacent skin. Left side: lesions on carapaces; right side: lesions on plastron and head.

Radiology (Fig. 3.40)

1. What is your interpretation of the radiographs in Fig. 3.40?

Clinical diagnosis laboratory examination

The results of the clinical diagnosis laboratory assays are shown in Tables 3.20 and 3.21.

Haematology was performed using a Diff Quik® stained blood smear as a quick overview instead of a detailed evaluation. Most of the heterophils and lymphocytes were toxic and some erythrocytes were vacuolized. There were some bacterial rods visible in the smear.

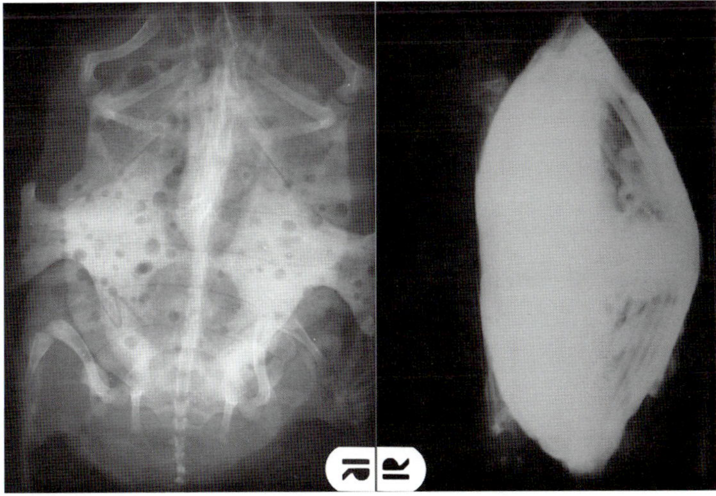

Fig. 3.40 Radiographs of the Chinese soft shell turtle. Left side: ventrodorsal plane; right side: craniocaudal plane.

Table 3.20 Refractometric blood analysis, basic haematology and haematocrit values of the Chinese soft shell turtle

Parameters	Results (absolute)	Reference values*
Specific weight (l/l)	1018	-
Plasma proteins (g/dl)	2	-
Hct (l/l)	0.31	0.29 (0.25–0.33)

**Reference values for soft shell turtles are not available. Therefore reference values of red-eared sliders* (Trachemys scripta) *were taken: Diethelm G (2001), Reptiles. In: Carpenter JW, eds. Exotic Animal Formulary, 3rd edn. Saunders Elsevier, St Louis, p. 108.*

Table 3.21 Blood chemistry values of the soft shell turtle

Analysis	Results	Reference values*
Total protein (g/dl)	<2.0	4.5 (3.4–5.6)
Albumin (g/dl)	<1.0	1.8 (1.3–2.3)
Globulin (g/dl)	<1.0	2.6 (1.7–3.5)
Potassium (mmol/l)	2.6	6.3 (4.3–8.3)
Sodium (mmol/l)	138	137 (133–140)
Calcium (mg/dl)	6.6	14 (14–15)
Phosphorus (mg/dl)	2.8	4.0 (3.7–4.3)
Ca:P ratio	2.36:1	-
Bile acids (μmol/l)	<35	-
AST (IU/l)	73	202 (0–419)
Glucose (mg/dl)	33	67 (20–113)
CK (IU/l)	4700	1288 (1093–1483)
Uric acid (mg/dl)	<0.3	1.2 (0.5–1.9)

**Reference values for soft shell turtles are not available. Therefore reference values of red-eared sliders* (Trachemys scripta) *were taken: Diethelm G (2001), Reptiles. In: Carpenter JW, eds. Exotic Animal Formulary, 3rd edn. Saunders Elsevier, St Louis, p. 108.*

2. What is your interpretation of the blood refractometry, blood chemistry, basic haematology and haematocrit analysis in Tables 3.20 and 3.21?

Results

- The results of the microbiological diagnostic from throat and cloaca:
  - + *Escherichia coli*, +++ *Citrobacter braaki*,
  - +++ *Staphyloccocus* spp., ++ *Streptococcus* spp.
  - + *Penicillium* spp.
- and the lesions:
  - +++ *Escherichia coli*, +++ *Citrobacter braaki*,
  - +++ *Staphyloccocus* spp., ++ *Streptococcus* spp.
- No fungal growth
- In radiographs, an opacification of the lung was visible, more pronounced on the left side than on the right. The circular lesions of skin and soft tissue were clearly visible on the radiograph indicating the severe tissue loss in those areas
- Using virology no virus was isolated on TH1-cells (Terrapene heart cells 1). A herpesvirus consensus PCR (originally designed for poultry) was negative for herpesvirus DNA
- The histology examination showed an acute to subacute, ulcerative and necrotizing dermatitis which was dominated by heterophil granulocytes. Although no intranuclear inclusion bodies were identified, a grey-patch disease could not be excluded by the pathologists

- Blood chemistry analysis revealed decreased protein levels (total protein, globulin, albumin), decreased levels of potassium, calcium, phosphorus and glucose, and increased level of creatine kinase, compared to reference values of red-eared sliders
- The basic haematology indicated a septicaemia and related reactions of leucocytes to the bacteria

Please evaluate the clinical history, Figs 3.39 and 3.40, the results of the physical examination and clinical diagnosis laboratory tests.

Q *3. List your differential diagnoses.*

Q *4. List your therapeutic strategy.*

Differential diagnoses for ulcerative shell lesions in turtles

- Bacterial infections (*Citrobacter* spp. [*C. freundii*], *Aeromonas* spp. [*A. hydrophila*], *Pseudomonas* spp., *Serratia* spp., *Beneckea chitonovora*)
- Viral infection (e.g. herpesvirus causing grey-patch disease in green sea turtles)
- Mycotic infection (e.g. *Aspergillus* spp., *Penicillium* spp., *Aphanomyces* spp., *Paecilomyces lilacinus*)
- Ectoparasitic infection (e.g. leeches)
- Algal infections
- Trauma (e.g. abrasions, bite wounds, gnawing of invertebrates)
- Impaired temperature (e.g. burns, frostbites), electricity or chemical agents
- Poor husbandry conditions (e.g. abrasive surfaces, inadequate hygienic conditions, inadequate size)

Differential diagnoses for cutaneous granulomas/ abscessation and similar swellings in the reptilian skin

- Gram-negative bacteria (such as *Pseudomonas* spp., *Edwardsiella* spp., *Enterobacter* spp., *E. coli*, *Klebsiella* spp., *Micrococcus* spp., *Salmonella* spp.)
- Gram-positive bacteria (such as *Streptococcus* spp., *Staphylococcus* spp., *Mycobacterium* spp., *Dermatophilus congolensis*)
- Anaerobic bacteria (such as *Bacteroides* spp., *Clostridium* spp., *Fusobacterium* spp., *Peptostreptococcus* spp.)
- Fungi (such as *Aspergillus* spp., *Penicillium* spp., *Paecilomyces lilacinus*, *Candida* spp., *Trichophyton* spp. and others)
- Foreign bodies
- Trauma
- Subcutaneous parasites (such as larvae of tapeworms, flukes, filarial worms)
- Papillomavirus infection
- Neoplasms (e.g. fibropapillomatosis, fibrosarcomas, melanomas, squamous cell carcinomas)

Therapy (Table 3.22)

Table 3.22 Therapy

Marbofloxacin 1%	10 mg/kg IM SID × 14 days
Itraconazole	10 mg/kg PO SID × 14 days prophylactically
Fluids	Ringer's lactate 20 ml/kg SC SID × 14 days
Forced feeding	First 3 days 2 ml Bioserin PO, later 5 ml ground fish mixed with water SID
Local treatment of lesions	Surgical debridement, cleaning and disinfection of the lesions under general isoflurane inhalant anaesthesia. Application of F10 and gentamicin-containing cream to the lesions

Post-mortem findings

Despite therapy the turtle died. A thorough post-mortem examination was performed (Fig. 3.41). Samples from different organs were collected for microbiology and histopathology analyses.

Q *5. What lesions can you observe in the post-mortem photograph (Fig. 3.41)?*

Q *6. What is your provisional post-mortem diagnosis?*

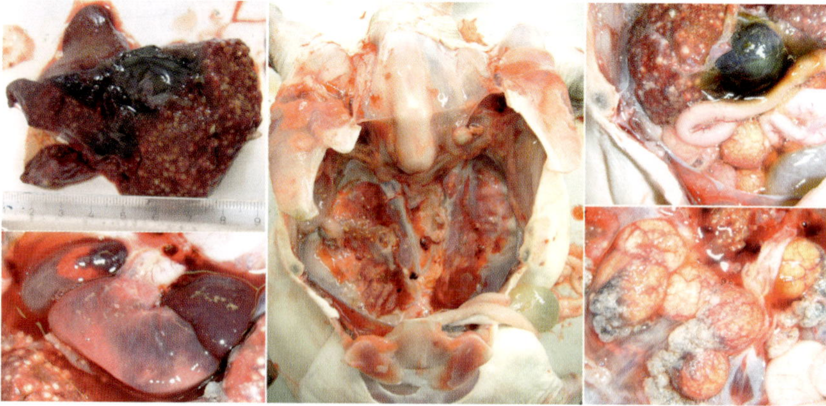

Fig. 3.41 Necropsy of the Chinese soft shell turtle. Left side top: liver with numerous nodules; left side below: heart and liver at the bottom; right side top: liver with gall bladder (above), intestinal loops (middle) and follicles (below); right side below: ovary and intestinal loop in right, lower corner; centre: ventral view on the coelomic cavity and the lung after removal of internal organs (heart, liver, gizzard, intestine, spleen).

Summary of post-mortem examination findings

- Coelomic cavity: filled with yellowish, clear fluid
- Pericardium filled with clear fluid
- Liver: multiple, pinhead-sized, solid, yellow nodules
- Urinary bladder: completely filled with green, granular content
- Lung: multiple, pinhead-sized, solid, yellow nodules
- Ovaries: multiple, pinhead-sized, solid, yellow to greyish-green coloured nodules
- Intestine: a 6 cm × 2 cm × 2 cm sized, growth in last third of intestinal wall

Provisional post-mortem diagnosis

- Ascites and pericardial effusion
- Granulomatous hepatitis
- Granulomatous pneumonia
- Urolithiasis
- Ovaritis
- Intestinal abscessation

Laboratory findings

- Microbiological examination using acid-fast stain (Ziehl-Neelsen stain)
  - Inside the lesions of all organs many acid-fast rods were detectable

Final diagnosis

- SCUD (septicaemic cutaneous ulcerative dermatitis)
- Systemic mycobacteriosis

Discussion

Shell infections, such as the ulcerative shell disease (USD), are known in a great variety of turtle species. Soft shell turtles are often affected by many kinds of dermatitis, varying from erosive to necrotizing and from peracute to chronic in character. The septicaemic cutaneous ulcerative dermatitis (SCUD) is a very complicated form of dermatitis in freshwater turtles. Different bacteria including *Aeromonas hydrophila, Citrobacter freundii* and *Serratia* spp. are described as causative agents, acting together with other pathogens (mainly Gram-negative bacteria), poor husbandry conditions (especially abrasive substrate and poor water hygiene) and invertebrate predation to culminate in SCUD. The bacterium *Beneckea chitonovora* is also suspected to contribute to SCUD after its ingestion with contaminated shellfish. Irregular caseated and crateriform ulcers of skin and shell, erythema of the scute suture lines, lethargy and collapse, due to septicaemia, are typical symptoms of SCUD. Moreover, hepatic necrosis, haemolysis, paralysis and death may occur. Systemic and local therapy with sensitive antibiotics is indicated beside surgical debridement of the ulcers and its obstruction with waterproof antibiotic paste. In addition, the authors successfully used low level laser therapy (LLLT) to improve and hasten the dermal healing process in a similar case.

Improvement of husbandry conditions, orientated towards the natural habitat, plays an important role in treatment and prevention of diseases. *Trionyx/Pelodiscus sinensis* lives in Asia (China, Hainan, Taiwan and Vietnam), in different waters with low flow, such as canals, rice fields, lakes and wetlands. It hibernates and is mainly carnivorous. Apart from swimming inside the water and burrowing inside mud, sunbathing on land is regularly performed, so that the tank should be sized and designed accordingly. As they are aggressive to conspecifics, the turtles should be housed singly.

In our case, the large amount of various bacteria isolated reflects the poor hygiene and the inadequate husbandry conditions the turtle was forced to live in. The isolated *Citrobacter* spp. was suspected as the main cause of SCUD in the soft shell turtle, so that treatment was adapted to this. No further investigations were done, so that an underlying and certainly predisposing infection with *Mycobacterium* spp. was not recognized until necropsy as the histopathological examination of the lesions had not led to suspicion of mycobacteriosis.

Mycobacterial infections are common in amphibians, fishes and reptiles. Although mycobacteriosis occurs comparatively rarely in turtles, it has been reported in soft shell turtles causing lesions in the skin, granulomatous pneumonia, hepatitis, splenitis and transudation in the coelomic cavity. In general, any treatment of mycobacteriosis should be refused and euthanasia should be elected in reptiles as it represents a potential zoonosis. The species of mycobacterium in the present case was not discriminated. However, different *Mycobacterium* species are known in turtles with *M. marinum* as the most common one, also known for opportunistic infections in man.

In this case, SCUD-inducing agents and *Mycobacteria* caused a long-acting and widely spread infection, including septicaemia and pneumonia, and making all treatment efforts unsuccessful.

Further reading

Cooper, J.E., 2006. Dermatology. In: Mader, D.R. (Ed.), Reptile Medicine and Surgery, second ed. Saunders Elsevier, St Louis, pp. 196–216.

Fraser, M.A., Girling, S.J., 2004. Dermatology. In: Girling, S.J., Raiti, P. (Eds.), BSAVA Manual of Reptiles, second ed. British Small Animal Veterinary Association, Gloucester, pp. 184–198.

Frye, F.L., Williams, D.L., 1997. Reptilien und Amphibien – Taschenatlas für Diagnose und Therapie. Schlütersche Verlagsgesellschaft, Hannover, p. 78.

Kraut, S., Fischer, D., Hampel, M.R., et al., 2011. Low-level-laser therapy (LLLT) in reptiles for the treatment of skin ulceration. J. Small Anim. Pract. submitted.

Orós, J., Acosta, B., Gaskin, J.M., et al., 2003. *Mycobacterium kansasii* infection in a Chinese soft shell turtle (*Pelodiscus sinensis*). Vet. Rec. 152, 474–476.

Case 3.11 *A. Montesinos*

Clinical history

A 4-year-old female red-eared terrapin or red-eared slider (*Trachemys scripta elegans*) weighing 1105 g was presented (Fig. 3.42) with the following clinical signs of 5 weeks' duration:

- Anorexia
- Clouds in both eyes
- Lack of stool production.

The terrapin was purchased when it was a baby and was kept in an aquarium with adequate gradient temperature and no supplement of UV light. The diet of the terrapin was based on raw meat and pieces of raw salmon. The owner reported that the terrapin was eating calcium stones ravenously one month before clinical signs. These calcium stones were provided by the owner as calcium supplement.

Clinical examination

On presentation, the terrapin had a body condition of 5/5 and was active and aggressive, and had a tacky white punctuate on both corneas. Abdominal and rectal palpation did not show masses compatible with eggs. Whole body radiographs were taken after administration of iodinated contrast medium and blood samples were collected for haematology, blood chemistry and plasma protein electrophoresis. The terrapin was kept at the hospital for observation. Radiographs were repeated 3 days after presentation.

Radiology (Fig. 3.43)

1. What is your interpretation of the radiographs of Fig. 3.43a, b?

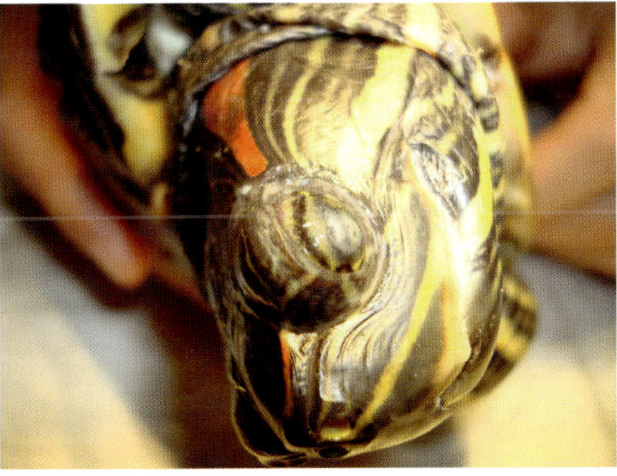

Fig. 3.42 A female red-eared terrapin or red-eared slider, presented with signs of anorexia, cloudy eyes and lack of stool production.

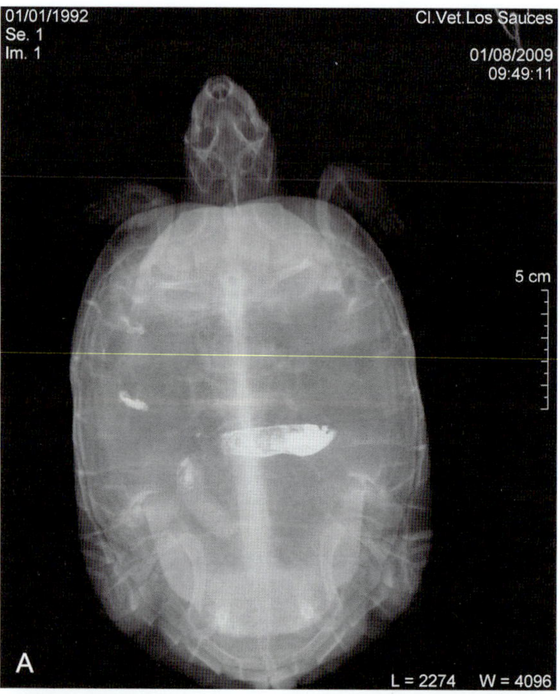

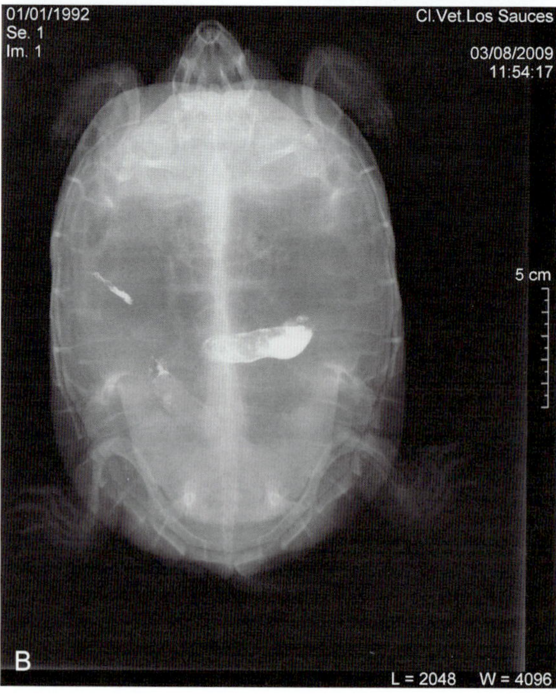

Fig. 3.43 (a) Ventrodorsal survey radiograph of a 4-year-old red-eared terrapin with constipation, day 1; (b) ventrodorsal survey radiograph of a 4-year-old red-eared terrapin with constipation, day 3.

Clinical diagnosis laboratory

The results of the clinical diagnosis laboratory assays are shown in Tables 3.23–3.25.

Table 3.23 Haematology values for the red-eared terrapin

Parameters	Results (absolute)	Results (%)	Reference values
RBC (×10^{12}/l)	0.45		0.3–0.8
Hb (g/dl)	6.2		7–10
Hct (l/l)	0.29	29	0.25–0.33
MCV (fl)	644		310–1000
MCH (pg)	137		95–308
MCHC (g/dl)	21.3		20–33
WBC (×10^9/l)	35		5–9
Heterophils (×10^9/l)	28	80	30–52%
Lymphocytes (×10^9/l)	7	2	15–35 %
Azurophils (×10^9/l)	0	0	0–3 %
Eosinophils (×10^9/l)	0	0	0–2 %
Basophils (×10^9/l)	6.3	18	20–40 %
Monocytes (×10^9/l)	0	0	0–1%

Table 3.24 Blood chemistry values of the red-eared terrapin

Analysis	Results	Reference values
Albumin (g/l)	7	6.1–18
ALKP (U/l)	560	81–343
Bile acids (μmol/l)	5	0–3
Calcium (mg/dl)	9	12–15
Cholesterol (mg/dl)	760	104–333
CK (U/l)	1200	900–1400
GGT (U/l)	12	
GOT (U/l)	479	0–400
Glucose (mg/dl)	121	20–113
Phosphorus (mg/dl)	9	3.7–4.8
Potassium (mmol/l)	4	2–5
Sodium (mmol/l)	135	133–140
Total protein (g/l)	30	24–49
Triglycerides (mg/dl)	1200	-
Urea (mg/dl)	18	10–59
Uric acid (mg/dl)	0.8	0–2

Table 3.25 Plasma protein electrophoresis of the red-eared terrapin

Parameters	Fractions (%)	Concentration (g/l)	Reference values (g/l)
Total protein	100	30	33.1±8.3
Albumin	40.3	12.1	10.3±4
Alpha globulins	36	1.9	8.5±2.3
Beta globulins	50	15	13.0±3.5
Gamma globulins	0.03	1	1.6±1.2
Globulins	79.6	26	22.8±3.5
A:G ratio	0.76	0.76	0.5±0.1

RBC, WBC and thrombocyte morphology

- Toxic heterophils +++
- Degranulated basophils
- Irregular population of red blood cells

2. What is your interpretation of the haematology, blood chemistry, and protein electrophoresis values shown in Tables 3.23–3.25?

Results

- Radiographic findings included halt of the contrast medium transit at the beginning and 48 hours later. This image was compatible with GI obstruction
- Haematology analysis showed high WBC count with toxic heterophilia
- Blood chemistry analysis showed elevated levels of bile acids, GGT, cholesterol and triglycerides. There is also low level of calcium
- Plasma protein electrophoresis showed normal total protein and low levels of albumin and increased A:G ratio and high levels of beta protein fraction

Please evaluate the clinical history, Fig. 3.43a, b, the results of the physical examination and clinical diagnostic tests.

3. List your differential diagnoses.

4. List your diagnostic strategy and possible further diagnostic testing.

Differential diagnoses

- Intestinal obstruction and generalized infection from intestinal flora
- Follicular stasis
- Hypocalcaemia and secondary nutritional hyperparathyroidism

Diagnostic plan

More imaging techniques were necessary to explore the possibility of an obstruction and to prepare an approach by inguinal fossa or by plastrotomy. The owner agreed to make an ultrasound study of the terrapin.

Echography (Fig 3.44)

5. What is your interpretation of the ultrasound image of Fig. 3.44?

Results of the ultrasound study

- There was no free fluid in the coelom of the terrapin
- There are follicles occupying the coelomic cavity and lack of intestinal movement
- With this ultrasound image, it was not possible to get more data about the intestinal obstruction

Therapy

Because the blood work was strongly suggestive of a generalized infection, treatment with a broad-spectrum antibiotic was started and surgery by the inguinal fossa was suggested to the owners to get a definitive diagnosis and resolution for the intestinal obstruction.

After an IV catheter was positioned in the right jugular vein, fluid therapy (Table 3.26) was started in order to avoid sepsis and to correct the ionic imbalances discovered in the terrapin.

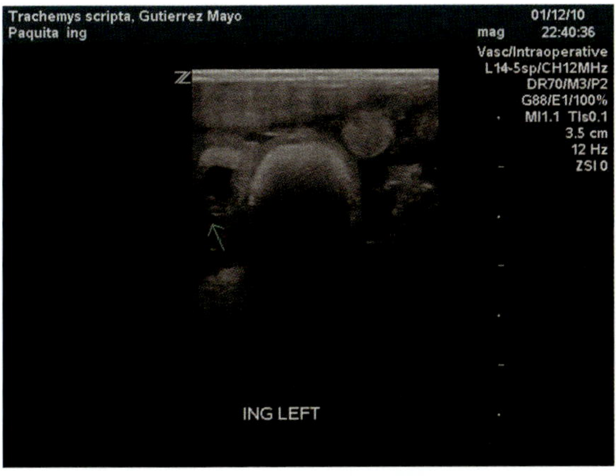

Fig. 3.44 Ultrasound view of the coelomic cavity of the red-eared terrapin.

Table 3.26 Therapy

Piperacilin–tazobactam 200 mg/ml	100 mg/kg IM SID, 3 weeks
Morphine 10 mg/ml	1.5 mg/kg IM SID, 1 week
Fluids	Ringer's lactate 10–25 ml/kg/day IV IRC during surgery and 1 day after

Surgery

The terrapin was anaesthetized with an induction dose of alfaxolone 10 mg/kg. Rectal temperature, haemoglobin saturation, blood pressure and end tidal CO_2 concentration were monitored during the surgical procedure. After left inguinal fossa incision (Fig. 3.45), the subcutaneous fat tissue was debrided (Fig. 3.46). After obtaining a clear view of the oblique abdominal muscles, access was gained to the coelomic cavity and the left ovary and the left oviduct were removed and haemoclips placed (Fig. 3.47). Two stay sutures were fixed to the intestine and the gut was exteriorized from the coelomic cavity as far as possible (Fig. 3.48). An incision was made over the obstruction. Compacted material was removed from the intestine and gentle flushing was done in order to remove and to soften the compacted material (Fig. 3.49). The intestine was closed with an inverting pattern 6/0 suture using absorbable suture material. The laparotomy incision was closed using standard techniques (Fig. 3.50) and the terrapin recovered uneventfully from anaesthesia (Fig. 3.51).

Final diagnosis

- Bacterial infection due to intestinal obstruction
- Intestinal obstruction from ingested calcium stone and low levels of calcium

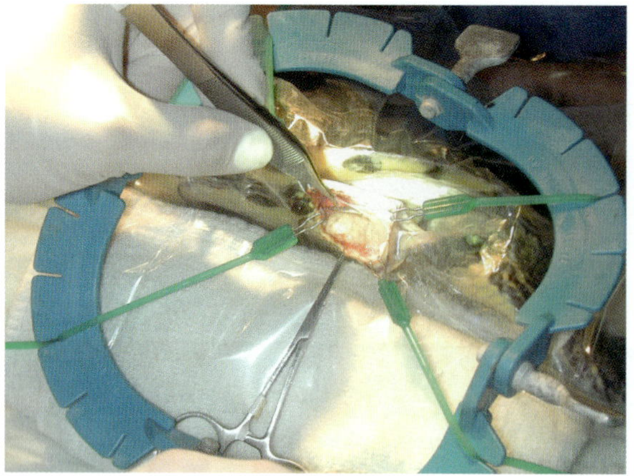

Fig. 3.45 View of the terrapin covered by a transparent surgical drape. The skin has been incised. The subcutaneous fat is covering the approach to the coelomic cavity. A ring surgical retractor was used to expose the surgical field as wide as possible.

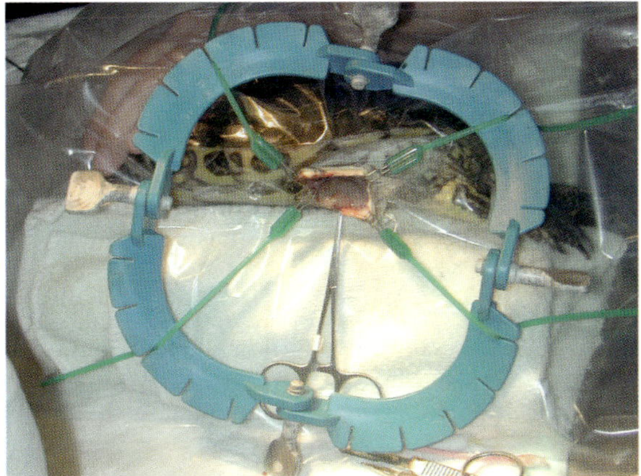

Fig. 3.46 After debriding the subcutaneous fat, a clear view of the oblique abdominal muscles was obtained to provide access to the coelomic cavity.

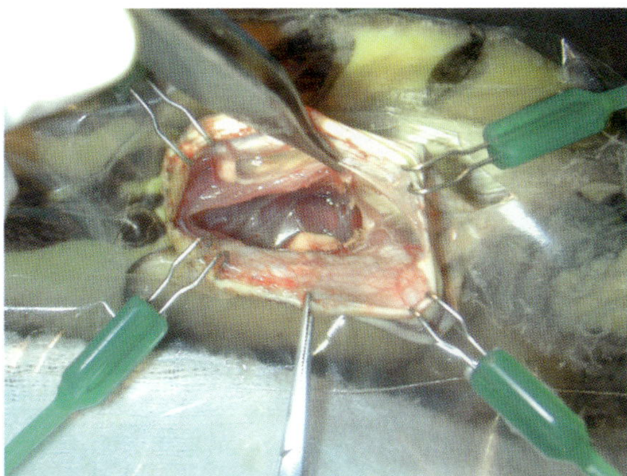

Fig. 3.47 After removal of the left ovary and left shell gland, the intestine became more accessible. Haemoclips were used to ligate the shell gland and ovarian blood vessels.

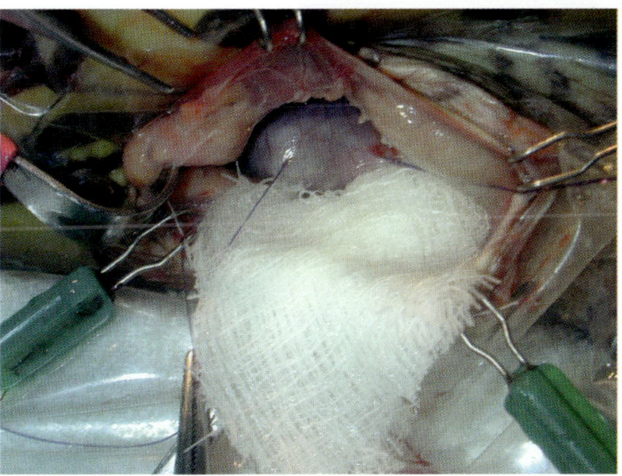

Fig. 3.48 Intraoperative view of the intestine. Two stay sutures were fixed over the obstruction area.

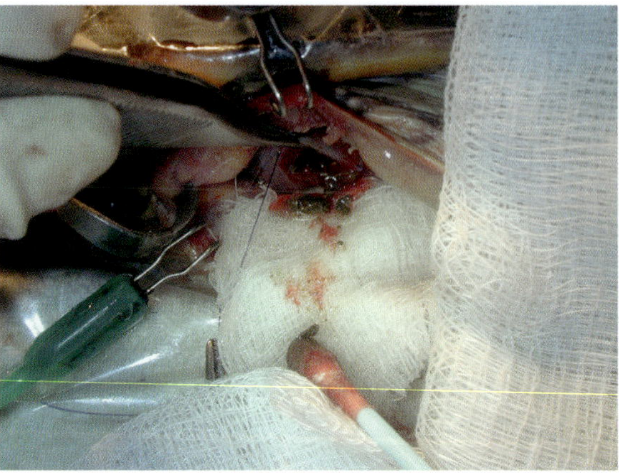

Fig. 3.49 After the longitudinal incision of the intestine, hard and compacted material was removed using forceps and surgical spoons.

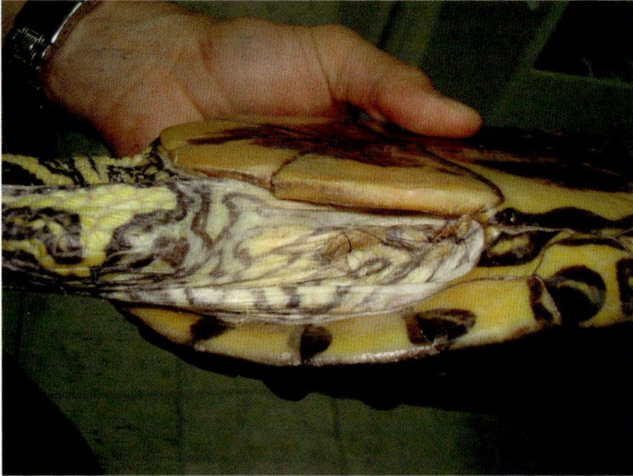

Fig. 3.50 The laparotomy was closed using routine techniques. This surgical approach leaves a wound that closes very fast and the terrapin can be returned to water in 2 days.

Follow up

After 2 days in hospital, the terrapin was permitted to return to the water and started to eat 1 day later. Soft stools were passed 12 hours after surgery. One week after the surgical procedure, the terrapin was sent home with antibiotic covering, and eating (turtle pellets) and defecating in a regular way. The corneal clouds disappeared when the terrapin started to eat. These were probably made of cholesterol deposition. Three weeks after surgery the terrapin was rechecked, including physical examination and blood analysis. All blood parameters were within reference ranges for the species and the corneal depositions were almost clear.

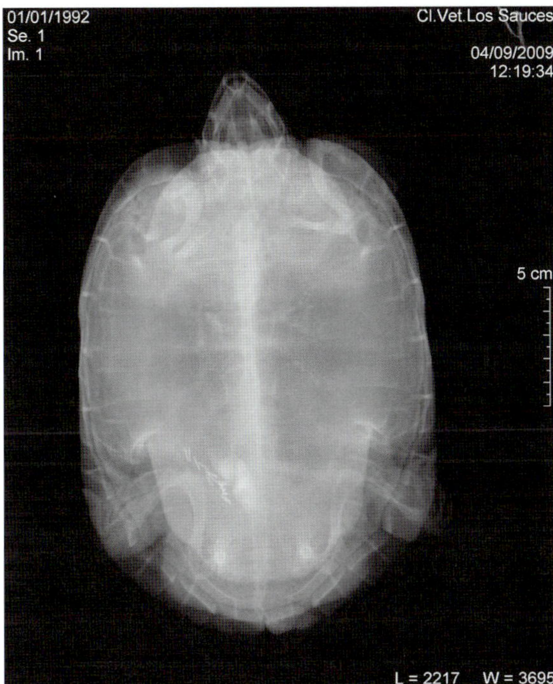

Fig. 3.51 Radiograph of the terrapin after surgery, the haemoclips used for vessels ligation are visible and the compacted material has disappeared.

Discussion

There are very few reports on enterectomy in terrapins in the reptilian literature. Descriptions of several techniques are found in reptilian medicine books but these are only reports from authors, not peer review studies. An inguinal approach has been described but advice on shearing serosa of the coelomic viscera is only lightly described. There are no reports on the best and safest suture material to close the intestine. This case describes the approach to the intestinal obstruction in a red-eared terrapin from a logical sequence of clinical events, similar to cases observed in other species during veterinary clinical practice.

Further reading

Branian, R.E., 1984. A soft tissue laparotomy technique in turtles. J. Am. Vet. Med. Assoc. 185 (11), 1416–1417.

Gimenez, M., Saco, Y., Pato, R., et al., 2010. Plasma protein EPH of *Trachemys scripta* and *Iguana iguana*. Vet. Clin. Pathol. 39 (2), 227–235.

Gould, W.J., Yaeger, A.E., Glenn, J.C., 1992. Surgical correction of an intestinal obstruction in a turtle. J. Am. Vet. Med. Assoc. 200, 705.

Innis, C.J., Hernandez-Divers, S.J., Martinez-Jimenez, D., 2007. Coelioscopic-assisted prefemoral oophorectomy in chelonians. J. Am. Vet. Med. Assoc. 230 (7), 1049–1052.

Mader, D.R., Bennet, A., Funk, R.S., et al., 2005. Surgery. In: Mader, D.R. (Ed.), Reptile Medicine and Surgery, second ed. Saunders Elsevier, St Louis, pp. 581–630.

McArthur, S., Hernandez-Divers, S.J., 2004. Surgery. In: McArthur, S., Wilkinson, R., Meyer, J. (Eds.), Medicine and Surgery of Tortoises and Turtles. Blackwell Publishing, Oxford, pp. 403–460.

Case 3.12 *C. Lloyd*

Clinical history

A 30-year-old female Mediterranean spur thigh tortoise (*Testudo graeca*) from a mixed sex outdoor colony presented with a suspected cloacal prolapse (Fig. 3.52). The tortoise was in good body condition (1.6 kg) and appeared bright and active. Hydration and mucous membranes were normal. The tortoise was admitted to the hospital for work up and stabilization.

Q *1. How would you identify the origin of the prolapsed tissue?*

Identification of the prolapsed organ is essential. It is helpful to know if urination and defecation are still continuing around the prolapse. The urinary bladder appears as a thin-walled, fluid-filled structure from which urine may be aspirated. A penile prolapse appears as a solid mass with no lumen and is often readily identified by its anatomy. Oviduct and rectal/colon tissue may appear similar as tubular structures with a lumen and identification may be complicated by tissue damage and swelling. In some cases, it is possible to aspirate faeces from the lumen of the mass confirming rectal or colon prolapse. In this case, manipulation of the prolapse produced faecal material which confirmed the mass as intestinal in origin. The prolapse was cleaned in 10% povodine–iodine solution and found to be devitalized and necrotic.

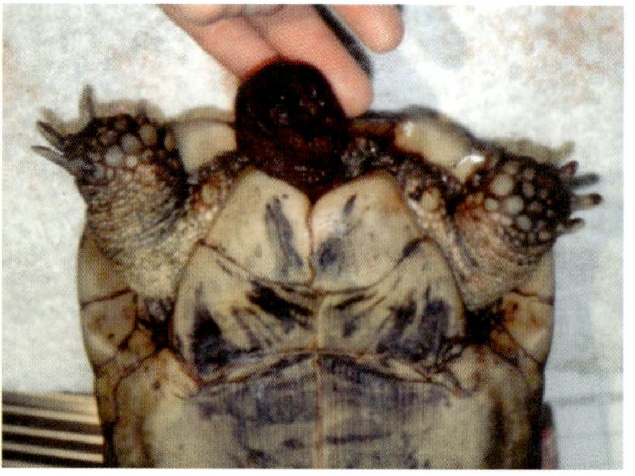

Fig. 3.52 Cloacal prolapse in the female *Testudo graeca*.

Clinical diagnosis examination

Haematology, biochemistry, radiography and direct faecal examination were performed. Blood work was unremarkable other than a mild elevation in CK. Radiographs were unremarkable. Findings of faecal examination are illustrated in Fig. 3.53.

Faecal parasitology revealed large numbers of *Oxyurid* spp. No other obvious cause for the prolapse could be found.

2. How would you interpret these findings and what are the causes of cloacal organ prolapse?

Differential diagnoses

Potential causes of cloacal organ prolapse in tortoises include:

- Debilitation or neurological dysfunction
- Any condition that results in tenesmus (intestinal foreign body, constipation, parasitism, space-occupying lesions such as uroliths or atopic eggs, dystocia)
- Obesity
- Hypocalcaemia
- Trauma during mating or mating displays. Male tortoises often protrude their penis during urination or defecation.

It could be hypothesized that the heavy *Oxyurid* load caused some colonic or rectal irritation and led to tenesmus and a prolapse that became damaged and unable to return. This may have resulted in further tenesmus and further progression of the prolapse.

3. How would you manage this case?

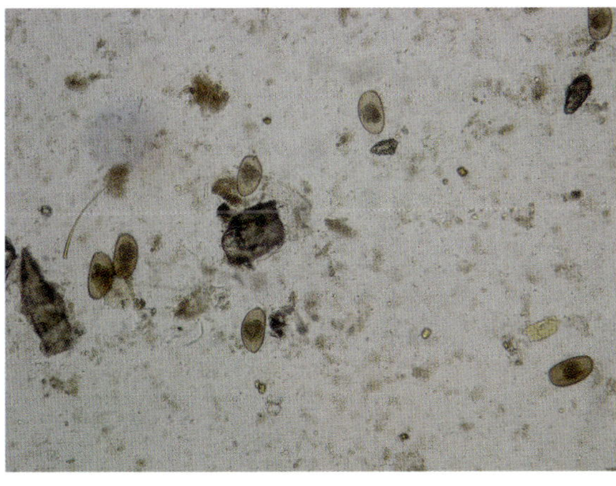

Fig. 3.53 Ova from direct faecal examination (10 × magnification).

Therapeutic management

Ceftazidime IM at 20 mg/kg every 72 hours and 2% bodyweight warm glucose saline solution was given intracoelomically once daily via the prefemoral fossa.

General anaesthesia induced with 10 mg/kg propofol given via a 24G 19 mm catheter placed in the right jugular vein. The tortoise was intubated and placed on a ventilator providing a mixture of oxygen and 3% isoflurane at a ventilation rate of two breaths per minute. The tortoise was placed in dorsal recumbancy on a table heated to 30 °C.

The outer casing from a disposable 10 ml syringe was inserted into the lumen of the prolapse to act as a stent while caudal traction was used until healthy mucosa was visible. Three 25 mm, 23G needles were placed perpendicular through the healthy tissue and stent to anchor the prolapse (Fig. 3.54). A circumferential incision was made in the viable tissue to resect the prolapse and 1.5 M PDS was used to place mattress sutures creating an inverting end-to-end anastomosis. On removal of the stent, the sutured colon invaginated and returned to the coelomic cavity. Recovery from anaesthesia was unremarkable.

The tortoise was discharged with nutritional support and ceftazidime injections. The animal was also treated with 20 mg/kg fenbendazole once daily for 7 days. The recovery was good and the tortoise was eating well 3 days post surgery.

After 16 days, the animal was returned to the clinic exhibiting signs of tenesmus and continued anorexia. No faeces had been passed since treatment of the prolapse. A dorsoventral radiograph was performed (Fig. 3.55).

Q *4. What can you see on the radiograph and how would you proceed with this case?*

The radiograph shows gas-distended loops of intestine in the coelomic cavity. Endoscopic examination of the cloaca and distal colon with saline insufflation and a 2.7 mm 30° rigid scope was suspicious for a stricture at the site of the previous colonic resection.

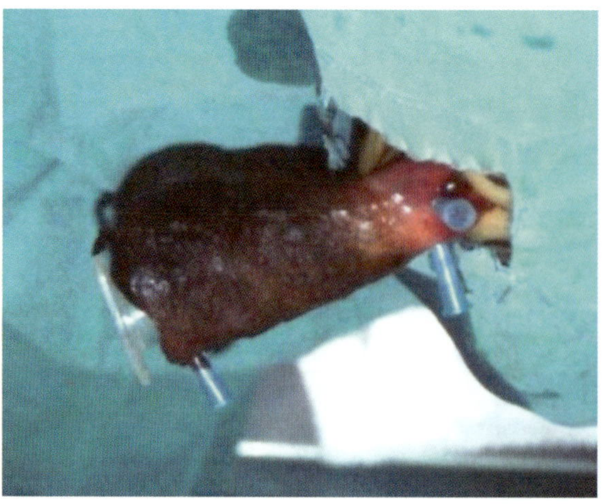

Fig. 3.54 Necrotic prolapse with syringe stent placed prior to resection.

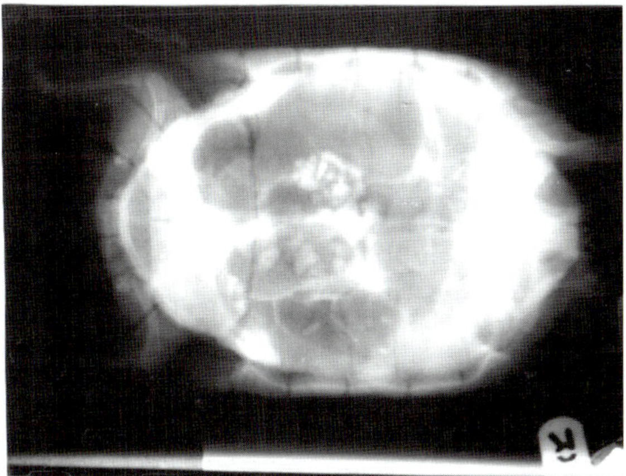

Fig. 3.55 Dorsoventral radiograph of the tortoise taken 16 days postoperatively.

Surgical procedure

It was decided that a coeliotomy was required to investigate and treat the obstruction. The tortoise was anaesthetized as described previously.

With the tortoise in dorsal recumbancy, the radiograph was used to identify margins of the pelvic girdle. A rectangular coeliotomy site was identified over the abdominal scutes and the area was prepared aseptically and then lightly scored using a low speed dental drill and tungsten carbide burr.

Bevelled plastron incisions were made using a high speed rotary dremel and diamond-edged cutting disc. A stream of Hartman's solution was used to minimize thermal necrosis. The caudal edge of the plastron flap was elevated and separated in a cranial direction from its abdominal muscle attachments using a periosteal elevator. Soft tissue attachments at the cranial edge of the flap were preserved. The flap was kept moist with saline swabs. The coelomic membrane was incised in the midline and the distended loops of bowel were palpated to a stricture associated with the previous surgery at the descending colon. A 2 cm incision was made perpendicular to and transecting the original anastomosis on the ventral surface of the colon. The incision was then closed in a transverse orientation using 1.5 M PDS in a Lembert suture pattern thus increasing luminal diameter. The coeliotomy incision was closed routinely and secured with large animal hoof acrylic. The tortoise was discharged on the same feeding and therapeutic protocol as previously described. Thirty days postoperatively, the tortoise was eating, defecating and gaining weight normally.

Discussion

A prolapse can often be easily replaced if detected before significant oedema and necrosis occurs and a purse string suture placed across the cloaca. In this case, the significant necrosis required that devitalized tissue was resected. Rectal and colonic prolapses carry a higher failure rate than oviductal problems and identification of the prolapse is essential.

An alternative to plastral coeliotomy in this case may have been coeliotomy via the prefemoral fossa. While this reduces healing time in a smaller chelonian it does limit access to the coelomic cavity.

Further reading

Girling, S.J., Raiti, P., 2004. BSAVA Manual of Reptiles, second ed. British Small Animal Veterinary Association, Gloucester.

Greiner, E., Mader, D., 2006. Parasitology. In: Mader, D.R. (Ed.), Reptile Medicine and Surgery, second ed. Saunders Elsevier, St Louis, pp. 360–364.

Jacobsen, E., 2007. Parasites and parasitic diseases of reptiles. In: Jacobsen, E. (Ed.), Infectious Diseases and Pathology of Reptiles. Taylor & Francis Group, Boca Raton, pp. 590–593.

McArthur, S.D., Wilkinson, R., Meyer, J., 2004. Medicine and Surgery of Tortoises and Turtles. Blackwell Publishing, Oxford.

Case 3.13 *P. Zucca*

Clinical history

A large sea turtle was found floating near the shore with a fishing line coming out of the beak. The animal was rescued by the Coast Guard and sent for treatment at a sea turtle rescue centre of the World Wildlife Fund (WWF).

Physical examination

The turtle was an adult female loggerhead sea turtle (*Caretta caretta*) with a carapace length of 76 cm and a weight of 75 kg. A thick nylon fishing line of 2 mm diameter was coming out of the beak (Fig. 3.56).

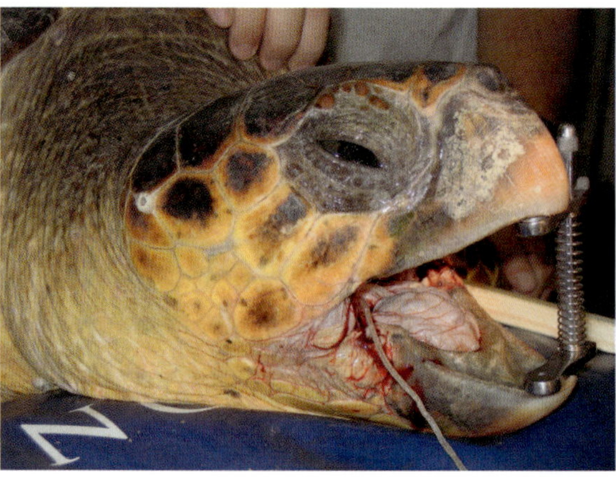

Fig. 3.56 Loggerhead sea turtle with a thick nylon fishing line of 2 mm diameter coming out of the beak.

Clinical diagnosis examination

A clinical examination revealed that the sea turtle was in good general condition and it was reactive to external stimuli. The margins of the oral cavity close to the beak were deeply wounded by the nylon line. The animal was not tagged and no other clinical signs were visible.

1. What is your diagnosis?

Radiography

The sea turtle was positioned in ventral recumbency and radiography of the area from the beak to the stomach was taken. The dorsoventral x-ray revealed that the sea turtle had swallowed a large 7 cm fish hook located deep in the middle-third of the oesophagus close to the anterior carapace margin as shown in Fig. 3.57.

Summary of clinical findings

- Fishing nylon line coming out of the oral cavity
- Deep wounds on the mouth
- Large fish hook deeply located in the middle-third of the oesophagus

Therapy

An attempt to remove the hook with a non-surgical procedure was decided. The sea turtle was sedated with ketamine administered intramuscularly at 40 mg/kg. The animal was placed on ventral recumbency and a cushion supported its head. A step-by-step description of the non-invasive procedure is reported in Fig. 3.58a–h.

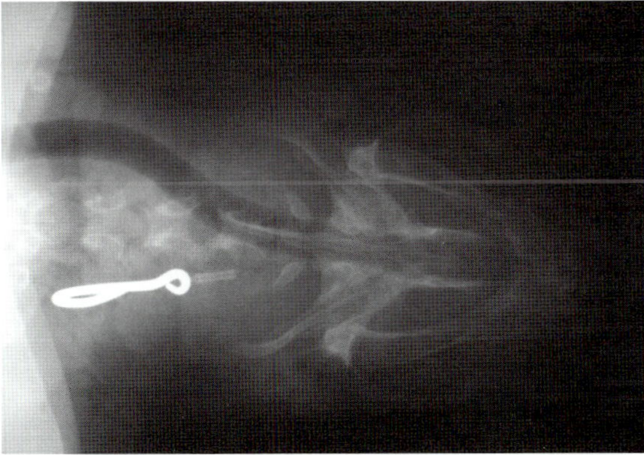

Fig. 3.57 The sea turtle had swallowed a large 7 cm fish hook located deep in the middle-third of the oesophagus close to the anterior carapace margin as seen on the dorsoventral radiography view.

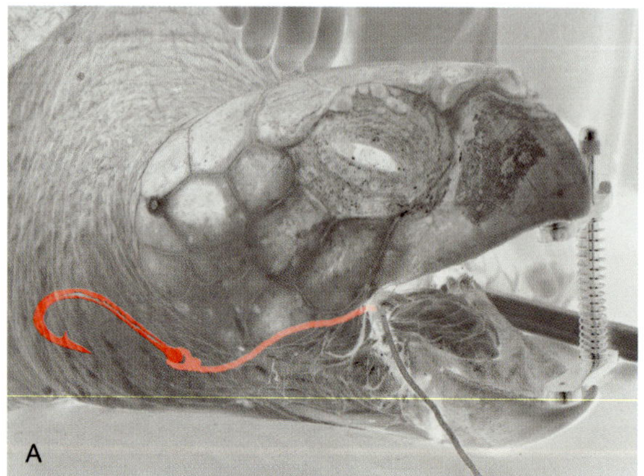

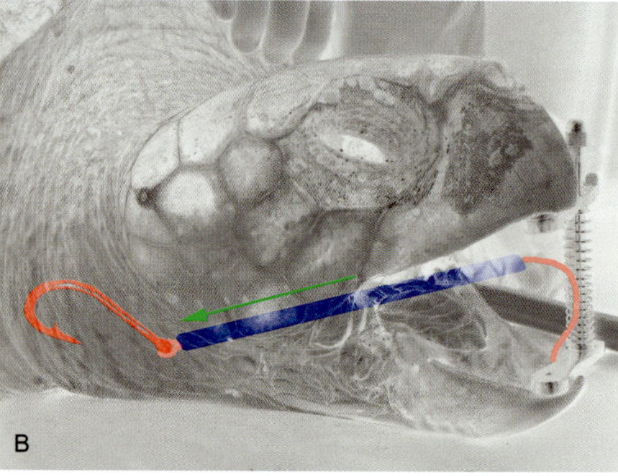

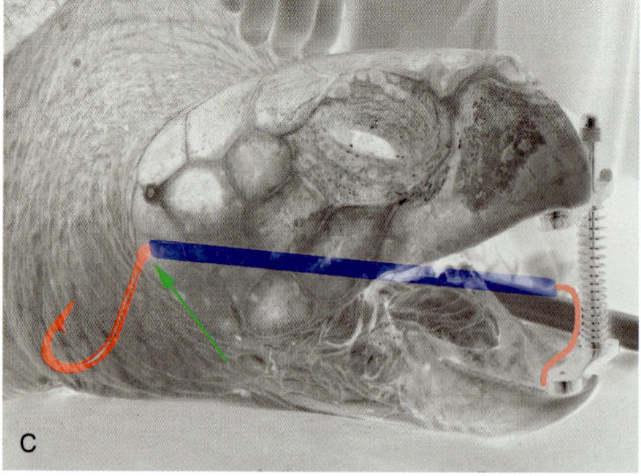

Fig. 3.58 (a) Although the hook was not visible from the oral cavity, radiography and palpation gave enough information about its position. (b) Step 1: pass the line inside the metal tube, slowly slide the tube down until reaching the hook. (c) Step 2: pull the line to keep the metal tube close to the hook, gently push/move the tube rotating the hook *in situ*.

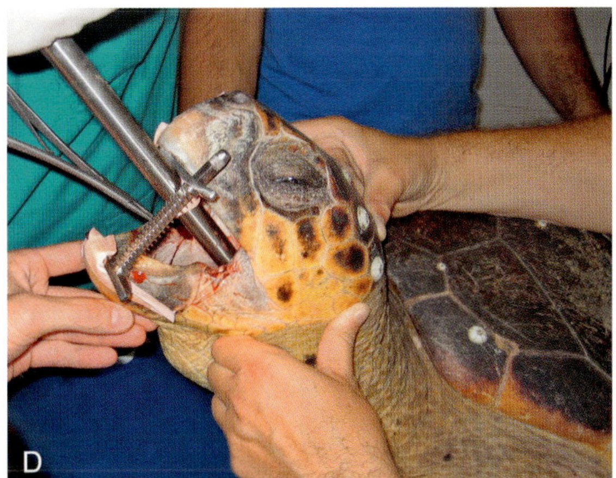

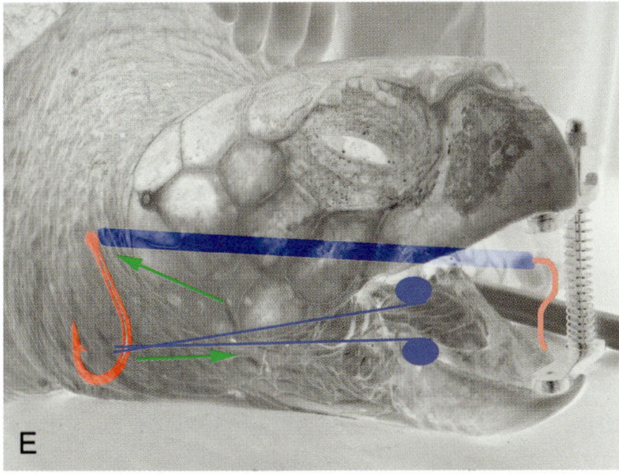

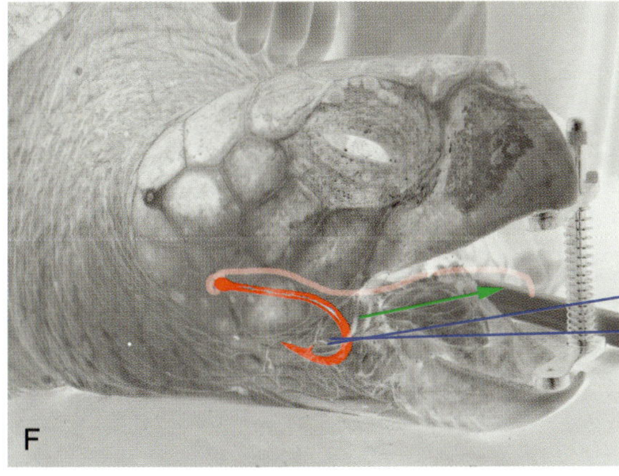

Fig. 3.58—cont'd (d) Keep the neck extended for increasing visibility inside the oral cavity. (e) Step 3: the metal tube works as a supporting axis and by means of a long surgical forceps grasps and rotates the hook. This process could be repeated one or more times for a complete rotation. (f) Step 4: when the hook is completely rotated, pull out the metal tube and gently remove the hook from the oesophagus.

(Continued)

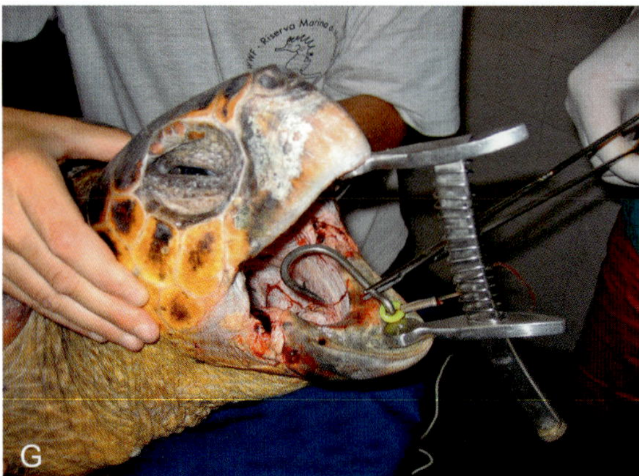

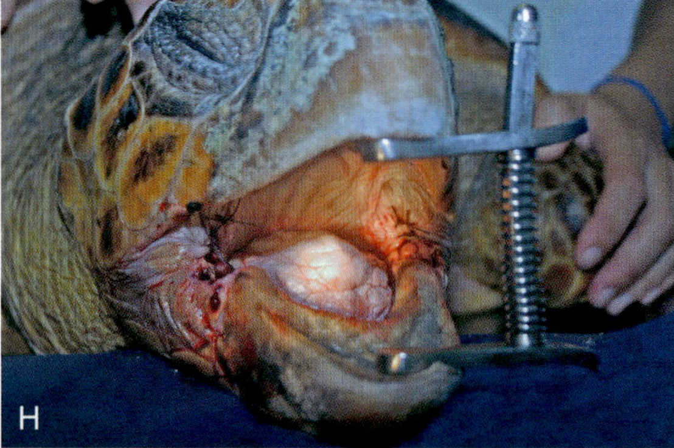

Fig. 3.58—cont'd (g) The free turned hook can be easily extracted from the oral cavity. (h) Step 5: the oral wounds caused by the line were treated and closed with simple interrupted sutures.

The head of the turtle was supported by a cushion and an assistant help was needed during the removing procedures.

During the first 24 hours postoperation, the sea turtle was maintained in an empty moist tank until its complete recovery from anaesthesia. The second day the turtle was moved to a larger tank filled with seawater, and antibiotic (enrofloxacin 10 mg/kg) diluted with normal saline solution was administered IM once daily for 10 days. Two days postoperation the sea turtle started to eat and it was released into the open sea after 30 days of hospitalization when it was completely recovered (Fig. 3.59).

2. Why during the de-hooking procedure is it necessary to rotate the hook before the extraction? Would it not be simpler to push the hook down with a de-hooker and then remove it?

Final diagnosis

- Oesophageal foreign body (fish hook and fishing line)

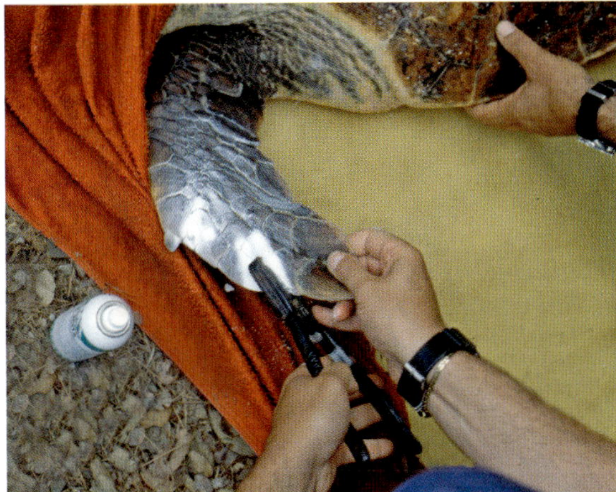

Fig. 3.59 Before release, the sea turtle was tagged on the left frontal flipper.

Discussion

Anthropic pressure on loggerhead sea turtle (*Caretta caretta*) populations has increased during the past decades and the ingestion of fishing hooks is a common injury that affects these marine reptiles. Suggested treatments vary from simple protocols to complicated and invasive surgery. Cutting the line as deep as possible without removing the hook is a protocol that should be avoided because in the long term a hook fixed with its line inside the digestive tract will affect the health and the hope of survival of an individual. On the other hand, oesophagostomy and even more invasive surgeries require longer postoperative hospitalization time and they are not always economically sustainable on a large scale. Therefore, non-invasive procedures should be used whenever possible. The technique described in this case is quite simple and does not require special medical equipment, although probably the same procedure could be better done by means of an endoscope. However, working with wildlife requires the development of simple, cheap and eco-sustainable veterinary techniques that could also be used in countries that do not have veterinary facilities or rescue centres for sea turtles. The only things you need are the injectable anaesthetic, some metallic tubes of different length, a canine mouth gag, a long forceps, gloves and a headlamp. Passing the line inside the metal tube that is gently pushed down the oesophagus can identify the location of the hook and therefore, when working in the field, radiography is not always necessary. The rotation *in situ* of the hook prior to extraction (see Fig. 3.58f.) is necessary because the oesophagus of the loggerhead sea turtle is very elastic (Fig. 3.60) and usually pushing down the hook with a de-hooker device simply extends the oesophagus without removing the hook from its fixing site (see Fig. 3.58d).

If the fish hook passes the oesophagus and fixes itself to the gastrointestinal mucosa, an invasive surgical approach is required. It is very important to remove the hook with the entire swallowed fishing line because, according to some authors, lethal injuries were related to the effect of strangulation and traction caused by the line inside the gastrointestinal tract rather than the presence of the hook.

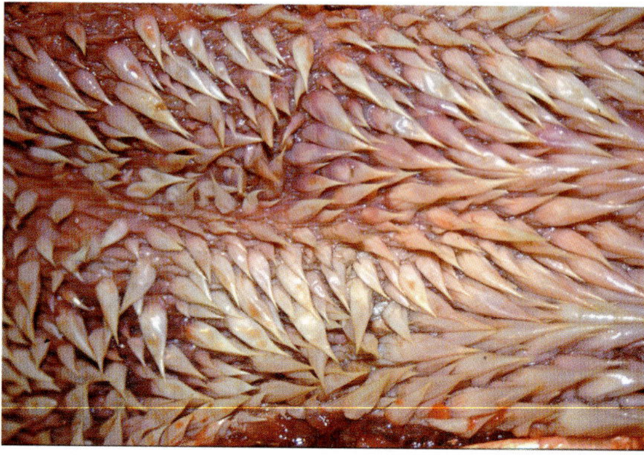

Fig. 3.60 The oesophageal mucosa of the loggerhead sea turtle (*Caretta caretta*) is very elastic and covered by several *papillae*. These anatomical features make the de-hooking procedure more difficult.

Further reading

Eckert, K.L., Bjorndal, K.A., Abreu-Grobois, F.A., et al., 1999. Research and Management Techniques for the Conservation of Sea Turtles. IUCN/SSC Marine Turtle Specialist Group Publication No. 4. Washington. Available online at the following URL: http://www.iucn-mtsg.org/publications/.

Epperly, S., Stokes, L., Dick, S., 2004. Careful release protocols for sea turtles release with minimal injury. NOAA Technical Memorandum NMFS-SEFSC-524. Available online at the following URL: http://www.nmfs.noaa.gov/sfa/hms/Protected%20Resources/TM_524.pdf.

FAO, 2004. Report of the expert consultation on interactions between sea turtles and fisheries within an ecosystem context. FAO Fisheries Report No. 738. Available online at the following URL: ftp://ftp.fao.org/docrep/fao/007/y5477e/y5477e00.pdf.

Phelan, S.M., Eckert, K.L., 2006. Marine Turtle Trauma Response Procedures: A Field Guide. Wider Caribbean Sea Turtle Conservation Network (WIDECAST) Technical Report No. 4. Beaufort, North Carolina. Available online at the following URL: http://www.widecast.org.

Valente, A.L.S., Parga, M.L., Velarde, R., et al., 2007. Fishhook lesions in Loggerhead sea turtles. J. Wildl. Dis. 43 (4), 737–741.

CHAPTER

Amphibians 4

Case 4.1 D. Fischer, M. Lierz

Clinical history

An Australian green tree frog (*Litoria caerulea*) was presented with the following clinical signs for one day:

- Swollen right thigh with boil-like distensions
- Inappetence.

The frog was acquired from a pet shop 2 years previously and it was unknown whether it was captive bred or wild caught. It was kept in a 60 cm × 40 cm × 60 cm sized aquaterrarium (1/4 water, 3/4 soil, pebbles and moss) together with a second Australian green tree frog of the same origin. The air humidity in the aquaterrarium was on average 60–80%, the air temperature about 26 °C and the water temperature about 22 °C. During the night the temperature decreased about 2 °C. Illumination and UV radiation were achieved by two 50 watt floodlit emitters over 12 hours daily. The food consisted of commercially-available larvae from darkling beetles (*Zophobas morio*), house crickets (*Acheta domesticus*), mealworms (*Tenebrio molitor*) and cockroaches (*Periplaneta americana*).

Clinical examination

On presentation, the frog had a good nutritional status (bodyweight 38 g). The animal was calm but alert and responsive. The general health and the animal's behaviour seemed to be unimpaired. The skin surface was smooth, moist and shiny. The mucous membrane in the mouth appeared pale pink-coloured and shiny. On the upper and lower surface of the right thigh were two 0.2 cm to 1.5 cm sized, whitish, round to oval, soft and elastic visible swellings. Similar distensions occurred on the frog's right foot and on its right body wall (Fig. 4.1).

Faecal examination and ultrasonographic examination (Fig. 4.2) were performed, followed by incision of the distensions.

Ultrasonographical examination

Ultrasonographic examination was done with a frequency of 12 MHz, using an examination glove filled with water as aqueous standoff. Several distensions were examined. Figure 4.2 shows a 1.39 cm × 0.92 cm sized, liquid-filled vesicle on the frog's right thigh.

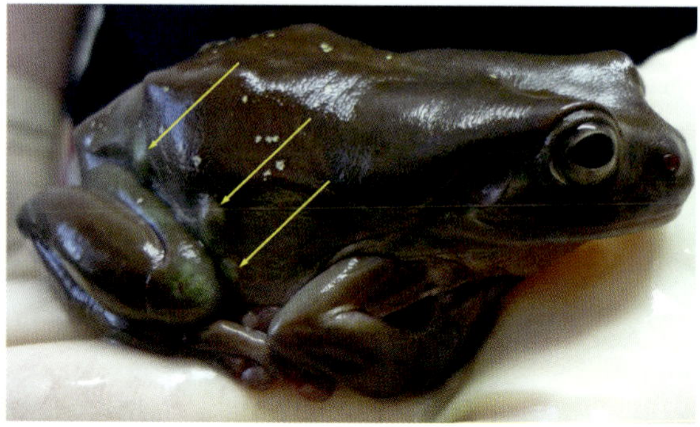

Fig. 4.1 Australian green tree frog (*Litoria caerulea*) with several boil-like distensions (yellow arrows) on its right body wall.

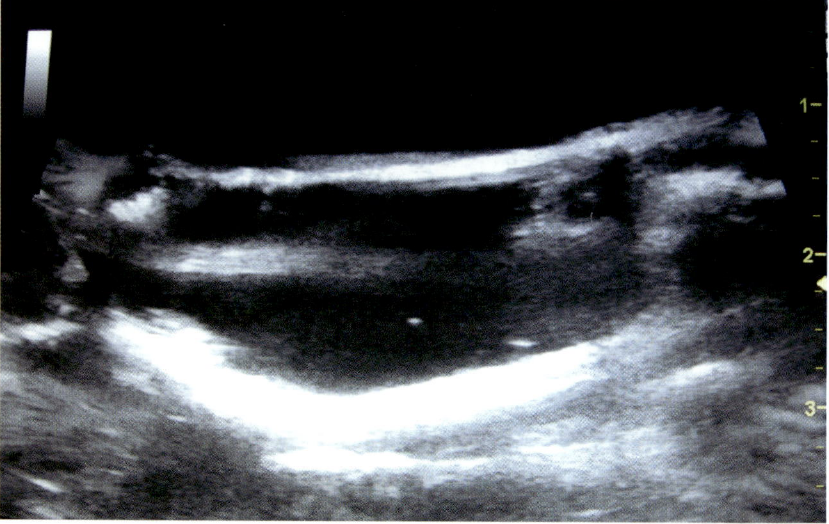

Fig. 4.2 Ultrasonographic examination of the frog's right thigh. A 1.39 cm × 0.92 cm sized vesicle is focused. An examination glove filled with water is used as aqueous standoff.

1. What is your interpretation of the sonograph?

Diagnostic lancing and laboratory examination

Incision of distensions

One vesicle at the frog's right foot and one on its abdominal wall were incised using a 23-G-needle. Several white objects were removed (Fig. 4.3) and microscopically evaluated.

A swab was taken out of one vesicle and subjected to a microbiological examination.

Q *2. What is your interpretation of the removed structures (see Fig. 4.3)?*

Results

- Ultrasonographic examination: in the subcutaneous, liquid-filled vesicles, several 0.2–0.4 cm sized hyperechogenic structures are visible
- Faecal examination using flotation and sedimentation techniques showed negative result for the presence of endoparasites
- Microbiological examination revealed a medium amount of *Enterobacter* spp., *Bacillus* spp. and *Staphylococcus* spp.
- In microscopic magnification (100×), the removed white structures showed peristaltic movement

Please evaluate the clinical history, Figs 4.1– 4.3, the results of the physical examination, diagnostic lancing and laboratory tests.

Q *3. List your differential diagnoses.*

Q *4. List your further diagnostic strategy.*

Q *5. List your therapeutic strategy.*

Differential diagnoses for subcutaneous swellings in frogs

- Subcutaneous larvae of cestodes or tapeworms, so called plerocercoids
- Subcutaneous stages of nematodes, e.g. filariae
- Subcutaneous larvae of acanthocephala or thorny-headed worms, so-called cystacantha
- Subutaneous larvae of trematoda or flukes, so-called metacercaria, e.g. *Clinostomum*

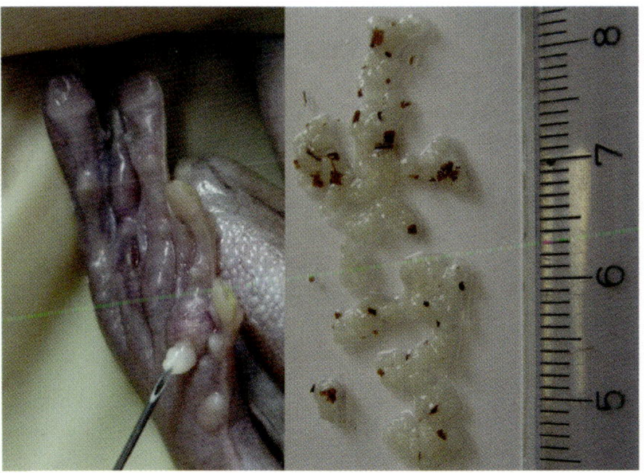

Fig. 4.3 Left side: using a 23 G needle, one distension on the frog's right foot was incised and several white objects were removed. Right side: in the procedure approximately 50 0.1–0.8 cm sized, irregularly shaped, white, partly transparent and tough objects were removed. Single objects were up to 3 cm long. The brown particles are soil from the aquaterrarium.

- Chronic, progressive myositis caused by microsporidia, e.g. *Pleistophora myotrophica*
- Myositis caused by *Ichthyophonus*-like protozoa
- Cysts and dermal nodules caused by *Amphibiocystidium (= Dermocystidium, Dermosporidium* and *Dermocystoides)*
- Dermal or subcutaneous granulomas, often caused by mycobacteria (e.g. *Mycobacterium xenopi, M. marinum, M. fortuitum*) or fungi like *Saprolegnia* (e.g. *S. parasitica*), *Basidobolus* (e.g. *B. ranarum*), *Mucor* (e.g. *M. amphibiorum*) or *Cladiosporum*
- Neoplasias, spontaneous or caused by viral agents like herpesviruses, e.g. Lucké tumour virus (LTHV or RaHV-1)
- Oedemas or dermal ulcers caused by ranaviruses from the family *Iridoviridae*

Further diagnostics

- Because of the morphology and the peristaltic movements, the structures were suspected to be of parasitic origin. To determine the family and/or genus of a parasitic structure, the removed structures were fixed in alcohol and submitted to specialized institutions (Fischer et al. 2010) for parasitology. A morphological, histological and molecular biological examination was performed
- Morphological and histological examinations revealed the structures as plerocercoids of pseudophyllid cestodes, termed spargana
- Molecular biological examination identified the parasite species as *Spirometra erinaceieuropaei*

Therapy (Table 4.1)

Table 4.1 Therapy

Praziquantel	15 mg/kg SC twice, every second week
Isoflurane	0.015 ml/g liquid isoflurane topically on the skin – to maintain anaesthesia during the surgery
Incision of the vesicles using a 23 G needle	In total about 50 0.1–0.8 cm sized, irregularly shaped, white, partly transparent and tough objects were removed from the vesicles. Some objects were up to 3 cm long
Quarantine	During the medication on wet towels
Disinfection of the aquaterrarium	Neopredisan® 135-1 (Menno GmbH, Norderstedt, Germany)

Discussion

Amphibians act as definitive hosts but more often as intermediate hosts of cestodes worldwide. In the two-phase life cycle of *Spirometra erinaceieuropaei*, amphibians, reptiles and rodents are common intermediate hosts. *Litoria cerulea* is also regularly reported as host of this tapeworm. The first larval stages of the cestode, the procercoids, develop in copepods as first intermediate hosts. If amphibians act as second intermediate host, the copepods may be already eaten by the tadpoles. Later, the plerocercoids develop inside the amphibians also during the metamorphosis. Cats, as preferred definitive host and other vertebrates get infected by eating the plerocercoid-containing intermediate host. As *Spirometra erinaceieuropaei* has no specific definitive host, humans may get infected too. However, the parasite infects humans not only by ingestion. In fact, the sparganosis is frequently transmitted to humans by applying raw meat on wounds and inflammatory processes, which is a routine treatment in Asia. Therefore, sparganosis is a common zoonosis in East Asia. The larval stages of the parasite are able to move from the raw meat and from contaminated water actively into the human.

In the tadpoles, an infection with plerocercoids results in prolonged growth. In the adult amphibian, they affect peritoneum, liver and other tissues. In the intermediate host, they cause boil-like distensions of skeletal muscles and skin by settling down in these tissues. If a frog is a definitive host, an infection may be clinically unapparent or unspecific. Symptoms like ileus, obstipation, cachexia, blood loss, necrosis and atrophy of the intestinal mucosa are described in immunosuppressed animals, after suffering transport or stress.

The faecal examination revealed negative results for endoparasites because only larval stages but no egg-producing adult cestodes were present in the frog. In general, tapeworm eggs can be demonstrated by using sedimentation techniques. The thorough examination of the removed structures was important to plan further steps of diagnosis and therapy. While the exact species diagnosis was done out of scientific interest, the identification and classification of the parasite was necessary to choose the right medication.

As therapy of a subcutaneous sparganosis, the surgical removal of plerocercoids is indicated. This should be performed under general anaesthesia to reduce potential pain and stress for the animal. As the larvae may also lie in deeper tissues and organs, praziquantel should be administered in parallel to treat cestodes. The literature provides a high dosage range (5–24 mg/kg) and different application intervals (once or twice every second week). Oral, subcutaneous, intracoelomical or topical administrations are described as application routes in amphibians. However, the dosage of 15 mg/kg SC twice every second week used in the present case did not lead to any side effects in the animal and was able to cure the disease in conjunction with surgical intervention.

In this case, the green tree frog probably was imported to Europe. It is most likely that the frog was infected for a long time before he came into the pet shop, especially as the second frog was without symptoms and should have been also affected if the aquaterrarium were contaminated. However, a later infection cannot be excluded but seems unlikely because the obligatory intermediate hosts in the parasitic life cycle must be present. The patient responded well on removal of the plerocercoids and two injections of praziquantel. No new distensions or swellings on the frog's body surface appeared and the animal recovered well from treatment.

Further reading

Berger, L., Skerratt, L.F., Zhu, X., et al., 2009. Severe sparganosis in Australian tree frogs. J. Wildl. Dis. 45, 921–929.

Fischer, D., Heuser, W., Pantchev, N. et al., 2010. Subcutaneous sparganosis in an Australian green tree frog (*Litoria caerulea*). Tierärztl. Prax. 38 (K), 249–253.

Mutschmann, F., 2010. Parasitosen der Amphibien. In: Mutschmann, F. (Ed.), Erkrankungen der Amphibien, 2. Aufl., Parey, Berlin.

Okamoto, M., Iseto, C., Shibahara, T., et al., 2007. Intraspecific variation of *Spirometra erinaceieuropaei* and phylogenetic relationship between *Spirometra* and *Diphyllobothrium* inferred from mitochondrial CO1 gene sequences. Parasitol. Int. 56 (3), 235–238.

Zhu, X.Q., Beveridge, I., Berger, L., et al., 2002. Single-strand conformation polymorphism-based analysis reveals genetic variation within *Spirometra erinacei* (Cestoda: *Pseudophyllidea*) from Australia. Mol. Cell. Probes 16 (2), 159–165.

Case 4.2 *L. Jepson*

Clinical history

Anderson's salamander (*Ambystoma andersoni*) (Fig. 4.4) is an aquatic, paedomorphic salamander closely related to the more commonly seen axolotl (*A. mexicanum*). An 18-month-old captive-bred Anderson's salamander (*Ambystoma andersoni*) was presented with the following signs:

- Swollen body that had developed over the course of around 4 days
- Increased respiratory (gill movements) rate
- Inappetance.

The salamander was one of two maintained with one albino axolotl in a 200 litre home aquarium. Filtration was with undergravel filtration. Water temperature was around 18 °C. pH was 7.5. Ammonia and nitrite levels were zero ppm and nitrates were 50 ppm. Other water quality parameters were not measured. They were fed primarily on defrosted frozen bloodworm and brine shrimp.

Physical examination

The salamander appeared swollen and oedematous to the touch. The gills were considered paler than expected. An increased respiratory rate was noted but the stress of capture and transport did mean that this was difficult to interpret.

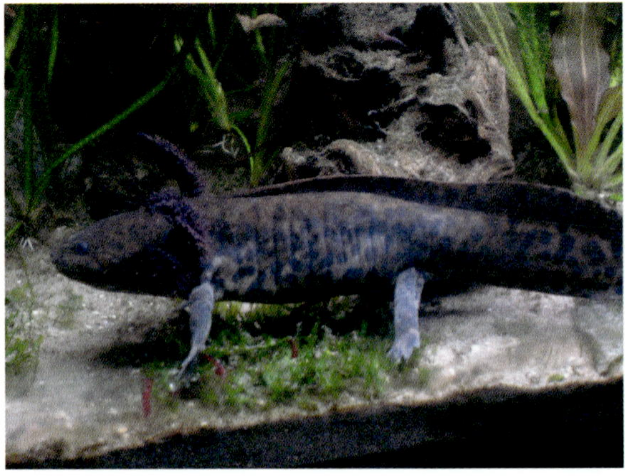

Fig. 4.4 The Anderson's salamander is an aquatic, paedomorphic salamander closely related to the more commonly seen axolotl.

After discussion with the owner it was decided to euthanase the salamander with MS222 on humane grounds.

1. In general terms, what would your provisional list of differential diagnoses be for a salamander showing such signs?

Post-mortem examination

The salamander weighed 72 g. The body cavity appeared swollen and oedematous (Fig. 4.5). A mid-line incision was made ventrally to open the coelomic cavity (Fig. 4.6). There was some coelomic fluid but this was not considered excessive.

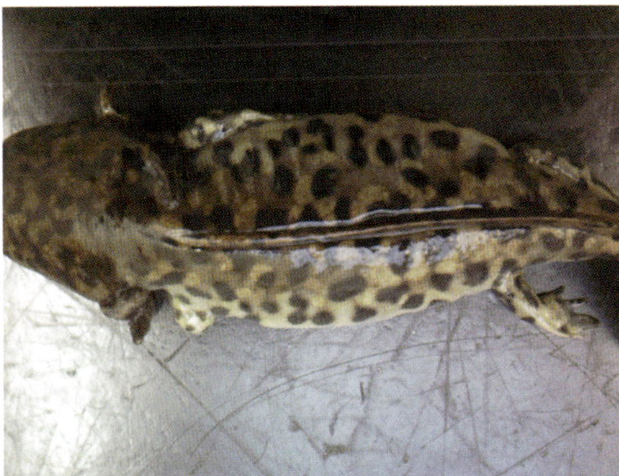

Fig. 4.5 The body cavity of the salamander appeared swollen and oedematous.

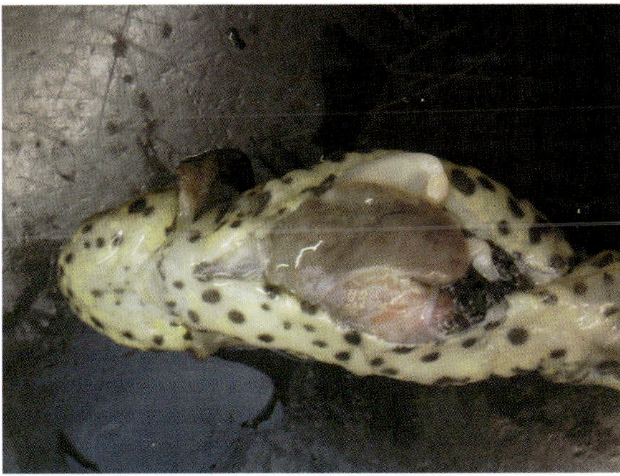

Fig. 4.6 Post-mortem examination. A mid-line incision was made ventrally to open the coelomic cavity.

2. Consider the post-mortem pictures. What is most strikingly obvious, especially in Fig. 4.6? Does this make you alter your differential list?

The carcass was placed into formal saline and submitted for histopathology.

Histopathology results

The main findings on histology were:

- The salamander was in good physical condition
- Gills: the gill filaments are lined with a variably simple to stratified squamous epithelium with a few goblet cells and a few presumed alarm cells. In the stroma, there is a rare deposition of fibrin, light infiltration of small round cells (presumed inflammatory leucocytes) and at the base of the filaments, expansion by clear space (oedema)
- The lungs have a focally mild heterophilic, histiocytic and lesser lymphoplasmacellular infiltration consistent with chronic suppurative and granulomatous pneumonia
- Spleen: there is a moderate, diffuse heterophilic, histiocytic and lesser lymphoplasmacellular infiltration. Moderate numbers of apoptotic cells are seen. Multifocal areas of acute coagulative necrosis are present (moderate diffuse chronic necrosuppurative and granulomatous splenitis)
- Small and large intestine: mild to moderate autolytic changes. Also a mild lymphoplasmacellular infiltration of the mucosa
- Liver: this is grossly abnormal with loss of normal architecture. The hepatic cords are widely separated and unusually compressed; the sinusoids and the space of Disse are greatly expanded by clear space (oedema). They are, however, also loosely infiltrated by spindle cells (fibrosis), along with fewer melanocyes and leucocytes. There are also bands of fibrous connective tissue, areas of necrosis and a moderate to diffuse heterophilic and lymphoplasmacellular infiltration. Bile canaliculi are prominent and frequently contain bile plugs. The subcapsular space is expanded by prominent haematopoeisis. No inclusion bodies are present
- There is a mild multifocal to diffuse interstitial heterophilic, histiocytic and lesser lymphoplasmacellular infiltration (chronic suppurative and granulomatous nephritis)

3. Based upon the above, would you consider asking the laboratory to undertake further staining techniques, and if so, which ones?

Differential diagnoses for coelomic swelling in aquatic amphibia

- Osmoregulation dysfunction (poor water quality, renal disease, gill disease, liver disease, cardiovascular disease, environmental intoxication)
- Renal disease (iridovirus, bacterial or fungal nephritis, neoplasia, *Entamoeba ranarum* [renal amoebiasis], myxosporea, parasitic trematodes)
- Cardiovascular, haematologic and/or lymphatic disease (cardiomyopathy, lymph heart failure, anaemia, neoplasia, endocarditis, trypanosomes, microfilaria)

- Hepatic disease (bacterial and fungal hepatitis, mycobacteriosis, neoplasia, amoebiasis)
- Renal disease (bacterial or fungal nephritis, iridovirus, neoplasia)
- Systemic disease (neoplasia, iridovirus, mycobacteriosis, bacteraemic infections, fungal infections)
- Gill disease (bacterial or fungal infections, ectoparasitic infections, poor water quality neoplasia)
- Lung disease (acute pulmonary emphysema)
- Gastrointestinal disease (gas build up secondary to intestinal disease or foreign body)
- Reproductive disorders (ovarian or uterine stasis)
- Environmental toxins

PAS reaction and Giemsa stains were non-contributory. However, Ziehl-Neelsen staining revealed moderate numbers of rod-shaped acid-fast bacilli, approximately 10 µm. They were present both in the interstitium and in macrophages.

Diagnosis

A diagnosis of systemic mycobacteriosis was made based upon histopathological findings and ZN staining. The most likely candidate was thought to be *Mycobacterium marinum*, which is the commonest cause of mycobacteriosis in fish and amphibia, and can also infect reptiles, although neither culture nor PCR was undertaken on this occasion.

In this salamander, the infection was systemic and, although it had primarily affected the liver producing a severe necrosuppurative and granulomatous hepatitis, the kidneys, intestines, liver, spleen and gills were also infected. The oedema was probably secondary to a combination of osmoregulatory dysfunction secondary to the liver, renal and gill disease, plus blood and lymphatic circulatory compromise as a result of localized vascular and lymphatic compression.

4. If mycobacteriosis had been diagnosed ante-mortem, for example on biopsy, how would you manage this case? What would you need to discuss with the owner?

Discussion

Mycobacteria are common pathogens of aquatic environments, and are frequently found as free-living constituents of the bacterial flora, either in the water column or as soil-associated saprophytes. Infection in amphibians is often linked to immune suppression typically secondary to environmental stressors such as poor water quality, high temperatures and poor nutrition. Super-exposure could also contribute such as being fed on mycobacteria-infected feeder fish.

Mycobacteria, including *M. marinum*, are both difficult to treat effectively and are potential zoonoses. One regimen suggested for ornamental tropical fish involved kanamycin at 50 mg/l every 48 hours for four treatments (Conroy and Conroy 1999).

Often euthanasia is recommended (Wright 2006) both as a means of managing animal welfare and to control contamination of the immediate environment. Depending upon where the mycobacterial granulomas are, infective organisms may be passed in the faeces or urine, or transmitted by cannibalism of dead or moribund individuals.

There are many potential causes of coelomic swelling and mortalities in Ambystomid salamanders, especially larvae and paedomorphic adults. In the context of unexplained mortalities in such salamanders, two diseases are worthy of further mention. The first is iridoviral infection, such as *Ambystoma tigrinum* ranavirus from Arizona (ATV) (Davidson et al. 2003a). The second is chytridiomycosis. Tiger salamanders (*A. tigrinum*) seem relatively resistant to *Batrachochytrium dendrobatidis*, although they can carry heavy skin burdens and act as possible reservoirs for this serious fungal infection (Davidson et al. 2003b).

Further reading

Conroy, G., Conroy, D.A., 1999. Acid-fast bacterial infection and its control in guppies (*Lebistes reticulatus*) reared on an ornamental fish farm in Venezuela. Vet. Rec. 144, 177–178.

Davidson, E.W., Jancovich, J.K., Borland, S., et al., 2003a. What's your diagnosis? Dermal lesions, hemorrhage, and limb swelling in laboratory axolotls. Lab. Anim. 32 (3), 23–25.

Davidson, E.W., Parris, M., Collins, J.P., et al., 2003b. Pathogenicity and transmission of Chytridiomycosis in tiger salamanders (*Ambystoma tigrinum*). Copeia 3, 601–607.

Wright, K.M., 2006. Overview of amphibian medicine. In: Mader, D.R. (Ed.), Reptile Medicine and Surgery, second ed. Saunders Elsevier, St Louis.

Case 4.3 *B. Gartrell*

Clinical history

A 3-month-old juvenile Japanese fire-bellied newt (*Cynops pyrrhogaster*) was purchased from a pet store approximately one month ago. The newt has a twisted back, which is getting worse as the animal grows. The growth of this animal is severely stunted in comparison to normal growth rates. The newt is kept in an indoor glass tank with access to natural sunlight provided by a nearby window. The substrate is a mix of damp moss, shelving gravel and water. The tank has a temperature range from 18 to 23 °C. The newt is fed whiteworms (*Enchytraeus albidus*) on a daily basis.

Physical examination

On physical examination, the newt weighs 0.8 g and has a marked curving lateral deviation of the vertebral column (Fig. 4.7). The newt is weak and has poor strength and movement in its limbs. Faecal examination by microscopic examination of a wet mount shows no evidence of parasites. The small size of the amphibian prevents further diagnostic testing.

Summary of diagnostic results

Please evaluate the clinical history, Fig. 4.7 and the results of the physical examination.

1. List your differential diagnoses.

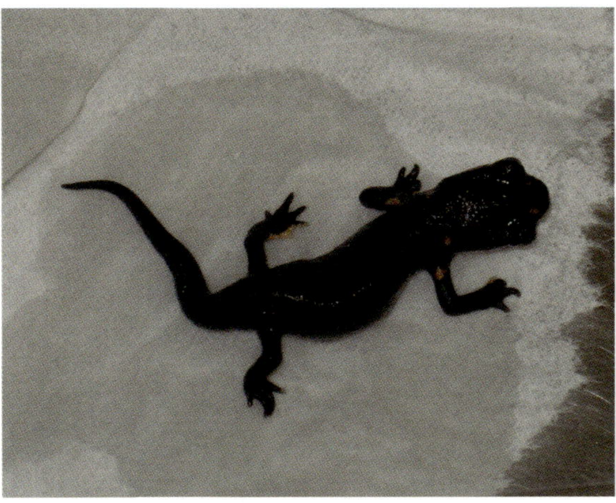

Fig. 4.7 On physical examination, the newt showed a marked curving lateral deviation of the vertebral column.

 *2. List your therapeutic strategy.*

Differential diagnoses

- Nutritional secondary hyperparathyroidism
- Congenital deformity of the spine
- Traumatic spinal fracture and remodelling
- Discospondylitis

Therapy

- Supplementary UVB light
- Calcium gluconate supplementation – 2% solution 1–2 hour bath SID
- Encourage greater dietary diversity of live and commercial foods to improve the calcium:phosphorus balance of the diet

The newt improved rapidly in strength and activity with this therapy, although the spinal deformity remained unchanged. The newt refused to eat food other than the whiteworms. Over the next 2 years the newt continued to grow more slowly than expected. The spinal deformity remained but the newt was otherwise well.

Final diagnosis

- Nutritional secondary hyperparathyroidism and hypocalcaemia

Discussion

This case presented challenges in that the small size of the patient precluded many diagnostic tests. The provisional diagnosis of nutritional secondary hyperparathyroidism and hypocalcaemia was made on the basis of the clinical history and clinical examination. The clinical response to a treatment trial with UVB light and calcium supplementation is strongly suggestive that hypocalcaemia was responsible for the poor growth and muscular weakness. In larger animals, radiographs, clinical pathology (ionized calcium, serum vitamin D concentrations) and bone densitometry can be useful in confirming a diagnosis.

Regular glass is impervious to UV light, so placing the tank near the window will not improve the newt's access to UV light. Many public websites state that newts do not require UV light, although most veterinary sources suggest that it is probably required. The newts in the wild show strong responses to photoperiod so natural light and its cycles are important in coordinating their endogenous cycles. UVB light is most important for the metabolism of vitamin D. Affordable light meters are now available and are the best option for keepers to check the UV output of commercially available bulbs. The UV output of these bulbs varies between and within brands and will diminish as bulbs age.

The monotonous whiteworm diet is also likely to result in calcium to phosphorus imbalance in the diet although the exact nutritional composition of the worms is not available. In the absence of specific nutritional recommendations, the use of diverse food items is recommended. Another strategy for improving the nutritional content of live food items is to gut-load them with a nutritional supplement.

Further reading

Hadfield, C.A., Whitaker, B.R., 2005. Amphibian emergency medicine and care. Seminars in Avian and Exotic Pet Medicine 14 (2), 79–89.

Marunouchi, J., Ueda, H., Ochi, O., 2000. Variation in age and size among breeding populations at different altitudes in the Japanese newt, *Cynops pyrrhogaster*. Amphibia-Reptilia 21 (3), 381–396.

Matsui, K., Mochida, K., Nakamura, M., 2003. Food habit of the juvenile of the Japanese newt *Cynops pyrrhogaster*. Zool. Sci. 20 (7), 855–859.

Nagai, K., Oishi, T., 1998. Behavioral rhythms of the Japanese newt, *Cynops pyrrhogaster*, under a semi-natural condition. Int. J. Biometeorol. 41 (3), 105–112.

Pough, F.H., 2007. Amphibian biology and husbandry. ILAR J. 48 (3), 203–213.

CHAPTER

Fishes 5

Case 5.1 L. Jepson

Clinical history

A telephone call was received from an aquarist who was concerned about one of his female Frontosa cichlids.

- A large, black swelling was visible on the first gill arch on the right hand side
- This female had a relatively recent history of not brooding her egg clutches to full term

This female *Cyphotilapia frontosa* was part of a breeding group consisting of two males and five females. The aquarium was 180 cm × 60 cm × 60 cm. Temperature was 28 °C. The pH was 8.1. Ammonia and nitrite were zero. Nitrate was 20 mg/l. *C. frontosa* are part of the cichlid species flock originating from Lake Tanganyika. They are maternal mouth brooders.

Physical examination

The cichlid was presented in a bucket of water that had been taken from its aquarium. The fish was showing atypical dark marking, probably as a result of the stress of transport.

The fish was netted and the gills briefly examined by alternately lifting the operculae with the fish restrained in the net. A dark mass could be seen associated with the gills on the right hand side (Fig. 5.1).

Clinical diagnosis examination

Examination under anaesthetic

The fish was subsequently examined under anaesthetic. A solution of tricaine methanesulphonate (MS222), dissolved in a saturated solution of $NaHCO_3$ to form a buffered stock solution of 10 g/l, was used to anaesthetize the fish. This was added incrementally until the cichlid began to show signs of induction, notably loss of the righting reflex.

Once the fish was failing to respond to external stimuli but respiration was still good (as judged by opercular movements), the cichlid was removed from the water and placed on a surface of damp tissue.

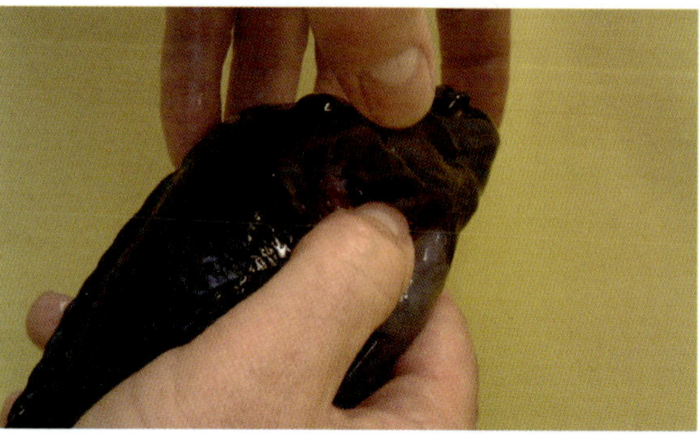

Fig. 5.1 A dark mass can be seen along the leading edge of the first gill arch, flanked by gill rakers at either end.

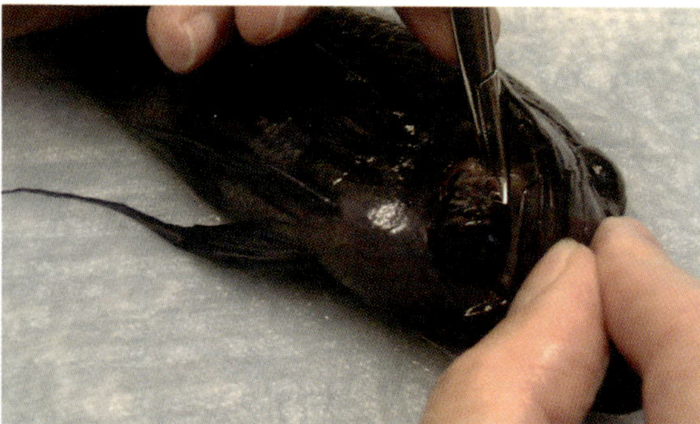

Fig. 5.2 The mass was hidden on the lingual side of the branchial arches.

Anaesthesia was continued by syringing oxygenated water into the mouth such that it flowed over the gills and out through the operculae. This mimics the physiologically normal direction of water flow so as not to short circuit the normal counter current gaseous exchange mechanism. Anaesthesia was maintained by alternating exposure either to water with MS222 if the fish appeared to be light or without if thought to be on a deep enough plane of anaesthesia.

The mass was examined. It appeared to be larger than initially thought, with the bulk of the mass hidden on the lingual side of the branchial arches (Fig. 5.2).

1. List your differential diagnoses.

Differential diagnoses for gill mass

- Parasitic cyst such as a cestode, or Microsporidial such as *Glugea*
- Granuloma (may be fungal such as *Ichthyophonus* or bacterial, for example *Epitheliocystis*)
- Neoplasia
- Foreign body granuloma
- Viral such as *Lymphocystis*

Therapy

2. What treatment options are available to you?

Treatment options are limited but would include:

- Biopsy and appropriate treatment for non-neoplastic conditions
- Surgical debulking. Possible but risky in view of the potentially highly vascular tissue involved
- Surgical resection
- Surgical debulking followed by weekly cisplatin injections may be considered for skin tumours, but again this mass is in a very vascular area and surgical debulking and chemotherapy may be highly risky.

It was elected to remove the mass surgically. This was achieved by resection of the first branchial arch. This was clamped at either end and ligated with PDS (Fig. 5.3). Antibiotic cover was provided with an intramuscular injection of 1 mg marbofloxacin. Recovery involved placing the cichlid back into water that did not contain MS222.

The mass was some 2.0 cm in diameter and was submitted for histological examination (Fig. 5.4).

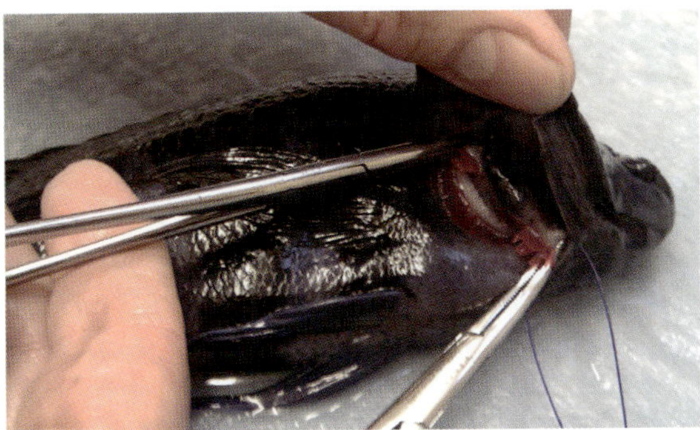

Fig. 5.3 The mass was surgically removed. This was achieved by resection of the first branchial arch. This was clamped at either end and ligated with PDS.

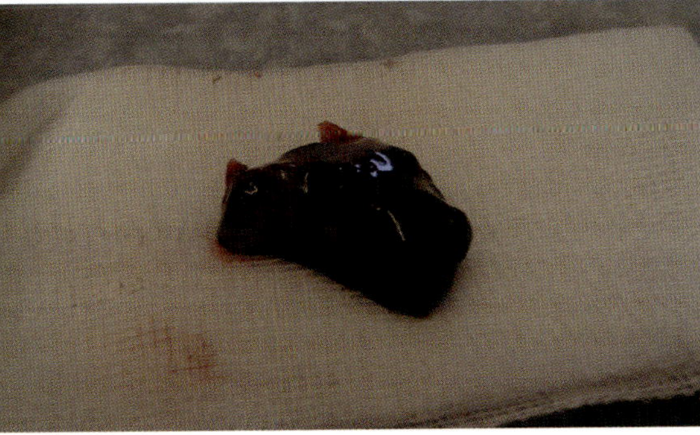

Fig. 5.4 The mass was 2 cm in diameter and was submitted for histological examination.

Histopathological diagnosis

The removed mass was histopathologically identified as a low-grade spindle cell sarcoma. No evidence for metastasis was noted.

Discussion

Spindle cell sarcomas are a wide group of mesenchymal malignancies that can originate from many different cells of origin and include fibrosarcomas, smooth muscle tumours and peripheral nerve sheath neoplasms. Typically, sarcomas prove to be locally invasive and destructive malignancies, although metastasis is rare. It is interesting here that this tumour also caused incubation difficulties in the previously successful mouth-brooding female. Whether this was a physical problem and she was unable to contain the full volume of the mass and her developing brood in the oral cavity, or whether it was because the mass was already compromising her respiration such that the presence of the brood proved one stressor too far, is unknown.

A variety of gill neoplasms have been recorded including papillomas, squamous cell carcinomas, branchioblastomas and chondromas (Childs and Whitaker 2001). Sarcomas have been well described in a variety of fish (Earnest-Koons et al. 1996, Lewbart et al. 1998, Schmale et al. 2002), although their presence in cichlids does not appear to have been widely reported. In the walleye, dermal sarcomas are due to a retroviral infection and can be transmitted (Earnest-Koons et al. 1996) – interestingly, other sarcomas in fish appear to be linked to viral agents or at least a virus-like agent (Schmale et al. 2002),

Surgical resection in this case should give a satisfactory outcome. There appears grossly to be several millimetres of normal gill tissue on either side of the tumour and, histologically, no evidence of metastasis was noted. No evidence of a viral infection was noted, although this cannot be excluded on histology alone.

Further reading

Childs, S., Whitaker, B.R., 2001. Respiratory disease. In: Wildgoose, W.H. (Ed.), BSAVA Manual of Ornamental Fish, second ed. British Small Animal Veterinary Association, Gloucester, p. 145.

Earnest-Koons, K., Wooster, G.A., Bowser, P.R., 1996. Invasive walleye dermal sarcoma in laboratory-maintained walleyes *Stizostedion vitreum*. Dis. Aquat. Organ. 24, 227–232.

Lewbart, G.A., Spodnick, G., Barlow, N., et al., 1998. Surgical removal of an undifferentiated abdominal sarcoma from a koi carp (*Cyprinus carpio*). Vet. Rec. 143 (20), 556–558.

Schmale, M.C., Gibbs, P.D.L., Campbell, C.E., 2002. A virus-like agent associated with neurofibromatosis in damselfish. Dis. Aquat. Organ. 49, 107–115.

Case 5.2 *L. Jepson*

Clinical history

Two common goldfish (*Carassius auratus*) were presented. The owner claimed that two or three fish per day were dying. Over the previous 3 weeks the owner had lost roughly half of his fish.

The pond is a butyl-lined formal pond with rough dimensions of 3 m × 2.5 m × 60 cm deep, and has been there for around 12 years. There are some marginal plants and it is filtered and has an extra pump installed to improve circulation. It held a mixture of goldfish and common carp and losses had been seen in both. The pond had been considered overstocked through natural breeding and so some had been re-homed previously. No new fish had been introduced in the last 2 years. A sample of his pond water had been checked by a local aquatics' retailer and he was told that it was fine, although he had no idea what had been checked. The water temperature was unknown.

The owner reported that the fish were trying to feed but were not ingesting the food; some were sluggish, some appeared to be quite swollen. They were not considered to be gasping at the surface and there were no obvious haemorrhagic lesions.

Physical examination

Both goldfish were considered to be in good physical condition. No haemorrhages or ulcers could be seen. The gills appeared pale and clogged with thick grey mucus.

Post-mortem diagnosis examination

Initially a skin scrape was taken, and then both fish were euthanased with intravenous pentobarbitone (Fig. 5.5). A post-mortem examination was then undertaken. The first goldfish weighed 179 g and had a standard length of 152 mm. The results for this first goldfish are:

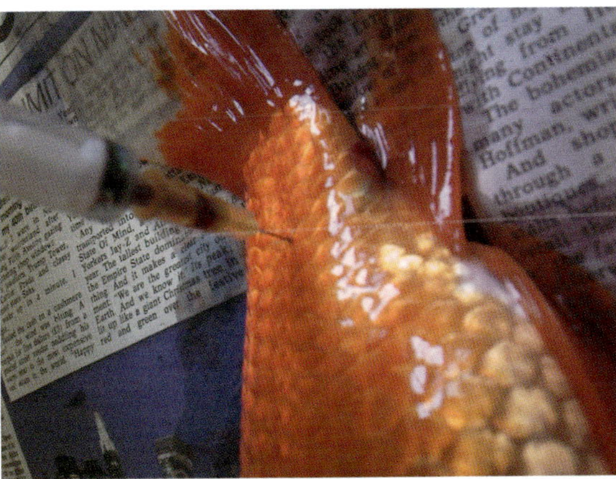

Fig. 5.5 A skin scrape was taken and both fish were euthanased with intravenous pentobarbitone.

Skin scrape

- Under 40× lens, a moderate number of flatworm-like parasites could be seen. The most distinguishing features of these were apparent hooks at the back end and four "eye spots" at the "head" end

Gill squash

- Huge numbers of these parasites were found
- Normal gill lamellar architecture disrupted. Significant clubbing of lamellae

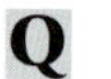 *1. What are these parasites likely to be?*

The parasites were identified as gill flukes – *Dactylogyrus* spp. They are readily distinguished from *Gyrodactylus* (skin flukes) by the characteristic four eye spots, plus *Gyrodactylus* are livebearers and the unborn fluke can frequently be seen inside the body of the adult. It was noted that the occasional protozoa *Ichthyobodo* spp. was seen at 100× magnification. Site of discovery is no real clue to identification – gill flukes, as in this case, will happily spread on to and survive on the skin, while skin flukes can occasionally infect the gills.

 *2. Why is it important to distinguish between* **Dactylogyrus** *and* **Gyrodactylus**?

On examination of the coelomic cavity, the fish was revealed to be female with well-developed ovaries showing evidence of asynchronous egg development. The carcass was very fatty and the caudal kidney appeared very soft with a loss of normal texture. The spleen appeared enlarged (Fig. 5.6).

The second goldfish weighed 151 g, and had a standard length of 162 mm and had a similar presentation.

To investigate the possibility of underlying disease, the following samples were taken from the first goldfish and submitted for histopathology:

- Heart
- Gills
- Hepatopancreas
- Spleen
- Head kidney.

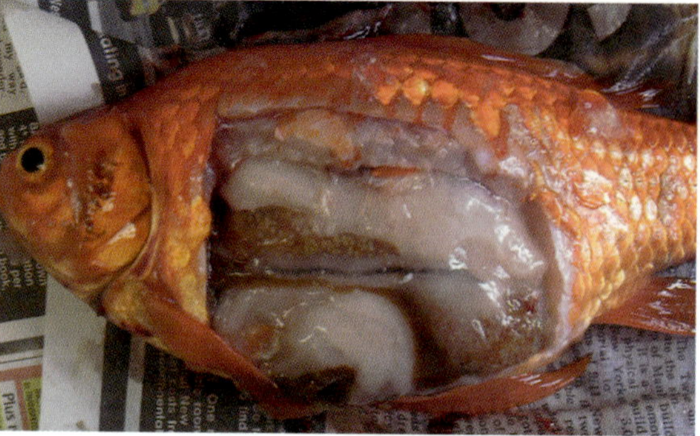

Fig. 5.6 Post-mortem examination. The fish was a female with well-developed ovaries. The carcass was very fatty and the caudal kidney appeared very soft with loss of normal texture. The spleen appeared enlarged.

Histopathology results

- Heart: no lesions visible
- Gills: severe hyperplasia of the branchial epithelium, from the base to the tip of the primary lamella. The basal filament epithelium is severely proliferative such that secondary lamellae are frequently obscured. The lamina propria is moderately infiltrated by mixed leucocytes and the vasculature is engorged. Between the filaments, there are innumerable, transverse to oblique to rarely longitudinal sections of metazoan parasites approximately 30–100 μm in diameter, with an eosinophilic cuticle, parenchymatous body, no visible digestive tract and occasionally visible sucker. Some of the organisms show either internal ova or internal spermatozoa
- Hepatopancreas: this section also contained free pancreatic tissue and adipose tissue. The hepatocytes contained occasional proteinaceous droplets. Two small granulomas were present in the serosa and adjacent adipose tissue near the free pancreas
- Spleen: free pancreatic tissue was attached here too. There were a few tiny granulomas in the interstitial tissue between the spleen and adjacent fragments of free pancreas
- Head kidney: tubular epithelial cells frequently contained proteinaceous material. Otherwise all appeared normal

Q *3. List your differential diagnoses.*

Q *4. Ziehl-Neelsen staining was negative. Does this change your differential diagnoses list in any way?*

Q *5. List your therapeutic strategy.*

Differential diagnoses

- Ectoparasitic infestation, e.g. with *Dactylogyrus* and *Ichthyobodo*
- Bacterial gill disease
- Fungal gill disease
- Peracute septicaemia
- Spring viraemia of carp
- Cyprinid herpesvirus 2
- Poor water quality
- Water-borne toxins

Therapy

This goldfish, and probably the other one too, had a severe proliferative branchitis associated with a heavy parasitic infestation. The parasite sections seen on histopathology are consistent with Monogenean flukes (Bruno et al. 2006) and were positively identified under light microscopy as *Dactylogyrus* species.

Failure for Ziehl-Neelsen staining to demonstrate acid-fast organisms does not absolutely rule out mycobacteriosis and should be borne in mind because of its zoonotic potential. However, the presence of a few granulomas which may indicate the low-level presence of what is considered a common pathogen, combined with the severe gill pathology, suggest that the fluke infestation is the primary cause of death.

Treatment with a proprietary soluble flubendazole preparation at a dose rate of 1 g per 386 litres (85 imperial gallons; 102 US gallons) was initiated. This was repeated after 4 weeks, by which time the mortalities had virtually ceased.

Discussion

This case demonstrates a severe case of *Dactylogyrus* infestation in an ornamental pond. The background to this case is that the month in which the problem arose was June, and it was an exceptionally warm June for local conditions. The pond was very highly stocked, plus it is relatively shallow and in an open situation, which would have predisposed to rapid temperature rises. The temperature was unknown, which is itself a mistake common to many pond owners, but it could be assumed to be in the mid-20°C, possibly peaking at higher temperatures. Gill flukes have a direct life cycle and the rate of reproduction of gill flukes is governed by water temperature. At 1–2°C the life cycle is 5–6 months, while it is reduced to only a few days at 22–24°C. In this case, a period of prolonged warm weather probably caused a rapid rate of fluke multiplication. The high stocking density would mean easy transfer of flukes between individuals, and a high survival and attachment rate of the newly hatched free-swimming oncomiracidium stage, such that all the fish would eventually carry a significant fluke burden.

Dactylogyrus are extremely common parasites of ornamental fish. Thilakaratne (2003) found that 47 out of 153 (30.7%) of goldfish and six out of 44 (13.6%) of carp farmed for the ornamental fish trade carried *Dactylogyrus*. Overall, 18.4% of all ornamental fish examined in this study had *Dactylogyrus* against 45.3% which were considered to harbour a parasitic infestation of some description.

Adult flukes feed upon the cells of the gill tissue, blood and the mucus produced in response to damage and irritation by the parasites. Therefore, respiration is eventually severely compromised with heavy infestations. In addition, the high water temperatures would hold less oxygen and so these fish are doubly compromised. In carp (*Cyprinus carpio*) infested with *Dactylogyrus vasator*, there was a direct correlation between parasite burden and mortality in water with low oxygen levels (Molnar 1994). It is of interest that the owner did not report typical signs of respiratory disease such as increased respiratory rate, marked flaring of the operculae, apparent gasping at the surface, especially in areas of high dissolved oxygen content such as filter outflows and airstones.

Dactylogyrus spp. are egg-layers and the egg stage is resistant to chemical attack. This is why it is important to differentiate *Dactylogyrus* species from *Gyrodactylus* – the live-bearing skin flukes can usually be eliminated with a single dose of treatment, but *Dactylogyrus* will need repeated application, usually at monthly intervals. Here, flubendazole was used; praziquantel would have been a suitable alternative and there are proprietary fluke medications, many of which rely on formalin as a flukicide.

The low incidence of the protozoan *Ichthyobodo necator* (formerly *Costia necatrix*) was considered incidental. Some consider it to be a skin commensal. Other potential sequelae would be bacterial or fungal gill disease secondary to fluke damage; this could potentially give rise to systemic disease secondary to haematogenous spread. This potentially could have accounted for the multiple small granulomas observed. Systemic viral infections such as spring viraemia of carp (SVC) or cyprinid herpesvirus 2 should also be considered. These would be diagnosed on histology (CHV-2) or virus isolation. SVC is a notifiable disease in the UK.

Further reading

Bruno, D.W., Nowak, B., Elliot, D.G., 2006. Guide to the identification of fish protozoan and metazoan parasites in stained tissue sections. Dis. Aquat. Organ. 70, 1–36.

Molnar, K., 1994. Effect of decreased water oxygen content on common carp fry with *Dactylogyrus vastator* (Monogenea) infection of varying severity. Dis. Aquat. Organ. 20, 153–157.

Thilakaratne, I.D.S.I.P., Rajapaksha, G., Hewakopara, A., et al., 2003. Parasitic infections in freshwater ornamental fish in Sri Lanka. Dis. Aquat. Organ. 54, 157–162.

Case 5.3 *L. Jepson*

Clinical history

A female pot-bellied seahorse (*Hippocampus abdominalis*) belonging to a small public aquarium was examined. The seahorse was losing condition and had progressively become anorectic.

The aquarium was a roughly triangular-shaped structure with cured concrete on two sides and glass as a viewing panel. The volume was approximately 1000 litres (220 Imperial gallons; 264 US gallons). Filtration was with an external filter. Temperature was 18°C. Ammonia was 0.0 mg/l, nitrite was 0.0 mg/l, nitrate was 25 mg/l and specific gravity was 1.025. The sides, rockwork and hitching ropes were covered with a combination of filamentous algae and a population bloom of small anemone-like cnidarians. Water changes were with locally collected natural seawater that was stored in black storage tanks for 8 weeks prior to use. The seahorses were fed on defrosted frozen and live mysid shrimp.

Physical examination

The seahorse was considered thin with some loss of muscle mass over the skull and a mild concavity of the abdomen. The respiratory rate was considered higher than those of the other seahorses although it was not measured.

Q *1. List your differential diagnoses*

- Incorrect diet (failing to initiate a feeding response)
- Poor water quality
- Mycobacteriosis
- Ichthyophonus
- Heavy parasitism
- Gill disease

- Pharyngeal obstruction
- Metabolic imbalance e.g. acidosis
- Hypoxia
- Copper toxicosis

There was a history of mycobacteriosis with this group of seahorses. Now only two females and one male were left. A presumptive diagnosis of mycobacteriosis was made and, because of the zoonotic potential, it was decided to euthanase this seahorse and undertake a post-mortem examination as part of disease surveillance in the collection.

Post-mortem diagnosis examination

A skin scrape was taken from the seahorse prior to euthanasia. The seahorse was euthanased with a solution of tricaine methanesulphonate (MS222) dissolved in a saturated solution of $NaHCO_3$ to form a buffered stock solution of 10 g/l. This was added incrementally until the seahorse was considered to be dead.

The coelomic cavity was incised into along the midline and the internal organs examined *in situ*. The seahorse was considered thin. The ovaries were slender strips with only a slight number of small undeveloped ova. The seahorse was then placed *in toto* into formal saline and submitted for histopathology.

Results

- No parasites were found on the skin scraping

Histopathological diagnosis

- No lesions were found in the brain or the bone of the skull, cartilage or eye. The head muscles had attenuated myocytes, with clear spaces between them that may have represented oedema
- The caudal pharynx around the gills appeared compressed and the base of the gill arches were slightly displaced and greatly expanded by proliferative thyroid follicles, which have a tall columnar epithelium and which contain variably none to abundant colloid. The gills showed no other obvious lesion
- Transverse section of the body wall showed no lesions
- Transverse section of the tail showed attenuated myocytes separated by clear spaces
- Autolysis prevented meaningful interpretation of the intestinal tract
- The hepatopancreas contained hepatocytes markedly distended, each with a single, clear lipid vacuole. No lesions present in the pancreatic portions
- Ziehl-Neelsen staining was negative

Q *2. What would your interpretation be based on the above results?*

Q *3. What is your list of differential diagnoses now? What readily available off-the-shelf test that is available in most aquatic retailers could you do to aid with your diagnosis?*

Revised differential diagnosis list

- Goitre secondary to absolute iodine deficiency
- Goitre secondary to relative iodine deficiency. High nitrate levels can interfere with the uptake of iodine from surrounding water
- Goitre secondary to neoplasia

Final diagnosis

- A diagnosis of thyroid follicular hyperplasia (goitre) was made

The water was tested for iodine concentration. It should be borne in mind that iodine exists as iodide, iodate, molecular iodine and hypoiodite in seawater and therefore one should use a test kit that measures *total* iodine. One was used here. Iodine level was found to be zero. The test kit used was a colorimetric test using liquid reagents. For comparison, another aquarium than this one, housing a large colony of a tropical species of seahorse *H. fuscus*, was measured. The total iodine level was 0.05 mg/l. Natural seawater is considered to have a total iodine concentration of 0.06 mg/l.

Discussion

Goitres are considered common in both elasmobranch fish and teleosts (Wildgoose 2001). Pathological enlargement of the thyroid follicles in response to low iodine would have altered the dynamics of the pharynx which, in seahorses, is a tightly enclosed space designed to enhance the rapid suction needed for feeding (Roos et al. 2009).

The atrophy of the myoctes and the hepatocellular lipidosis are probably in response to prolonged anorexia induced by the inability to feed, or the endocrinological effects of hypothyroidism.

The occurrence of goitre raises some interesting questions. The two seahorse aquaria tested for total iodine in this collection differed primarily in that one was temperate where the pot-bellies were housed, and one was tropical. The management of the two groups of seahorses was considered identical with regard to diet and water sources and water changing regime.

However, each aquarium is a small ecosystem and the lack of iodine suggests a degree of sequestration of any available iodine thereby making it inaccessible to the seahorses. The most obvious potential cause of the situation was either the excessive algal growth or the small anemone-like organisms. Algae are present in other aquaria which do not suffer iodine loss, therefore, the small cnidarians may have been the culprit. Certainly, anemones are considered to have a definite, but ill-defined iodine requirement (Delbeek and Sprung 1997) and it is possible that large numbers could strip the water of its iodine supply. We were unable to find a laboratory that was confident that they could measure iodine content in collected cnidarians so that question remained unanswered.

Early stages of goitre can be reversed by supplementing the diet or directly into the water, for example with potassium iodide (Wildgoose 2001). Both were instigated here but, unfortunately, the other two seahorses eventually succumbed. The second female showed a similar picture on histology. The male was not examined.

Further reading

Delbeek, J.C., Sprung, J., 1997. The Reef Aquarium: A Comprehensive Guide to the Identification and Care of Tropical Marine Invertebrates. Ricordea Publishing, Miami.

Delbeek, J.C., Sprung, J., 2005. The Reef Aquarium: Science, Art, and Technology. Ricordea Publishing, Miami.Roos, G., Van Wassenbergh, S., Herrel, A., et al., 2009. Kinematics of suction feeding in the seahorse *Hippocampus reidi*. J. Exp. Biol. 212 (21), 3490–3498.

Wildgoose, W.H., 2001. BSAVA Manual of Ornamental Fish, second ed. British Small Animal Veterinary Association, Gloucester.

Case 5.4 *L. Jepson*

Clinical history

A koi (*Cyprinus carpio*) was one of approximately 90 medium to large koi belonging to an elderly lady. The fish had originally been managed by her late husband but now she, with the help of a neighbour, continued to care for them. These koi were considered quite old, with many of them well over 20 years old, although this one was said to be 9 years old. The pond was an 8 m × 2 m × 1 m deep concrete-lined structure that appeared well filtered and had multiple air stones *in situ*.

The owner was concerned that one of the larger koi was showing a marked distension of the body cavity, accompanied by abnormal swimming patterns. This koi tended to spend much time resting on the bottom of the pond and when roused swam with an exaggerated waddling motion. The koi was said to be still feeding well. On initial examination the following points were noted:

- The koi had a pronounced, asymmetric caudal coelomic swelling greater on the right than left side
- This fish swam with an exaggerated movement of the tail and caudal fin plus it did appear regularly to rest on the bottom of the pond
- Water quality was found to be non-remarkable.

1. List your differential diagnoses for (a) coelomic swelling and (b) abnormal swimming.

Differential diagnoses for coelomic swelling in koi

- Parasitic such as heavy worm burden, e.g. cestode such as *Bothriocephalus*, or microsporidial granuloma such as *Glugea*
- Granuloma (may be fungal such as *Ichthyophonus* or bacterial, e.g. mycobacteriosis) or abscess
- Neoplasia (such as renal, hepatic or gonadal)
- Foreign body granuloma
- Ascites
- Cardiovascular disease
- Renal disease. In goldfish (*Carasius auratus*) also consider renal enlargement secondary to *Hoferellus carassii* or polycystic renal disease
- Hepatic disease
- Ovarian stasis (egg retention)
- Spring viraemia of carp (SVC)

Differential diagnoses for abnormal swimming pattern in koi

- Poor water quality
- Neurological disease, e.g. CNS infection/granulomas
- Swimbladder disease or compromise, including swimbladder torsion
- Musculoskeletal disease
- Cardiovascular disease
- Neoplasia
- Electrocution (spinal fractures)
- Myxosporidial infections such as *Sphaerospora renicola*
- Poisoning, e.g. zinc toxicity from galvanized products

Investigative procedures

2. What investigative procedures are potentially available to you?

- Radiography
- Ultrasonography
- Coelomic tap
- Advanced diagnostic imaging such as CT scan
- Biopsy
- Haematology and biochemistry
- Water quality analysis

Physical examination

The koi was netted and placed upon a wet towel for examination purposes. A second wet towel was placed over the head of the koi to reduce stress and inhibit violent escape reactions.

A general examination was undertaken. Skin scrapes were negative. Gills and oropharynx appeared normal. A firm mass was palpable in the caudal coelomic cavity, particularly on the right side (Fig. 5.7). The skin over the swelling appeared slightly

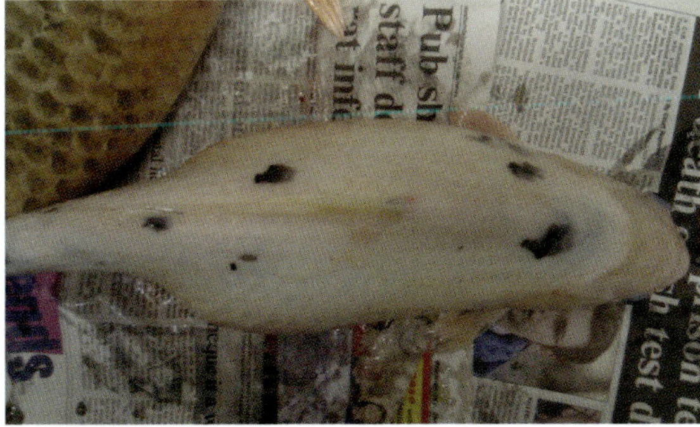

Fig. 5.7 A firm mass was palpable in the caudal coelomic cavity, particularly on the right side.

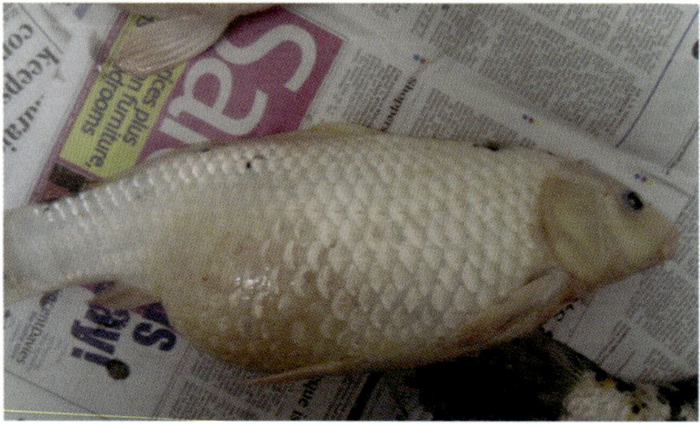

Fig. 5.8 The skin over the swelling appeared slightly oedematous and distended with separation of the overlying scales.

oedematous and distended with separation of the overlying scales (Fig. 5.8). A midline, coelomic aspirate was non-productive.

After discussion with the owner, euthanasia of the koi on welfare grounds was decided upon. The koi was euthanased with intravenous pentobarbitone administered into the ventral tail vein.

Post-mortem diagnosis examination

The koi weighed 950 g and had a standard length of 325 mm. Following a midline incision a large, firm, off-white mass was revealed in the caudal coelom (Fig. 5.9). The margins were not clearly definable and the mass appeared to merge progressively with the surrounding tissues including fat and hepatopancreas. When incised, the mass appeared as amorphous white tissue with a necrotic centre (Fig. 5.10). The veterinarian felt that this was sufficiently different from more typical koi coelomic masses that samples were submitted for histopathology.

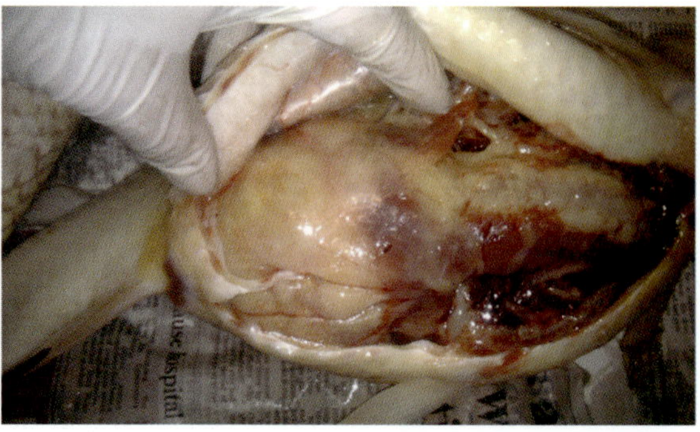

Fig. 5.9 Following a midline incision a large, firm, off-white mass was revealed in the caudal coelom.

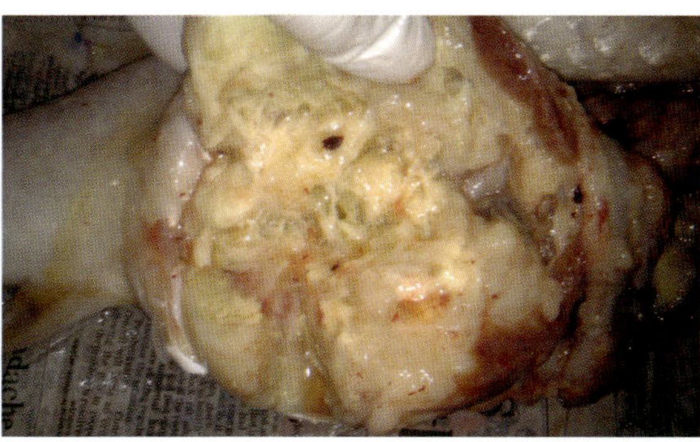

Fig. 5.10 The mass appeared as amorphous white tissue with a necrotic centre.

Histopathological diagnosis

Renal, splenic and hepatopancreas and coelomic mass tissue samples were submitted for histopathology. The samples of the first three were considered normal. Two sections of the coelomic mass were examined. The first was entirely necrotic, with just a tiny amount of neoplastic tissue along one edge. The other sample also contained necrotic tissue, but consisted mainly of neoplastic tissue. This appeared as a fairly loose, oedematous-looking, fibrocellular stroma-surrounded irregular island, cords and trabeculae of rather pleomorphic, spindloid to polyhedral cells with variably abundant, often vacuolated cytoplasm and medium to large, moderately hyperchromatic nuclei – some with a distinct nucleolus. Occasional mitotic figures could be seen. The growth pattern was highly infiltrative.

- ➤ Ziehl-Neelsen staining proved negative
- ➤ Histologically, the tissue appeared anaplastic with no recognizably normal tissue to give a clue as to its exact origin. A diagnosis of an unidentified malignant neoplasm was made

Discussion

Coelomic tumours are a common cause of coelomic swelling in captive fish (Wildgoose 2001) and are frequently of renal or gonadal origin.

Potential treatment options are limited but would include:

- Biopsy and appropriate treatment for non-neoplastic conditions
- Surgical debulking
- Surgical resection
- Chemotherapy, although possible, would be speculative at best
- Euthanasia.

In this case, there were limited investigative procedures undertaken, primarily due to financial restrictions. A coelomic tap was performed which, although unhelpful in this case, can be useful in diagnosing some cases of neoplasia, ascites and certain infections such as mycobacteriosis. Ultrasonography of the coelom would certainly have helped to characterize the mass; radiography less so, although the position of the swimbladder relative to the viscera (and the inferences one can gain) could have been a useful finding. Coelomic masses frequently displace the swimbladder causing swimming and positional disturbances. Other local consequences can be ulceration of the overlying abdominal wall, either from within by the tumour itself (May 1993) or by external trauma. Continual contact with abrasive surfaces may also contribute.

In some cases, coelomic tumours can be amenable to surgical resection (Lewbart et al. 1998, Raidal et al. 2006) but, in reality, barriers to surgical intervention are as much financial as practical. The poor differentiation and infiltrative nature would probably have made this a poor candidate for surgery, however.

The overall pattern was considered epithelial in origin (carcinoma) rather than mesenchymal (sarcoma). Suggested origins included intestinal, pancreatic or biliary adenocarcinoma or possibly even a gonadal tumour. No obvious gonad was detected on gross post-mortem so this would be a possibility.

Further reading

Lewbart, G.A., Spodnick, G., Barlow, N., et al., 1998. Surgical removal of an undifferentiated abdominal sarcoma from a koi carp (*Cyprinus carpio*). Vet. Rec. 143 (20), 556–558.

May, E.B., 1993. Goldfish, koi and carp neoplasia. In: Stoskopf, M.K. (Ed.), Fish Medicine. WB Saunders, Philadelphia, p. 490.

Raidal, S.R., Shearer, P.L., Stephens, F., et al., 2006. Surgical removal of an ovarian tumour in a koi carp (*Cyprinus carpio*). Aust. Vet. J. 84, 178–181.

Wildgoose, W.H., 2001. Internal disorders. In: Wildgoose, W.H. (Ed.), BSAVA Manual of Ornamental Fish, second ed. British Small Animal Veterinary Association, Gloucester, p. 130.

Index

Note: Page numbers followed by *f* indicate figures, and *t* indicate tables.

C

K

L

M

N

O

P

V

W

X

Y

Z